MENTAL HEALTH AND CHIROPRACTIC

This book is dedicated to the memory of

GEORGE W. HARTMANN, PH.D.

HENRY GUZE, PH.D.

WILLIAM A. WATKINSON, D.C.

These three great men have during a period of thirty years been a major force in helping to make this book a reality.

MENTAL HEALTH AND CHIROPRACTIC

A MULTIDISCIPLINARY APPROACH

HERMAN S. SCHWARTZ, D.C.
EDITOR

SESSIONS PUBLISHERS
NEW HYDE PARK · NEW YORK, N.Y. 11040

Library of Congress Catalog Card No. 73-84037
SBN 0-911366-02-4

Published by
SESSIONS PUBLISHERS
48 Nassau Drive
New Hyde Park, New York, N.Y. 11040

PRINTED IN THE UNITED STATES OF AMERICA
BY VAIL-BALLOU PRESS, INC., BINGHAMTON, N.Y.

"Since no one theory or method of diagnosis or treatment can as yet conclusively be called superior, we can all agree that dogmatism and rigid adherence to a particular system have no place in the immediate future of services to the mentally ill. . . . At this state of knowledge, it is important that new ideas not be rejected automatically because their proponents do not wear the conventional garb of workers who have traditionally been involved with mental health problems. Regardless of their source, serious proposals and efforts deserve serious scrutiny and evaluation."

ACTION FOR MENTAL HEALTH *

* ACTION FOR MENTAL HEALTH, is the Final Report of the Joint Commission on Mental Illness and Health (1961, p. 168). It was created under Federal Law 182. Grants from the U.S. National Institute of Mental Health of $1,410,600 went into research studies which are reported in this and several other volumes. These extensive studies were made under the sponsorship of 36 leading health organizations comprising the commission.

FOREWORD

For me it is a singular privilege to be asked to write a foreword to this anthology. I consider the theme of this book to be of great importance and of considerable clinical significance. It is both encouraging and rewarding to know that here is a text that succinctly explores the biological and clinical implications of the idea that structural changes may condition attitudes; and in turn, mental attitudes can disturb structure. The organism, in response to a stimulus, normal or abnormal, acts or reacts as a whole. The relations between the emotional and the physical and the intimacy of the dynamics of structural and psychological interaction are distinctly emphasized in this volume.

Man, homo-sapiens, is structurally and phylogenetically a biped. In man, frequent postural fatigue, the strain and stress of postural incompetence, the high incidence of spinal architectural defects, as well as the asymmetrical activities of work and play may tend to inflict an undue and aberrant volley of stimulations upon the brain, causing a possible buildup or expansion of some type of psychological problem. The converse, however, is also possible. Extended, nagging emotional strain will frequently mirror itself in neuromuscularskeletal tensions. The emotionally and mentally harassed individual often develops physical tensions. Once this sequence of pathological interreaction has been established, it becomes possible to influence it in a number of different ways.

Into this picture of one stress factor leading to another, chiropractic care is projected as a normalizing, relaxing, tension-dissipating and reflex regulating therapy. This text relates information demonstrating benefits to people in distress.

I should like to extend my personal appreciation to the noble and dedicated pioneer of this concept, Dr. Herman S. Schwartz, who is to be encouraged and commended. To those who worked with Dr. Schwartz as advisors and contributors, a most sincere expression of gratitude. Their contributions have provided the text with a sophistication and depth that make it truly a unique publication.

National College of Chiropractic JOSEPH JANSE, D.C.
President

PREFACE

In 1922, shortly after I began my career in chiropractic, I had the experience of preventing the hospitalization of a young man with a severe emotional disturbance, whose commitment papers were already signed. The patient's emotional disturbance was caused by a physical trauma, resulting in a neuromuscularskeletal distortion (subluxation). The chiropractic structural adjustment was largely responsible for the recovery of his emotional equilibrium, making it possible for him to finish his semester at Harvard. The family of the patient was of enormous help. They eagerly cooperated, and gladly provided all the facilities, including nursing and custodial care and the consultation with a specialist. In retrospect, what this procedure actually involved was the establishment of an interdisciplinary approach in the home.

A national survey of *350 Nervous and Mental Cases Under Chiropractic Care,* which I conducted with the assistance of the late Dr. George W. Hartmann of Teachers College, Columbia University, revealed similar reductions in manifest emotional distress as a consequence of applied chiropractic, in the home as well as in general office practice.

Fifty years of practice have also taught me that many factors, such as social, biochemical, or environmental, may enter into the etiology and management of psychological distress. It must be assumed that, when indicated, a total approach to the treatment of psychological problems, employing diverse methods of healing, might well contribute to more effective and lasting benefits.

My motives in compiling this volume were several:

to share some of my experiences in chiropractic;

to present a basic organismic principle of chiropractic—that there is always a reciprocal relationship between body structure and various types of behavior;

to explore in depth the concepts and implications of chiropractic, based upon empirical evidence and neurophysiological data as to the effectiveness of its manipulative techniques for mental health;

to present general ancillary aids to be implemented, when necessary, by the practitioner or the family to buttress chiropractic, and also to indicate the occasional need for consultations, cooperation, or referrals;

to present to students of the healing arts and to concerned laymen the challenge of unprejudiced inquiry into chiropractic as one of the relevant disciplines for emotional disorders.

I have included contributions from such varied fields as anthropology, biochemistry, biology, education, psychology, psychiatry, and sociology, as well as chiropractic. Although some of the contributors have lent credence to the proposition that chiropractic is deserving of impartial investigation as to its possible value for better mental health, this does not necessarily imply that they all endorse the chiropractic premise.

I want to express my deepest appreciation and profound gratitude to all the scholars and renowned scientists who have contributed to this anthology.

I am also deeply indebted to my wife and son, to my consultants, to the contributors, research workers, editorial assistants, secretaries, publishers and the printers who have sustained my efforts and helped greatly in the production of this work. It is not possible to list all the fine persons who aided me in various ways. To mention only a few would be unfair to the rest. They all have my full appreciation and gratitude. The memory of their generous spirit of helpfulness will always remain with me.

Special appreciation is extended to the Foundation for Chiropractic Education and Research without whose encouragement this book would not have been possible.

It would be presumptuous to believe that this or any other book holds the final answers to the problems of mental illness. However, I hope that a sturdy foundation has been laid for the cooperation of the various healing disciplines to make a united contribution towards mental health.

HERMAN S. SCHWARTZ, D.C.

CONTRIBUTORS

DE RUSHA, J. LAMOINE, D.C.
Dean, Northwestern College of Chiropractic, Minneapolis, Minnesota. Member of the Basic Science Board of Examiners, University of Minnesota.

DUBOS, RENÉ, Ph.D., Nobel Laureate
Professor Emeritus, Rockefeller Institute of New York. Author of: *Biochemical Determinants of Microbial Diseases; The Unseen World; Bacterial and Mycotic Infections of Man; Dreams of Reason: Science and Utopias; The Torch of Life; Man Adapting; The Mirage of Health; A God Within.*

*GUZE, HENRY, Ph.D.**
Lecturer in physical anthropology, Drew University; Psychotherapist; Fellow Academy of Psychosomatic Medicine. Director of Publications—American Academy of Psychotherapists.

HALDEMAN, SCOTT, D.C., Ph.D.
Completing the Ph.D. degree in Synaptic Transmission. Author of: *The Antagonism of Glutamate Induced and Synaptic Excitations of Thalamic Neurons; Interactions Between the Somatic and Visceral Nervous Systems; The Evolution of Neurology and the Concept of Chiropractic.*

*HARTMANN, GEORGE W., Ph.D.**
Professor of Educational Psychology, Teachers College, Columbia University; Chairman Department of Psychology, Roosevelt College, Chicago; Author of: *Educational Psychology* and *Gestalt Psychology.*

HOCKMAN, LEONARD, Ph.D.
Director of Counseling Services, Fairleigh Dickinson University; Associate Professor of Psychology, Fairleigh Dickinson; U.R.A. Fellow, Texas Tech College.

HOMEWOOD, A. E., D.C.
Dean Emeritus Canadian Memorial Chiropractic College. Associate Dean, Los Angeles College of Chiropractic. Secretary of the Council on Chiropractic Education. Author of: *The Neurodynamics of the Vertebral Subluxation; The Chiropractor and the Law.*

* *Deceased.*

JANSE, JOSEPH, D.C.

President, the National College of Chiropractic. Former Secretary, The Council on Chiropractic Education. Officer dans l'Ordre des Palmes Academiques, Ministere de L'Education Nationale, Republic of France.

KIMMEL, EDWIN H., D.C.

American Council of Mental Health, New York Academy of Science; former faculty member of Chiropractic Institute of New York. Regional Research Director, N.C.A. Council on Psychotherapy.

LEMESHOW, SEYMOUR, D.C., Ed.D.

Professor of Special Education, Trenton State College. Formerly Chairman, Department of Special Education, Director of Educational Development Clinic, Jersey City State College.

LEVINE, MORTIMER, D.C.

Former Chairman, Department of Chiropractic, Chiropractic Institute of New York. Author of: *The Structural Approach to Chiropractic.*

LOWEN, ALEXANDER, M.D.

Director of Bio-Energetic Institute. Author of: *The Betrayal of the Body; Physical Dynamics of Character Structure; Love and Orgasm; Pleasure; Depression and the Body.*

MOULTON, DWAYNE R., D.C.

Past President, National Chiropractic Association. Past President of the Ada County (Idaho) Mental Health Association. Advisory Board Member of the Ada County Mental Health Center.

PAULING, LINUS, Ph.D., Nobel Laureate, 1954, 1962.

Professor of Chemistry, California Institute of Technology. Author of: *Introduction to Quantum Mechanics; The Structure of Line Spectra; General Chemistry; Molecular Psychiatry; Vitamin C and the Common Cold.*

PLUTCHIK, ROBERT, Ph.D.

Director of Program Development, Department of Psychiatry, Albert Einstein College of Medicine; Adjunct Professor, L.I. University, Department of Psychology; former Director, Evaluation Research Program, Bronx State Hospital; formerly Associate Research Scientist N.Y. State Psychiatric Institute. Author of: *The Emotions; Facts, Theories and a New Model; Small Group Discussion in Orientation and Teaching.*

PRESSMAN, RALPH, Ph.D.

Director of Research, American Chiropractic Association. Author of: *The Bacterial Efficiency and Toxicity of Creosote and its Components; The Isolation of Pathogenic Bacteria from the Air; Detection of Tubercule Bacilli in Suspected Environments.*

QUIGLEY, W. HEATH, B.S., D.C.

President of the ACA Council on Mental Health; Associate Professor of Diagnosis, Palmer College of Chiropractic; former Director of the Clearview (Mental) Sanatorium.

RULE, COLTER, M.D.

Former research fellow, Rockefeller Institute; American Board of Internal Medicine; American Psychiatric Association; Former member of governing council for New York Academy of Medicine; Author of: *A Theory of Human Behavior Based on Non-Human Primates.*

SCHWARTZ, HERMAN S., D.C.

President Emeritus of the ACA Council on Mental Health; Author of: *Nervous and Mental Cases Under Chiropractic Care; The Art of Relaxation; Home Care for the Emotionally Ill.*

SULZER, JEFFERSON L., Ph.D.

Head, Department of Psychology, Newcomb College, Tulane University. Author of: *Empirical Test of Heider's Levels in Attribution of Responsibility; Goal and Error Training Methods in the Learning of a Positioning Response; Nutrition and Behavior in Head Start Children; The Effect of Frustration upon Imitation of Aggression.*

SZASZ, THOMAS S., M.D.

Professor of Psychiatry, State University of New York; Upstate Medical Center; Editorial Board of the Journal of Nervous and Mental Disease; Fellow of the American Psychiatric Association; Consultant to the Committee on Mental Hygiene, N.Y. State Bar Association; author of: *The Myth of Mental Illness; Law, Liberty and Psychiatry;* and *Ideology and Insanity.*

VEAR, HERBERT J., D.C.

Dean, Canadian Memorial Chiropractic College; Toronto, Ontario, Canada.

WEIANT, C. W., D.C., Ph.D.

Dean Emeritus of the Chiropractic Institute of New York. Author of *Medicine and Chiropractic*. Co-author of: *Rational Bacteriology*. Many articles on Anthropology and on Chiropractic.

WENDLAND, HARRY

Director of Nutritional Research, Vitaminerals, Inc. Expert research-science writer on biochemical subjects.

CONTENTS

* *Deceased.*

* *Deceased.*

INTRODUCTION

by W. HEATH QUIGLEY, D.C.

There never has been a book comparable to MENTAL HEALTH AND CHIROPRACTIC. Working against many disappointments, with a minimum of encouragement, and a burden of many personal responsibilities, Dr. Schwartz was unyielding in his determination to bring this book to the world of the serious unbiased reader—a reader with a genuine concern for better mental health.

The book is now available both to the chiropractic profession and to the general public. It is therefore with real, as well as vicarious relief, mixed with pride, that I can now write this introduction. It is a book which has at last brought together two major loves of Dr. Schwartz—chiropractic and mental health. The chapters in this book are not mere readings from these disciplines, but are concerned with the meaningful relationships found to exist between them. This is the real message of MENTAL HEALTH AND CHIROPRACTIC.

The field of mental health is broad-based, and it follows most naturally that the contents of this anthology are similarly broad-based. The areas of: biology, neurology, psychology, and nutrition; are represented. Each author was selected with great care for the specific contributions he could make to the understanding of the relationships between mind and body. Many chapters flash brilliant messages, each different but held together by a common bond which integrates these messages into a greater whole.

Dr. Schwartz and those of us who have worked in this field of chiropractic and mental health for many years, are well aware that the image of a chiropractic doctor working with a mental patient in a patient-doctor relationship is difficult to consider seriously. However, it is well to be reminded that in many universities, the stereotype of the psychoanalyst with his patient on the couch is not taken seriously. It has become for many therapists an unjustifiable anachronism. This comparison was not made to downgrade any particular discipline, but simply to emphasize the point that, that which is acceptable today may be replaced tomorrow. It is clear that MENTAL HEALTH AND CHIROPRACTIC is a most serious effort to present some key facts and concepts which will make the relationships between mental health and chiropractic more understandable.

This anthology derives its life force from clinical experience. Early in the history of the chiropractic movement, every type of patient and disease was brought to chiropractors for cure. This variety also included the range of mental disorders. Although no controls existed and no standard measurement was employed, except the rule of thumb—"social recovery," chiropractors reported successes with a variety of mental disorders. Eventually in the early twenties, chiropractic mental hospitals (sanatoriums) were built for the care of the violent and disturbed patient. The results from one such sanatorium in Davenport, Iowa, was so impressive to a Judge in a nearby State, that he consistently refused to commit a patient to the State mental hospital unless the patient had at least three months care in the chiropractic sanatorium first. He had attempted to persuade the officials of the State institution to allow a chiropractor to treat patients who so desired it within the hospital, but it became apparent no such opportunity would be allowed.

These experiences are presented to provide a brief historical note to indicate why chiropractors have been interested in mental health. Chiropractic is not a late entry into the mental health field; it does have an established record.

Driven by these facts, by the results of his own practice, and by long hours of study, Dr. Schwartz worked to educate the chiropractic profession as to the meaning of the concept: chiropractic and mental health. He has written a great deal of material in chiropractic journals. He has been a most faithful servant of his self-appointed task. This drive has never ceased to motivate him in behalf of the profession and in behalf of the mentally ill.

Dr. Schwartz has a great dedication. He is well aware that even though chiropractic has afforded great relief to many sufferers of mental health problems, no single claim can be made for exclusiveness. He has seen the role of the family in helping, the need for the conventional psychiatrist and the psychotherapist, the value of the clinical psychologist, the educator, the minister, priest and rabbi. He has clearly perceived the patient's need for help from different sources, and has not been concerned with labels. He ardently desires to see the role of the authoritarian mental hospital or ward changed, a role many investigators are beginning to consider a major cause of the persistence of maladjusted lives. Dr. Schwartz's message tells why the transition from disturbed states to mental health can be more effective when there is a multidisciplinary analysis and approach. Among the participating disciplines, chiropractic must be included, not only for what it has done, but for what it can do; not only for itself, but especially as an essential part of an integrated team.

It is fitting that a man of Dr. Schwartz's experience and compassion has compiled this volume, and it is highly appropriate that the first chapter was written by a major critic of the present day mental health philosophy. It will be most gratifying if the role of chiropractic in mental health can be recognized and accepted.

As chiropractors, we wish to help. No single discipline is adequate to solve the massive personal-social problems of mental illness. However, MENTAL HEALTH AND CHIROPRACTIC provides evidence of the benefits likely to be achieved when chiropractic is added to the efforts of the mental health team.

* * *

PART I

THE MENTAL HEALTH PROBLEM

CHAPTER

CHAPTER 1

THE MENTAL HEALTH ETHIC*

THOMAS S. SZASZ, M.D.

LET US BEGIN with some definitions. According to *Webster's Third New International Dictionary* (unabridged), ethics is "the discipline dealing with what is good and bad or right and wrong or with moral duty and obligation. . . ."; it is also "a group of moral principles or set of values . . ." and "the principles of conduct governing an individual or a profession: standards of behavior. . . ."

Ethics is thus a distinctly human affair. There are "principles of conduct" governing individuals and groups, but there are no such principles governing the behavior of animals, machines, or stars. Indeed, the word "conduct" implies this: only persons conduct themselves; animals *behave,* machines *function,* and stars *move.*

Is it too much to say, then, that any human behavior that constitutes conduct—which, in other words, is a product of choice or potential choice, and not simply of a reflex—is, *ipso facto,* moral conduct? In all such conduct, considerations of good and bad, or right and wrong, play a role. Logically, its study belongs in the domain of ethics. The ethicist is a behavioral scientist par excellence.

If we examine the definition and practice of psychiatry, however, we find that in many ways it is a covert redefinition of the nature and scope of ethics. According to Webster's, psychiatry is "a branch of medicine that deals with the science and practice of treating mental, emotional, or behavioral disorders esp. as originating in endogenous causes or resulting from faulty interpersonal relationships"; further, it is "a treatise or text on or theory of the etiology, recognition, treatment, or prevention of mental, emotional, or behavioral disorder or the application of psychiatric principles to any area of human activity (social psychiatry)"; thirdly, it is "the psychiatric service in a general hospital (this patient should be referred to psychiatry)."

The nominal aim of psychiatry is the study and treatment of mental disorders. But what are mental disorders? To accept the existence of a class of phenomena called "mental diseases," rather than to inquire into the conditions under which some persons may designate others as "mentally ill," is the decisive step in the embracing of the mental health ethic.[1] If we take the dictionary definition of this discipline seriously, the study of a large part of human behavior is subtly transferred from ethics to psychiatry. For while the ethicist is supposedly concerned only with normal (moral) behavior, and the psychiatrist only with abnormal (emotionally disordered) behavior, the very distinction between the two rests on ethical grounds. In other words, the assertion that a person is mentally ill involves rendering a moral judgment about him. Moreover, because of the social consequences of such a judgment, both the "mental patient" and those who treat him as one become actors in a morality play, albeit one written in a medical-psychiatric jargon.

Having removed mentally disordered behavior from the purview of the ethicist, the psychiatrist has had to justify his reclassification. He has done so by redefining the quality or nature of the behavior he studies: whereas the ethicist studies moral behavior, the psychiatrist studies biological or mechanical behavior. In Webster's words, the psychiatrist's concern is with behavior "originating in endogenous causes or resulting from faulty interpersonal relationships." We should fasten our attention here on the words "causes" and "resulting." With these words, the transition from ethics to physiology, and hence to medicine and psychiatry, is securely completed.

Ethics is meaningful only in a context of self-governing individuals or groups exercising more or less free, uncoerced choices. Conduct resulting from such choices is said to have reasons and meanings, but no causes. This is the well-known polarity between determinism and voluntarism, causality and free will, natural science and moral science.

Defining psychiatry in the above way leads not only to a reapportionment of disciplines taught in universities, but also promotes a point of view about the nature of some types of human behavior, and about man in general.

By assigning "endogenous causes" to human behavior, such behavior is classified as *happening* rather than as *action*. Diabetes mellitus is a disease caused by an endogenous lack of enzymes necessary to metabolize carbohydrates. In this frame of reference, the endogenous cause of a depression must be either a metabolic defect (that is an antecedent chemical event) or a defect in "interpersonal relationships" (that is, an antecedent historical event). Future events or expectations are excluded as possible "causes" or a feeling of depression. But is this reasonable? Consider the millionaire who finds himself financially ruined because of business reverses. How shall we explain his "depression" (if we so want to label his feeling of dejection)? By regarding it as the result of the events mentioned, and perhaps of others in his childhood? Or as the expression of his view of himself and of his powers in the world, present and future? To choose the former is to redefine ethical conduct as psychiatric malady.

The healing arts—especially medicine, religion, and psychiatry—operate within society, not outside it. Indeed, they are an important part of society.

It is not surprising, therefore, that these institutions reflect and promote the primary moral values of the community. Moreover, today, as in the past, one or another of these institutions is used to mold society by supporting certain values and opposing others. What is the role of psychiatry in promoting a covert system of ethics in contemporary American society? What are the moral values it espouses and imposes on society? I shall try to suggest some answers by examining the position of certain representative psychiatric works and by making explicit the nature of the mental health ethic. And I shall try to show that in the dialogue between the two major ideologies of our day—individualism and collectivism—the mental health ethic comes down squarely on the side of collectivism.

II

Men desire freedom and fear it. Karl R. Popper speaks of the "enemies of the open society,"[2] and Erich Fromm of those who "escape from freedom."[3] Craving liberty and self-determination, men desire to stand alone as individuals, but, fearing loneliness and responsibility, they wish also to unite with their fellow men as members of a group.

Theoretically, individualism and collectivism are antagonistic principles: for the former, the supreme values are personal autonomy and individual liberty, for the latter, solidarity with the group and collective security. Practically, the antagonism is only partial: man needs to be both—alone, as a solitary individual, and with his fellow man as a member of a group. Thoreau at Walden Pond and the man in the gray flannel suit in his bureaucratic organization are two ends of a spectrum: most men seek to steer a course between these extremes. Individualism and collectivism may thus be pictured as the two shores of a fast-moving river, between which we—as moral men—must navigate. The careful, the timid, and perhaps the "wise" will take the middle course: like the practical politician, such a person will seek accommodation to "social reality" by affirming and denying both individualism and collectivism.

Although, in general, an ethical system that values individualism will be hostile to one that values collectivism, and vice versa, an important difference between the two must be noted: In an individualistic society, men are not prevented by force from forming voluntary associations, nor are they punished for assuming submissive roles in groups. In contrast, in a collectivistic society, men are forced to participate in certain organizational activities, and are punished for pursuing a solitary and independent existence. The reason for this difference is simple: as a social ethic, individualism seeks to minimize coercion and fosters the development of a pluralistic society; whereas collectivism regards coercion as a necessary means for achieving desired ends and fosters the development of a singularistic society.

The collectivist ethic is exemplified in the Soviet Union, as in the case of Iosif Brodsky. A twenty-four-year-old Jewish poet, Brodsky was brought to trial in Leningrad for "pursuing a parasitic way of life." The charge stems from "a Soviet legal concept that was enacted into law in 1961 to permit the exiling of city residents not performing 'socially useful labor.' "[4]

Brodsky had two hearings, the first on February 18 and the second on March 13, 1964. The transcript of the trial was smuggled out of Russia and its translation published in *The New Leader*.[5] In the first hearing Brodsky was vaguely accused of being a poet and of not doing more "productive" work. At its conclusion, the judge ordered Brodsky to be sent "for an official psychiatric examination during which it will be determined whether Brodsky is suffering from some sort of psychological illness or not and whether this illness will prevent Brodsky from being sent to a distant locality for forced labor. Taking into consideration that from the history of his illness it is apparent that Brodsky has evaded hospitalization, it is hereby ordered that division No. 18 of the militia be in charge of bringing him to the official psychiatric examination."[6]

This point of view is characteristic of the collectivist ethic. It is also indistinguishable from that of contemporary American institutional psychiatry. In both systems, a person who has harmed no one but is considered "deviant" is defined as mentally ill; he is ordered to submit to psychiatric examination; if he resists, this is viewed as a further sign of his mental abnormality.[7]

Brodsky was found guilty and sent "to a distant locality for a period of five years of enforced labor."[8] His sentence, it should be noted, was at once therapeutic, in that it sought to promote Brodsky's "personal well-being," and penal, in that it sought to punish him for the harm he had inflicted on the community. This, too, is the classic collectivist thesis: what is good for the community is good for the individual. Since the individual is denied any existence apart from the group, this equation of the one with the many is quite logical.

Another Russian man of letters, Valeriy Tarsis, who had published a book in England describing the predicament of writers and intellectuals under the Khrushchev regime, was incarcerated in a mental hospital in Moscow. It may be recalled that the American poet Ezra Pound had been dealt with in the same way: he was incarcerated in a mental hospital in Washington, D.C.[9] In his autobiographical novel, *Ward 7,* Tarsis gives the impression that involuntary mental hospitalization is a widely used Soviet technique for repressing social deviance.[10]

It seems clear that the enemy of the Soviet state is not the capitalist entrepreneur, but the lonely worker—not the Rockefellers, but the Thoreaus. In the religion of collectivism, heresy is individualism: the outcast par excellence is the person who refuses to be a member of the team.

I shall argue that the main thrust of contemporary American psychiatry—as exemplified by so-called community psychiatry—is toward the creation of a collectivist society, with all this implies for economic policy, personal liberty, and social conformity.

III

As was pointed out earlier, mental health and illness are but new words for describing moral values. More generally, the semantics of the mental health movement is but a new vocabulary for promoting a particular kind of secular ethic.

This view may be supported in several ways. Here I shall try to do so by citing the opinions expressed by the Scientific Committee of the World Federation for Mental Health in the monograph, *Mental Health and Value Systems,* edited by Kenneth Soddy.

In the first chapter, the authors candidly acknowledge "that mental health is associated with principles dependent upon the prevailing religion or ideology of the community concerned." [11]

There then follows a review of the various concepts of mental health proposed by different workers. For example, in Soddy's opinion, "A healthy person's response to life is without strain; his ambitions are within the scope of practical realization. . . ." [12] While in the opinion of a colleague whose view he cites, mental health "demands good interpersonal relations with oneself, with others, and with God" [13]—a definition that neatly places all atheists in the class of the mentally sick.

The authors consider the vexing problem of the relation between social adaptation and mental health. They succeed admirably in evading the problem that they claim to be tackling: "[M]ental health and social adaptation are not identical. . . . [This] can be illustrated by the fact that few people would regard a person who had become better adjusted as a result of leaving home and moving into a different society as having thereby become mentally healthy. . . . In the past, and still today in some societies, adaptation to society has tended to be highly valued . . . as a sign of mental health; and failure to adapt has been even more strongly regarded as a sign of mental ill-health. . . . There are occasions and situations in which, from the point of view of mental health, rebellion and non-conformity may be far more important than social adaptation." [14] But no criteria are given for distinguishing, "from the point of view of mental health," the situations to which we ought to conform from those against which we ought to rebel.

There is much more of this kind of sanctimonious foolishness. Thus we are told, "While it is unlikely that agreement could be reached on the proposition that all 'bad' people are mentally unhealthy, it might be possible to agree that no 'bad' person could be said to have the highest possible level of mental health, and that many 'bad' people are mentally unhealthy." [15] The problems of who is to decide who the "bad" people are, and by what criteria they are to decide, are glossed over. This evasion of the reality of conflicting ethics in the world as it exists is the most outstanding feature of this study. Perhaps one of the aims of propounding a fuzzy, yet comprehensive, mental health ethic is to maintain this denial. Indeed, the true goal of the community psychiatrist seems to be to replace a clear political vocabulary with an obscure psychiatric semantic, and a pluralistic system of moral values with a singularistic mental health ethic. Here is an example of the way this is accomplished:

"Our view is that the assumption of an attitude of superiority by one social group towards another is not conducive to the mental health of either group." [16] Some simplistic comments about the Negro problem in America then follow. No doubt, the sentiment here expressed is admirable. But the real problems of psychiatry are bound up not with abstract groups but with concrete individuals. Yet nothing is said about actual relations between people—for example, between adults and children, doctors and patients, experts and clients; and how, in these various situations, the attainment of a relationship that is both egalitarian and functional requires the utmost skill and effort of all concerned (and may, in some cases, be impossible to realize). Self-revealing as the mental health ethicist is when he discusses mental health and illness, his moral stance is even clearer when he discusses psychiatric treatment. Indeed, the promoter of mental health now emerges as a social engineer on the grand scale: he will be satisfied with nothing less than gaining license to export his own ideology to a world market.

The authors begin their discussion of the promotion of mental health by noting the "resistances" against it: "The principles underlying success in attempts to alter cultural conditions *in the interest of mental health,* and the hazards of such attempts, are very important considerations for practical mental health work. . . . The introduction of change in a community may be subject to conditions not unlike those which obtain in the case of *the child* . . ." (italics added).[17] We recognize here the familiar medical-psychiatric model of human relations: the client is like the ignorant child who must be "protected," if need be autocratically and without his consent, by the expert, who is like the omnicompetent parent.

The mental health worker who subscribes to this point of view and engages in this kind of work adopts a condescending attitude toward his (unwilling) clients: he regards them, at best, as stupid children in need of education, and, at worst, as evil criminals in need of correction. All too often he seeks to impose value change through fraud and force, rather than through truth and example. In brief, he does not practice what he preaches. The egalitarian-loving attitude toward one's fellow man, which the mental health worker is so eager to export to the "psychiatrically underdeveloped" areas of the world, seems to be in rather short supply everywhere. Or are we to overlook the relations in the United States between white and black, or psychiatrist and involuntary patient?

The authors are not wholly oblivious of these difficulties. But they seem to think it sufficient to acknowledge their awareness of such problems. For example, after commenting on the similarities between Chinese brainwashing and involuntary psychiatric treatment, they write:

"The term brain-washing has . . . been applied with unfortunate connotations to psychotherapeutic practice *by those who are hostile to it.* We consider that the lesson of this needs to be taken to heart by all who are responsible for securing psychiatric treatment of non-volitional patients. The use of compulsion or deceit will almost certainly *appear, to those who are unfriendly to or frightened of* the aims of psychotherapy, to be wicked" (italics added).[18]

The "benevolent" despot, whether political or psychiatric, does not like to have his benevolence questioned. If it is, he resorts to the classic tactic of the oppressor: he tries to silence his critic, and, if this fails, he tries to degrade him. The psychiatrist accomplishes this by calling those who disagree with him "hostile" on "mentally ill." Here we are told that if a person admits to the similarities between brain-washing and involuntary psychiatric treatment he is, *ipso facto, hostile* to psychotherapy.

The statement about "the lesson . . . to be taken to heart by all who are *responsible* for securing psychiatric treatment of nonvolitional patients" (italics added) requires special comment. The language used implies that involuntary mental patients exist in nature—whereas, in fact, they are created, largely by psychiatrists. Thus, after raising the vexing problem of involuntary psychiatric treatment, the authors fail to deal with it in a clear and forthright manner; instead, they impugn the emotional health and moral intentions of those who would dare to look at the problem critically.

This antagonism to a critical examination of his doctrines and methods may be necessary for the mental health worker, just as it is for the missionary or the politician: the aim of each is to conquer souls or minds, not to understand human problems. Let us not forget the dangers of trying to understand another person: the effort invites disproof of one's views and questioning of one's beliefs. The thoughtful person who is content to teach by the example of his own conduct must always be ready to acknowledge error and to change his ways. But this is not what the mental health worker wants: he does not want to change his ways, but those of others.

In an analysis of the mental hygiene movement written nearly thirty years ago, Kingsley Davis has suggested this and more. Commenting on the "family clinic," Davis observed that such agencies offer not medical treatment but moral manipulation: "Before one can cure such patients, one must alter their purpose; in short, one must operate, not on their anatomy, but on their system of values." [19] The trouble is, of course, that people usually do not want to *alter* their goals—they want to *attain* them. As a result, "Only those clients whose ends correspond to socially sanctioned values may be expected to come voluntarily to such a clinic. Other troubled persons, whose wishes are opposed to accepted values, will stay away; they can be brought in only through force or fraud." [20] Nor does Davis shirk from stating what many know but few dare articulate—namely, that ". . . many clients are lured to family clinics by misrepresentation." [21] Similarly, many more are lured to state mental hospitals and community-sponsored clinics. Community psychiatry thus emerges, in my opinion at least, as a fresh attempt to revitalize and expand the old mental hygiene industry.

First, there is a new advertising campaign: mental health education is an effort to lure unsuspecting persons into becoming clients of the community mental health services. Then, having created a demand—or, in this case, perhaps merely the appearance of one—the industry expands: this takes the form of steadily increasing expenditures for existing mental hospitals and clinics and for creating new, more highly automated factories, called "community mental health centers."

Before concluding this review of the ethics of mental health work, I want to comment briefly on the values advocated by the authors of *Mental Health and Value Systems.*

They promote change as such; its direction is often left unspecified. "The success of mental health promotion depends partly upon the creation of a climate favorable to change and a belief that change is desirable and possible." [22] They also emphasize the need to scrutinize certain "unproven assumptions"; none of these, however, pertains to the nature of mental health work. Instead, they list as unproven assumptions such ideas as ". . . the mother is always the best person to have charge of her own child." [23]

I believe that we ought to object to all this on basic logical and moral grounds: if moral values are to be discussed and promoted, they ought to be considered for what they are—moral values, not health values. Why? Because moral values are, and must be, the legitimate concern of everyone and fall under the special competence of no particular group; whereas health values (and especially their technical implementation) are, and must be, the concern mainly of experts on health, especially physicians.

IV

Psychiatry is a moral and social enterprise. The psychiatrist deals with problems of human conduct. He is, therefore, drawn into situations of conflict—often between the individual and the group. If we wish to understand psychiatry, we cannot avert our eyes from this dilemma: we must know whose side the psychiatrist takes—the individual's or the group's.

Proponents of the mental health ideology describe the problem in different terms. By not emphasizing conflicts between people, they avoid enlisting themselves explicitly as the agents of either the individual or the group. As they prefer to see it, instead of promoting the interests of one or another party or moral value, they promote "mental health."

Considerations such as these have led me to conclude that the concept of mental illness is a betrayal of common sense and of an ethical view of man. To be sure, whenever we speak of a concept of man, our initial problem is one of definition and philosophy; What do we mean by man? Following in the tradition of individualism and rationalism, I hold that a human being is a person to the extent that he makes free, uncoerced choices. Anything that increases his freedom, increases his manhood: anything that decreases his freedom, decreases his manhood.

Progressive freedom, independence, and responsibility lead to being a man; progressive enslavement, dependence, and irresponsibility, to being a thing. Today it is inescapably clear that, regardless of its origins and aims, the concept of mental illness serves to enslave man. It does so by permitting —indeed commanding—one man to impose his will on another.

We have seen that the purveyors of mental health care, especially when such care is provided by the government, are actually the purveyors of the moral and socioeconomic interests of the state. This is hardly surprising. What other interests could they represent? Surely not those of the so-called patient, whose interests are often antagonistic to those of the state. In this way, psychiatry—now proudly called "community psychiatry"—becomes largely a means for controlling the individual. In a mass society, this is best accomplished by recognizing his existence only as a member of a group, never as an individual.

The danger is clear, and has been remarked on by others. In America, when the ideology of totalitarianism is promoted as fascism or communism, it is coldly rejected. However, when the same ideology is promoted under the guise of mental health care, it is warmly embraced. It thus seems possible that where fascism and communism have failed to collectivize American society, the mental health ethic may yet succeed.

REFERENCES AND NOTES

1. See Szasz, T. S.: *The Myth of Mental Illness: Foundations of a Theory of Personal Conduct* (New York: Hoeber-Harper, 1961).

2. Popper, K. R.: *The Open Society and Its Enemies* (Princeton, N.J.: Princeton University Press, 1950).

3. Fromm, E.: *Escape from Freedom* (New York: Rinehart, 1941).

4. Quoted in *The New York Times,* August 31, 1964, p. 8.

5. "The trial of Iosif Brodsky: A transcript." The New Leader, 47:6–17 (August 31), 1964.

6. *Ibid.,* p. 14.

7. For a comparison of Soviet criminal law and American mental hygiene law, see Szasz, T. S.: *Law, Liberty, and Psychiatry: An Inquiry into the Social Uses of Mental Health Practices* (New York: Macmillan, 1963), pp. 218–21.

8. "The trial of Iosif Brodsky," op. cit., p. 14.

9. See Szasz, *Law, Liberty, and Psychiatry,* supra, Chap. 17.

10. Tarsis, V.: *Ward 7: An Autobiographical Novel,* transl. by Katya Brown (London and Glasgow: Collins and Harvill, 1965).

11. Soddy, K., ed.: *Cross-Cultural Studies in Mental Health: Identity, Mental Health, and Value Systems* (Chicago: Quadrangle, 1962), p. 70.

12. *Ibid.,* p. 72.

13. *Ibid.,* p. 73.

14. *Ibid.,* pp. 75–76.

15. *Ibid.,* p. 82.

16. *Ibid.,* p. 106.

17. *Ibid.*, p. 173.

18. *Ibid.*, p. 186.

19. Davis, K.: "The application of science to personal relations: A critique of the family clinic idea." *Amer. Sociological Rev.*, I:236–47 (April), 1936, p. 238.

20. *Ibid.*, p. 241.

21. *Ibid.*

22. Soddy, op. cit., p. 209.

23. *Ibid.*, p. 208.

CHAPTER 2

CHIROPRACTIC AND MENTAL HEALTH IN THE WORLD OF THE FUTURE

C. W. WEIANT, D.C., PH.D.

THE IMAGE OF THE FUTURE

The most exciting phenomenon on the horizon today is a quiet revolution in human thinking about the nature of man. Harman (1969) reports that:

> "There are many signs that man may be undertaking a systematic exploration of the vast, imperfectly known universe of his own being, a step as epochal as his construction of a science of the galaxies."

As might be expected, it is such outstanding psychologists as Henry A. Murray, the late Abraham Maslow, J. F. T. Bugental, Erich Fromm, and Roberto Assagioli, who figure most prominently in this dynamic movement.

The new science of man seeks to bridge the gap between what C. P. Snow called "the two cultures," the culture of science and the culture of the humanities, in the hope of creating a true science of man.

HUMAN POTENTIAL AND MENTAL HEALTH

The image which a human being acquires of himself and of his own future tends to be self-fulfilling. What has been envisaged comes to pass. Moreover, there is evidence that this principle holds true for societies as well as for the individual. Whether or not we are prepared at this time to accept the premises of a new science of man, this concept has already enormously enriched the raw materials of mental health. Its findings give substance to beliefs, attitudes, and modes of thinking generally taken to characterize the healthy mind. They are ego-strengthening, altruistic, exhilarating, and charged with hope. One's first task should be to take stock of *all* available resources from all the healing arts and then to formulate a program for their judicious use. I emphasize the word *all,* because the present state of our knowledge points to a whole category of resources long ignored in this undertaking; namely, the physical organism which is the vehicle of all psychic manifestation.

As research continues, new and better techniques for accomplishing this purpose will surely be developed. But who would deny that even the most ingenious techniques are likely to flounder if applied to a brain which by reason of adverse physical or chemical influence, is functioning at subnormal [or less than optimal] physiological levels? Clearly, then, the prime requisite, the *sine qua non,* for releasing the enormous potentialities of the brain is to make certain that it is a healthy brain functioning in a healthy body.

Within the inventory of resources which deserve serious consideration is a system of healing which has already been abundantly evaluated by repeated demonstrations of its effectiveness. Such a system of healing is chiropractic. It has been used for 75 years and has won the adherence of millions of people who have found therein the answer to problems for which orthodox procedures were no match.

Direct relevance to our concern may be found in the engaging and thoroughly objective book *The Case of Unorthodox Medicine* (Inglis, 1965), especially the chapter on "osteopathy and Chiropractic." It is to the latter discipline that we shall now address ourselves in somewhat greater detail.

THE ROLE OF CHIROPRACTIC

Inglis (op. cit.), in his discussions of the various schools of unorthodox medicine, divides them into three categories according to whether the emphasis is on the body, the mind, or the spirit. Within the body category at least, chiropractic easily stands out as preeminent. It is the world's second largest healing art in point of numbers: some 20,000 doctors of chiropractic in the United States alone, with an estimated clientele on the order of 30,000,000. It is officially recognized and regulated in 48 of the states, as well as in the District of Columbia and the Commonwealth of Puerto Rico. Elsewhere in the Americas licenses to practice chiropractic have been issued by most of the provinces of Canada and by Mexico, Nicaragua, Bolivia, and Uruguay. The same is true of every canton of Switzerland in which doctors of chiropractic are located. (In fact, Geneva is the principal center of chiropractic research in Europe.)

A degree of recognition exists also in Germany and Denmark, and while official recognition is lacking in Britain, no serious obstacles to the practice exist in the United Kingdom, where, in fact, many of the more affluent citizens seem to prefer it to the socialized medical services available to them. In Greece the late Dr. K. Ligeros, a medical physician who became a chiropractor, was designated official chiropractor to the royal family. In at least half a dozen other European countries chiropractors have received wide public acceptance. This is true also of South Africa. In Japan chiropractic enjoys prestigious patronage which extends even to the imperial household. Both New Zealand and Australia have given official recognition to the practice.

THE CRUX OF CHIROPRACTIC THEORY

While its ramifications are as wide as the whole of human biology and ecology, the focal concern of chiropractic as a science is the interrelationship between skeletal-muscular structure (more especially spine and pelvis) and the nervous system. The goal of chiropractic as an art is the establishment, primarily by manual techniques, of optimal functional relations between the body structure and the nervous system. It should come as no surprise to the anatomist or the neurophysiologist that a discipline with this dual orientation has discovered a solid foundation on which to build a health system.

As for the spine, biologists have long recognized that it represents something less than an ideal adaptation to the upright posture. The eminent British physician and anthropologist Sir Arthur Keith (1923) pointed out that "human spines were not evolved to withstand the monotonous and trying postures entailed by modern education and by many modern industries." Indeed, the multiple functions which the spine is called upon to fulfill, the accidents to which it is prone, occupational strains, malnutrition, and biochemical changes accompanying the aging process all contribute to its impairment. Moreover, its musculature, repeatedly bombarded by volleys of motor impulses responding to excessive stimuli from within and without, is beset by spasms which effectively immobilize one or more of its articulations. The dyskinesis of one joint is compensated by the hyperkinesis of another, but both become the foci of damaging nerve irritation. One can hardly quarrel with the anatomist MacKensie, who is reported (Wilbur 1932) to have said that "if generalizations are to be made about the causes of human diseases, it would be along the line of failure of accommodation to the erect posture."

The specific lesion sought by the doctors of chiropractic is traditionally referred to as the vertebral subluxation. Even before the discovery of chiropractic, this term had been used in medical literature, and, despite repeated assertions by medical writers that no such lesion exists, it has steadily gained currency in medical literature over the past half century (Weiant and Goldschmidt, 1966). The term subluxation implies minor displacement, a structural concept. Though this aspect has never been abandoned, clinical experience (including radiographic studies) has shifted the emphasis from a structural to a functional criterion. The really significant feature is restriction of the range of vertebral movement, often amounting to a complete locking of the articulation. Movement palpation to detect such limitations in joint mobility (now commonly referred to as *fixations*) has become a standard part of the chiropractic examination of the patient.

How much importance does the chiropractor assign to vertebral subluxations or fixations? The irritative character of this lesion is at once apparent in acute situations. It is accompanied by localized changes in skin temperature, surface hyperemia, and contractures of small paravertebral muscles; moreover, tenderness is readily elicited in the area. More impressive still are the data obtained by dissection and *in vivo* observations made by surgeons in the course of spinal operations. In this connection special importance attaches to the investigations of Dr. Peter Duus, neurologist and professor at the Johann Wolfgang Goethe University in Frankfurt, Germany. What follows is a condensed version of the account of Duus' work published in the book *Medicine and Chiropractic* (Weiant and Goldschmidt, 1966).

One of Duus' patients was a woman suffering from numbness and tingling of the fingers. The patient's neck presented an exaggerated anterior curvature (lordosis). Suspecting a herniated disc, Duus operated, but he found no disc herniation. Subsequently the symptoms disappeared, and much to the surgeon's surprise, so had the curvature. The cutting of ligaments and muscular attachments had eliminated the abnormal pulls which had distorted the cervical spine. What had happened suggested to Duus that there might be some truth in the chiropractic hypothesis that reduction in the size of the intervertebral foramen interferes with nerve conductivity. To test the hypothesis further, he decided to make a detailed microscopic study of intervertebral foramina and their contents. Using autopsy material, he prepared thousands of frozen sections of the area to be investigated. First of all, he noticed certain blank spaces which he assumed had formerly been occupied by nerves that had degenerated. Further probing, however, convinced him that these spaces were not the shells of degenerated nerves, but spaces formed by serum and solidified fibrin forced out of tiny blood vessels by the compressed foramen. This conclusion was reinforced by the finding of flattened blood and lymph vessels. The damage to these vessels was considerable; there was evidence of inflammatory changes and thrombi formation.

Moreover, in some of his preparations, he detected changes in the substance of the spinal cord at the level of the involved foramen. Since these were of the same nature as those seen in cases of multiple sclerosis, it occurred to Duus that subluxations may be one of the factors in the etiology of that disease.

Duus was able, also, to demonstrate the role of subluxations in initiating pathological processes which by their very nature lead to a reduction in the size of the foramen; for example, the degeneration and thinning of intervertebral discs and the growth of bony spurs which project into the foramen and give its cross-section an hour-glass form.

It must, however, be borne in mind that the work of Duus was directed to but one facet of chiropractic theory, namely, nerve interference at the intervertebral foramen. It is now generally recognized by the profession that other facets are equally pertinent and probably more important. A. E. Homewood, D.C. (1961) as Dean Emeritus of the Canadian Memorial College of Chiropractic, made this point very clearly in a brilliant paper requested by and published in the *University of Toronto Medical Journal* from which we quote:

> "While the attention of the chiropractor of some years ago was directed to proving that the vertebral subluxation caused direct interference to the spinal nerve as it makes its exit through the intervertebral foramen, the present day

doctor of chiropractic, backed by the neurological research of the past century, has turned his attention to the more subtle influences of the reflex arc and the neural bed of the associated holding elements. Hence the theory of chiropractic is no longer simple and direct nerve pressure, but as complicated as the central nervous system itself, with recognition of the fact that the last word cannot be said in the field of explanation for the success of chiropractic technique until the last words have been said in explanation of the complexities of the nervous system."

It is something of a paradox to be able to say that in the writings of Edgar Cyriax, one of the leading *medical* exponents of mechanical therapeutics, a statement can be found which neatly summarizes and defends the major contentions of chiropractic theory. He has this to say:

"I hold the following, based on the experience of over 1,000 cases:
a) Minor displacements of the vertebrae . . . are quite common . . .
b) Symptoms of disease are readily traceable to them
c) The displacements can, in the great majority, be reduced quite painlessly;
d) Their replacement is a material factor, a *sine qua non,* in curing or ameliorating the disease of which they are the cause." (Cyriax, 1924).

Ussher (1933 and 1940) attributes visceral disease to derangements of the vertebral column. In the second paper, referring to the first, he says:

"Typical cases were presented in which symptoms of appendicitis, gall-bladder disease, ureteral colic or other manifestations of visceral disease were apparently relieved by correction of a spinal curvature or of the associated myositis. In the main I was convinced that the variations in the visceral symptomatology depended on the various spinal levels involved. Gall-bladder colic and cardiospasm, for example, were shown in some instances to be related to myositis in the middle dorsal area. Symptoms of appendicitis or pelvic inflammation were shown to be definitely associated with irritation of the lower dorsal segments. They were treated without success by one or more physicians who had used the standard medical procedures."

After fifteen years of research on some 400 cases of visceral disease, he was more than ever convinced that he could restore patients with visceral disease to health without recourse to drugs, but purely by mechanical measures aimed at the correction of mechanical defects in the spine.

Hundreds of similar reports by American physicians could be cited. In nearly every instance, however, no matter how much the technique employed may have simulated chiropractic, no mention is made of that fact. The situation is different in Germany, where a great many physicians and surgeons have experimented with chiropractic and have frankly so stated in their reports. For example, Cramer, after a four year study of some 6,000 clinic patients handled chiropractically, wrote a textbook of chiropractic for medical doctors (1955). Both in this book and in a series of technical papers published in medical journals, he cites cases of colitis, constipation, cardiac irregularities, urethritis, thyroid dysfunction, menstrual disturbances, and many other types of visceral disease which responded well to vertebral adjustment.

Cramer is but one of many German medical doctors who have made similar reports. (For other references see Weiant and Goldschmidt, 1966). One in particular, however, deals with such a remarkable piece of research that it calls for special attention. Sollman and Worner (see Weiant 1966) used as their subjects 150 cases of very ill, bedfast, and non-ambulatory patients. Excluding every other therapy, they limited their procedure to the adjustment of the first two cervical vertebrae. The progress of each case was followed by recourse to frequent blood tests and other laboratory examinations. In their report they evaluate their results as follows:

> "Summing up, we would draw from this sample of 150 of the most thoroughly studied patients the following conclusions: according to the most stringent medical—and, in our case, surgical—indications, the answer to the question as to whether there is or is not a vertebral-therapeutic influence on serologically proved events is yes . . . In the majority of the cases studied an improvement in both the objective and the subjective findings was obtained."

The special importance of this study is that it goes beyond the question of the effectiveness of spinal correction in the management of specific visceral disease; it answers the broader question of the relation of such correction to general systemic disturbances. This is not the whole of chiropractic theory. It does not go into the intricacies of spinal and pelvic mechanics, the larger explanation and rationale of chiropractic, but it is, as we say, the crux of the matter. Implicitly, we have therein the answer to our question: "What importance does the chiropractor attach to vertebral subluxations?"

A BIT OF HISTORY

In the perspective of world history spinal manipulation has a very ancient heritage. That it was practiced in Greece in the time of Hippocrates has been made evident by K. Ligeros, M.D., D.C. (1937). Early visitors to Polynesia found that it was common practice among the natives to have the children walk upon the backs of ailing adults, a practice still in vogue among many cultures. The Mexican scholar Leon Portilla cites Aztec codices as authority for saying that the Aztecs distinguished between true doctors and witch-doctors, one of the criteria for recognizing the former being that they knew how "to concert the bones." The German surgeon Zukschwerdt, (1953) in a paper on the problems of chiropractic maintains that practices resembling chiropractic have long been part of the folk medicine of many lands and he states that this kind of folk medicine still exists in parts of Germany, notably in the Bavarian Alps, Westphalia, and Friesland.

The Discoverer. Dr. A. E. Homewood, in his already cited paper in the *University of Toronto Medical Journal,* gives this terse account of the discovery of chiropractic: "The rebirth of Hippocrates' rachiotherapy under the name of chiropractic occurred in Davenport, Iowa, in 1895, by D. D. Palmer of Port Perry, Ontario. D. D. Palmer was a self-educated man, similar to many of his day, who achieved prominence and fame despite their lack of formal education and degrees.

At first glance it is difficult to conceive how a man of such humble origin could have started a movement that was to blossom into a full-fledged healing art of worldwide renown. But Palmer was no ordinary man. He was an avid student with a passion for knowledge about the body and human welfare. He collected animal skeletons and set up a small museum of natural history. He accumulated a library of as many of the standard works of his day as he could get hold of dealing with the biological and natural science,—a library said to have been worth $5,000 (no small sum in those days).

"D. D. Palmer taught that the cause of all disease is irritation (stress), either mechanical, chemical, or mental, which overcomes the natural resistance of the body to produce distortion, interference to normal nerve transmission, functional change, and the tissue changes causing pathology. Palmer was not unmindful of the detrimental effects of pathogenic micro-organisms, the psychomatic background of many conditions, the ill effects of unsanitary conditions, the adverse influence of faulty diet, the stress of occupation, the irritation of chemicals taken into the body either through the digestive or respiratory systems, and, of course, the evils of mechanical trauma. D. D. Palmer had in many areas of his book stressed the diversity of cause, and further, emphasized that the resistance of the individual was governed to a considerable degree by hereditary factors, environmental circumstances, and the previous history of his nervous system. Thus the distortion of the vertebral segments, or other anatomical disrelations, produce varying responses within the individual which may be quite different from those observed in another person with like disrelations, and that the manner in which the victim of a spinal distortion responds varies with the circumstances and his general condition."

THE FUNDAMENTAL NATURE OF CHIROPRACTIC

In the light of our discussions up to this point it should be apparent that chiropractic is a neuro-mechanical approach to the problems of health and disease. It cannot be viewed from the same frame of reference as orthodox medicine. It does not look upon a disease as an entity to be combated; the disease is physiology gone wrong, a process in which the body is reacting to a bad situation. The subluxation perpetuates the disease. To overcome the disease one must get rid of the perpetuating factor, rather than treat the effects. Once the pernicious foci of nerve irritation at the spine have been removed, the body cures itself, in accordance with what the famous Harvard physiologist Walter B. Cannon called *The Wisdom of the Body*. Thus the role of the chiropractor is to mobilize the biological resources of the organism,—to allow it to do for itself as much as it is able to do. He does not whip a tired organ into activity by stimulants, nor squelch over-excited nerves with sedatives and narcotics. What he accomplishes is not accomplished at the expense of masking the symptoms, side-effects, and the general physical deterioration that so often follows dependence upon drugs.

There are, of course, limitations to the body's capacity to respond. All human beings do not have identical biological resources. Some are handicapped by hereditary endowment; some have been damaged by years of unhealthful living and the ravages of disease. Yet many of these handicaps can be reversed by a return to hygienic modes of life, and barring irreversible degeneration in parts of the nervous system, we have in that system the greatest of all biological resources, a system frequently referred to as the most marvelous product of organic evolution in existence.

Obviously chiropractic is not a panacea. It cannot turn an idiot into a genius, cure a bleeder of his hemophilia, make the colorblind see colors, nor reverse the irreversible. Records in many thousands of cases, however, point to spectacular successes, not just with backaches and the various other neuromuscular disturbances with which a large segment of the public associates chiropractic, but with a wide variety of visceral disturbances as well. Oddly enough, some of the finest evidence has been supplied by German physicians who have been using chiropractic procedures in clinical research for the past twenty years. For example, Albert Cramer, M.D. (1955), in a textbook of chiropractic for physicians, lists successfully handled cases of asthma, colitis, constipation, cardiac anomalies, hemorrhoids, impotence, menstrual disturbances, thyroid dysfunction, urethritis, varicosities, and many others. In a book the English title of which would be *Chiropractic as Rational Therapy,* he mentions circulatory disturbances to the point of angina, digestive disorders, kidney and bladder disturbances, and unexplained rises in body temperature.

The matter of communicable disease deserves at least brief mention, since people who learn for the first time that chiropractors frequently attend patients thus afflicted, infer that chiropractors deny any role to microorganisms and viruses in disease production. This is not at all the case. The position of the chiropractor is simply that, since the mechanism of immunity and all other physiological reactions involved in resisting infection are under nerve control, there is reason to suspect that nerve irritation of vertebral origin is at least partly responsible for the disease manifestation. Clinical successes in this field appear to validate this contention. It is recognized, however, that situations arise in which the invading organisms are so numerous and of such virulence that medical intervention becomes necessary.

Many people are equally startled upon learning that chiropractic can point to some degree of success in the management of psychic disturbances. We have already presented the theoretical considerations underlying this experience, and we can again cite Gutmann (op. cit.) for medical substantiation. Some of the symptoms which he mentions as having responded to chiropractic technique are the following: loss of will power and desire, uncontrollable inner restlessness and insecurity, excessive sensitivity to climactic influences, feeling of insecurity on the street in heavy traffic and in crowded rooms and theatres, *globus hystericus,* a compulsion to clear the throat, depression, inability to concentrate, hesitancy and indecision, and labored attention to performances ordinarily requiring little thought. Some of the clinical experiences of chiropractors in this field are presented elsewhere in this book.

Again let it be emphasized, however, that the chiropractor's task is to restore the integrity of the body to normal nerve transmission he can no more claim to have treated the disease than can the psychoanalyst whose patient gets rid of his ulcer claims that he was treating the ulcer. This is not mere sophistry; it is the principle which differentiates chiropractic from medicine.

CORROBORATIVE EVIDENCE FROM EXPERIMENTAL PATHOLOGY

Evidence of the ability of spinal nerve irritation to produce not only head pain but severe psychological disturbance is to be found in experiments carried out a quarter of a century ago (Campbell and Parsons, 1944). Using forty medical students and doctors as subjects, these investigators scratched the periosteum and periarticular structures of the cervical spine and occipital condyles and injected small amounts of 6% sodium chloride in sterile solution. This procedure invariably produced head pain, and it was possible to relate the distribution of the pain to the specific points irritated. Various other concomitants were noted in particular cases: giddiness, sweating, nausea, alterations of pulse, ptosis, and tinnitus.

In their discussion of their findings, Campbell and Parsons explain in considerable detail the anatomical relationships which readily indicate the mechanisms of the pain production. They point out that hypertension of the long, hypoaxial back muscles may be caused by irritation at any spinal segment. It is especially likely to occur with irritation in the cervical region, but "thoracic and even lumbosacral lesions such as luxations, postural malalignments, and arthritis or myofascitis from local or remote (visceral) causes have been shown to produce cephalalgia and its concomitants."

Commenting in particular on the importance of the suboccipital muscles, they state: "The direction of gaze, the visual axes, and accompanying head, neck, and trunk posturing are produced and maintained by movements among which these small suboccipital muscles play a major role. They might be considered, as a functional unit, the concert master of the postural symphony."

What is the relevance of this for mental health? Campbell and Parsons focus on the vicious circles involving pain and muscle spasm, especially in the presence of local ischemia due to reflex spasm. Neuropsychic affective states such as fear and anger may also be present or, indeed, may be aroused by the somatic disturbance, via the cortico-diencephalic mechanism. "In individuals of low pain threshold and prone to neurotic anxiety, a vicious circle is more quickly established . . . Morphological, physiological, and psychological stresses form a field of reciprocal relations."

They note that one type of case where such psychosomatic mechanisms are frequently found is the post-traumatic "head syndrome," probably because of the special symbolic significance the head and neck have had throughout human history. They conclude: "The investigation and treatment of referred head pain and its concomitants involves the search for mesodermal lesions as a fundamental step and the conjoint management of psychosomatic factors."

In the light of these studies, it goes without saying that the influence of the chiropractic adjustment is far-reaching indeed. It is obvious that such profound physical effects cannot fail to be accompanied by equally profound and beneficial psychological changes. Millions of distress signals from the soma which formerly bombarded the higher centers have been reduced or disposed of. They no longer clutter and muddle the sensorium. The way is cleared for more rational thinking and greater self-control.

We have made no attempt here, of course, to survey more than a small fraction of the literature pertinent to the subject. It would require several volumes, no doubt, to list even a comprehensive bibliography. Our purpose has been simply to document that workers in such varied disciplines as anatomy, physiology, kinesiology, psychology, chiropractic, osteopathy, medicine, psychiatry, and pathology have all documented the substantiating evidence that chiropractic has a definite place in the control or in the alleviation of many forms or facets of mental or physical pathology.

CHIROPRACTIC AND THE HISTORY OF IDEAS

If we are to take advantage of the resources of chiropractic in harnessing the human potential, the time is now to follow the admonition of a distinguished sociologist, V. F. Calverton (1931).

In the introductory chapter of his book *The Making of Man,* Calverton traced the effects of societal pressures on the formation and the acceptance or rejection of certain anthropological theories. After using the ideas of Westermarck and Morgan as examples, he concluded . . .

> "There is no other way, as far as I know, of explaining idea-sets or fixations of a social character such as are represented in the influence of Westermarck and Morgan, than by resort to what I have called the theory of *cultural compulsives.* By use of this theory we are better able, I believe, to understand something of the social mechanism at work in the rise and fall of ideas and their authors. *It is not what has usually been called the truth of their doctrine which makes them so powerful, but their adaptability to other interests, class interests in the main, which they subserve.* It is these other, these more basic, interests that turn these ideas into *cultural compulsives,* invest them with social meanings which are more important than their intrinsic content.

Social history is full of such cultural compulsives. The influence of Rousseau is just as excellent an illustration as that of Westermarck or Morgan. The cultural compulsive represents the group interest in its psychological form. It is a compulsive because the ideas it represents are dependent for their influence upon the strength of the interests they represent, and not upon the abstract accuracy or inaccuracy of their sequence or structure. Its content . . . is more emotive than intellectual. It can be destroyed only by the removal of the interests which constitute its origin. But since those interests will be with us until we organize a new kind of society in which they can no longer function, and since we are all affected by those interests, however objective we may try to be, the task that confronts us is not to deny the presence of such *cultural compulsives,* but to attempt to keep them from blinding us to the facts that are of importance to our intellectual heritage."

If Calverton were alive today, he would no doubt see the controversy over chiropractic as another illustration of his theory. We cannot afford, at this juncture of history to allow cultural compulsives to blind us from the truth of chiropractic. It can be rich grist for the mill of harnessing the human potential.

REFERENCES

Assagioli, Roberto. *Psychosynthesis: a Manual of Principles and Techniques.* New New York: Hobbs, Dorman, 1965.

Bechgaard, Paul (et al.). *Manipulation av ryggradon.* Copenhagen: Munksgaard, 1963.

Bucke, Richard M. *Cosmic Consciousness.* New York: Dutton, 1923.

Bugental, James F. T. *The Search for Authenticity.* New York: Holt, Rinehart & Winston, 1965.

Campbell and Parsons. "Referred Head Pain and Its Concomitants," *N.Y. Journal of Nervous and Mental Diseases,* 1944.

Calverton, V. F. *Modern Anthropology and the Theory of Cultural Compulsives, in the Making of Man.* New York: The Modern Library, 1931.

Christensen, Finn. "Chiropractic in Danish Medicine," *Journal of Clinical Chiropractic* (New York, 1969), 2:1, and 2.

Cramer, Albert. *Lehrbuch der Chiropraktik der Wirbelsaule.* Stuttgart, 1955.

Cyriax, Edgar. *Collected Papers on Mechano-Therapeutics.* London, 1924.

Encyclopedia Britannica. "Manipulative surgery." Chicago-London-Toronto (1952), 14:810.

Fromm, Erich. *The Revolution of Hope.* New York: Harper and Row, 1968.

Gutmann, G. *Die Chiropraktik im Rahmen der Gesamtmedizin.* Hippokrates: August 31, 1957.

Harman, Willard W. "The New Copernican Revolution," *Stanford Today.* Palo Alto: Winter, 1969.

Homewood, A. E. "Chiropractic," *University of Toronto Medical Journal* (February, 1961).

Huxley, Aldous. *The Perennial Philosophy*. New York: Harper and Brothers, 1945.

Inglis, Brian. *The Case for Unorthodox Medicine*. New York: G. P. Putnam's Sons, 1965.

James, William. *Varieties of Religious Experience*. New York: Longmans. Green & Company, 1902.

Keith, Sir Arthur. "Man's Posture, its Evolution and Disorders," *British Medical Journal* (March, 1923).

Ligeros, K. *How Ancient Healing Governs Modern Therapeutics*. New York: G. P. Putnam's Sons, 1937.

Maslow, A. H. *Toward a Psychology of Being*. New York: Van Nostrand, 1962.

Mellor, Ethel. *Manipulation as a Curative Factor*. London: Methuen, 1933.

Myers, F. W. H. *Human Personality and its Survival of Bodily Death*. New York: Longmans, Green & Company, 1903.

Otto, Herbert A. "New Light on the Human Potential," *Saturday Review* (December 20, 1969).

Penfield, Wilder. "Oriental Renaissance in Education and Medicine," *Science* (September 20, 1963).

Planck, Max. The Philosophy of Physics. London: George Allen & Unwin, Ltd. (1963).

Teilhard de Chardin, P. *The Future of Man*. New York: Harper and Row, 1964.

Ussher, Neville T. "Spinal Curvatures," *California & Western Medicine* (1933), pp. 423–428.

———. "The Viscerospinal Syndrome," *Annals of Internal Medicine* (May, 1940).

Wardwell, Walter I. "A Marginal Professional Role: The Chiropractor," *Social Forces* (1952), 30:339–348.

———. "The Reduction of Strain in a Marginal Social Role," *American Journal of Sociology* (July, 1955), 61:16–26.

———. "Public Regulation of Chiropractic," *Journal of Clinical Chiropractic*. Summer, 1968.

Weiant, C. W. *et al. Opportunities in a Chiropractic Career*. New York: Universal Publishing and Distributing Corporation, 1967.

Weiant, C. W. and S. Goldschmidt. *Medicine and Chiropractic* (4th ed.). New York and Glueckstadt, Germany: J. J. Augustin, 1966.

Zukschwerdt, L. *Probleme der Chiropraktik,* in *Neuralmedizin* (May, 1953).

CHAPTER 3

MENTAL HEALTH—A TOTAL PROFESSIONAL PROBLEM

SEYMOUR LEMESHOW, D.C., ED.D.

ALL PROFESSIONALS TRAINED in the many disciplines have special mandates to render services consistent with their preparation and competencies. Such services are multiple and varied, and when available can make a difference in the solution of the total mental health problem. Its magnitude is staggering. Based on this awareness and the realization that mental health is a psycho-bio-social problem, responsibility will rest upon all the professionally trained individuals who have a considerable contribution to make toward total health, to become increasingly involved in the problem. They include not only the medically trained psychiatrist, but also psychologists, social workers, educators, physical and occupational therapists, as well as physicians—allopathic, chiropractic and osteopathic.

The "job" descriptions presented are intended to help explain the scope of contribution of the various practitioners. Although there seems to be an overlapping of services in many respects, each discipline presents an approach peculiar to its orientation and training and to the need of the patient. Differences in approach would tend to broaden the base of comprehensive services and also to provide desirable choice to the patient.

THE PSYCHIATRIST

The psychiatrist is a medically trained practitioner whose additional education and training usually in residence at a psychiatric setting, prepares him to diagnose and treat mental and emotional illness. He may employ drugs, shock therapies and where indicated, surgery in the treatment of mental afflictions, in addition to psychotherapeutic procedures. His psychotherapeutic approaches may be peculiar to a specialized philosophic and therapeutic orientation such as psychoanalysis or he may employ other therapeutic approaches as Neo-Freudian, Adlerian, Gestalt or Rogerian techniques singly or in combination, to name a few.

Many psychiatrists, particularly those who are psychoanalytically oriented, seem to rely essentially upon psychotherapeutic approaches, while others may rely extensively on adjunctive drugs and shock treatments. Certain therapists may use drugs only minimally or not at all, while some have repudiated a chemotherapeutic approach to treatment for certain mental patients. Other psychiatrists are now using orthomolecular techniques in conjunction with various procedures.

Psychiatrists in private practice may see patients on an individual basis or in groups (group therapy). Recently "Marathon" and "Encounter" group techniques have also emerged. Historically, psychiatrists were the administrators of mental hospitals and had the supervisory responsibility of the institution. In recent years, the supremacy of the psychiatrist in the hierarchy of management and supervision has somewhat receded. Observation would suggest that now, greater equality of responsibility has emerged with the advent of the sophistication of the other professional disciplines interested in mental health.

While the psychiatrist may no longer be the sole dominant professional resource in the diagnosis and treatment of mental illness, his medical license places major legal responsibility upon his judgments in legal definitions in many states and communities. Since the psychiatrist has the legal responsibility for diagnosis, treatment and institutional commitment, he would be the logical choice of referral or for consultation where his expertise is indicated.

PSYCHOLOGISTS

The work of the psychologist is varied and broad. Depending upon his interest and training he may perform services in a clinical setting, in industry and business, in the community affairs, in the military, or in a school setting, to mention a few. At the time of this writing, there were thirty-one divisions of the American Psychological Association reflecting a diversity of preparation and interest of the professionally trained psychologist.

All psychologists are trained in the understanding of behavior. Although not medically trained, they have preparation in problems of human growth and development, normal and abnormal personality development and an understanding of the assessment and measurement of developmental characteristics.

Many psychologists have demonstrated interest and received specialized training in counseling and psychotherapy and perform such services in an agency or institutional setting or on a private basis. The clinical psychologists specialize in the use of psychological tools and techniques in a clinical setting. In the past, they often performed restricted services on request of the psychiatrist which may have included personality and intellectual assessment. He provided information to the psychiatrist to assist him with diagnosis and treatment of patients.

Today the clinical psychologist may still continue to employ such projective techniques as the *Rorschach* and *Thematic Apperception Test* for personality assessment and specialized individual mental abilities tests such as the Wechsler Scales, but his scope of practice and responsibility has considerably expanded in recent years. Experience reveals that the psychologist now performs many of the services formerly the major domain of the psychiatrist as described above. For example, he employs psychotherapy and in a number of situations, has the administrative and supervisory responsibility of agencies and institutions. In private practice he deals with the emotionally ill patient and performs any of the range of non-medical psychotherapeutic procedures. He is the doctor of choice for referral when specialized testing and assessment of human personality characteristics are required. His expert knowledge in human psychodynamics renders him an excellent consultant in such matters.

SOCIAL WORKERS

Social workers are trained for a minimum of two years of graduate study in an approved school of social work. They help individuals adjust to themselves, their families, their communities, and to society. The usual degree awarded the social worker at the completion of their training is the MSSW or MSW.

The social worker has gained considerable status during recent years. His services have proved to be of considerable value in a variety of situations. He may act as the intake interviewer in psychiatric, child guidance or family counseling agencies. He may supervise welfare departments and activities. His competence may lead him to serve as an officer of the courts dealing in a number of capacities in the areas of crime and delinquency. He may be involved in parole, probation, and other rehabilitation procedures.

The social worker may specialize in medical and psychiatric social work with a responsibility to collect, through the interview and other means, all pertinent family, social, medical, and psychiatric information needed for the management of the medical or psychiatric problems of patients.

The work of the social worker has extended far beyond his early identification as a "welfare worker." He now has the training and experience to perform psychotherapeutic services in an institution or on a private basis. The "case worker" has come into his own as a capable and most useful counselor of individuals with emotional problems.

In school settings, the social worker is indispensable to the "team." In addition to providing needed background information for children with problems in a school setting, he frequently works directly with families to help interpret the school and its program to them. He may counsel members of the family to facilitate their adjustment and alleviate certain problems which may be having deleterious affects upon the student. In some situations the case worker has taken the major responsibility for the therapeutic counseling of the emotionally disturbed individual in a school setting.

EDUCATORS

Many emotional disorders manifest themselves in school settings. In certain instances, emotional disturbances are school induced. Most frequently, however, they are precipitated in other circumstances and become evident during the school situation, due to the many demands for social interaction and other requirements imposed in the learning situation. The emotionally disturbed child frequently presents learning and behavior problems directly related to the underlying emotional difficulties. Possibly at no other time during the child's day is his behavior so intensely observed as in the schools. The classroom also provides, in many instances, optimum circumstances for desirable social and emotional learning to take place.

The school is in an ideal position to meet many of the emotional and social needs of the child and youth. Adverse school experiences may also exacerbate previous disturbance in vulnerable individuals. The classroom teacher, guidance counselor, learning disabilities specialist, remediation teacher and school psychologist all have vital roles to play in the mental health of children and are frequently consulted for this purpose. Appropriate counseling and guidance, desirable student-teacher relationships, suitable curriculum assignments, and corrective remediation procedures may make the difference between mental well being and emotional disturbance of children and youth.

Special classes are generally available for severely disturbed students in many communities. The specially trained teacher is equipped not only to meet the academic but also the emotional needs of the individual.

Many special classes now provide a "therapeutic milieu" for positive change to take place. In certain instances of schizophrenic and autistic children the educational setting constitutes the treatment of choice to effect behavioral change. The "educational therapist" is emerging as a critical professional in the total management of emotionally disturbed children and youth.

PHYSICAL AND OCCUPATIONAL THERAPISTS

Physical and occupational therapists have historically performed services in a hospital, clinic or agency setting under medical supervision to help rehabilitate individuals whose incapacitation was usually secondary to medical or surgical problems. Retraining old (rehabilitation) and introducing new (habilitation) skills for the impaired patient has demonstrable values. Applying physical manipulation of tissues and limbs and the application of massage, heat and light provide many patient benefits.

In recent years the use of physical procedures, corrective exercises, relaxation techniques with mentally and emotionally affected individuals have provided many desirable therapeutic consequences. Certain institutions for the mentally retarded have found that physical therapy rendered its recipients more alert and responsive to environmental demands.

Occupational therapists have recently expanded their scope of practice to include perceptial-motor techniques directed at the alleviation and remediation of a number of behavioral and learning difficulties. The occupational therapists emphasis on developmental and postural problems and the correction and remediation thereof, promises much for the solutions to problems of mental health. Psychiatric occupational therapy seems to be an approach to the management of many psychiatric patients. Although occupational and physical therapists have, in the past, offered their services under the prescription and supervision of medical doctors, observations suggest that private practices seem to be emerging with increasing frequency.

THE PHYSICIAN

It is recognized that the life experiences of an individual do affect his general health and that physical problems often mask psychological events. It is frequently said, that the majority of problems confronting the general practitioner are not physical but emotional in origin. Although it is difficult to establish reliable estimates of the incidence of emotionally based physical difficulties, one can rely however upon the premise that they do occur with sufficient frequency to warrant attention.

In addition to the masking of emotional symptoms through the physical complaint, there are those patients who present demonstrable physical disorders which are psychologically induced. Physical disease and pathologic tissue change can be and are psychogenic in a number of instances.

The physician is frequently the first line of defense or perhaps confrontation for the psychologically disturbed patient. He must therefore deal with the emotional as well as the physical health of the patient. He must be prepared to identify the variety of emotionally based problems confronting his practice.

The physician may employ medical procedures to help palliate the symptoms. Often however, this procedure may tend to further mask the symptoms. Certain drugs may have the effect of reducing the perceived severity of emotional stress while other drugs may render the patient more amenable to psychotherapeutic procedures.

Current writings encourage the doctor in general practice to assume a more active role in the management of emotionally ill patients. Frequently the sophisticated physician with the drug and supportive psychotherapeutic procedures apparently could and should manage such patients without the need for psychiatric referral. The physician may supply the necessary psychological "crutch" to help the patient over certain critical emotional events. The family physician is being encouraged to become increasingly sophisticated in psychological dynamics and management. The physician may refer to community mental health centers when indicated for additional assistance.

THE DOCTOR OF CHIROPRACTIC

The chiropractic physician also encounters a number of patients who present a variety of physical manifestations of emotional stress. Because of the nature of his orientation and practice, many patients seek his services for the reduction of neuromuscular and other somatic disorders induced by tensions and stress. Many of the tensions prove to be structural as well as emotional in origin.

There apparently are many structurally based physical problems which are frequently overlooked by those doctors who are not oriented to view pathologic changes as having structural etiology. Frequently, psychological causes are erroneously attributed to undiagnosed neurologically based problems.

The orientation of the chiropractic doctor directs his attention to the neural basis for psychological malfunctioning. Because of his awareness and sensitivity to neurologic etiologies, a number of patients who may be otherwise uncorrectly diagnosed, are treated successfully through chiropractic adjustive procedures. By reducing interference of nervous activity by manual means and helping to restore the body to normal functioning beneficial behavioral changes do occur.

The chiropractic physician, as the allopathic physician, finds that he must deal with the many emotionally based difficulties presented by patients in his daily practice. The doctor of chiropractic's sophistication, sensitivity and concern for the patient's welfare prepares him to effect the necessary referrals or for additional consultations, diagnosis, or specialized treatments, where indicated.

COOPERATION OF THE HEALING ARTS

Schwartz as early as 1947, suggested the need for cooperation among professionals to cope with the mental health problem. He advocated that community hospitals be available to all professionals. He contended that a community hospital belongs to all the people. Every effort should be made to develop it to the highest degree of efficiency as a public service institution. This accomplishment would necessitate incorporation and correlation in hospital service of the best skills of the modern healing arts.

He points out that in many forward-looking institutions, a therapeutic "team" consists of a psychiatrist, psychologist, general medical practitioner, psychiatric nurse, occupational therapist, social worker, and clergyman, all combined on the principle that the diversity of patient problems require an organization of specialized skills. Schwartz advocated that, adding a doctor of chiropractic to the lineup would make the "team" complete. Then a patient would receive medical care, psychiatric guidance, spiritual help and environmental manipulation, as well as requisite neurological and structural aid for the alleviation of adverse transmission of spinal nerve impulses due to structural changes.

He holds that those patients whose mental disturbances stem only from neurospinal distortions when placed under chiropractic care, would require little, if any, attention by the other specialists. Consequently, greater mental health services could be given to those patients most needful of these highly specialized skills.

In the historic and expansive report by the Joint Commission on Mental Illness and Mental Health "ACTION FOR MENTAL HEALTH" (1961) Page 247, certain comments may be pertinent here.

> "In the name of helping patients we must guard against employing high professional standards simply to maintain a guild or monopoly. This point is particularly compelling in view of the imprecise state of our knowledge of functional mental illness, its diagnosis and treatment, and the fact that the typical mental patient is different in certain fundamental aspects from those seeking help from the physical branches of medicine. The therapeutic truth boils down then to what the public action slogan suggests. Mental illness is 'everybody's business.' This is the potentiality we must exploit as a means of resolving the man-power problem."

"Mental health is everyone's job." There are many professional disciplines concerned with the staggering problems of ministering to the emotional health needs of individuals. The chiropractic doctor has a special interest and facility in dealing with a variety of emotionally based disorders. In this regard he has a vital role to play in the total mental health problem.

This book points out that doctors of chiropractic are making a valuable contribution to public mental health. The massive problem of mental illness calls for greater cooperation among the healing arts. In discussing the difference between the psychiatrist and the psychologist over their respective and competitive roles in the field of mental hygiene and related services, Robert White, Ph.D., head of the Harvard Psychological Clinic remarks: "This . . . kind of controversy . . . a struggle for professional prestige . . . obscures the real issue, which has to do not with the interest of the two professions but with the interest of the public."

REFERENCES

Action for Mental Health. The final report of the joint commission on mental illness and health. New York: Basic Books, 1961.

Brower, Eli M. *Early Identification of Emotionally Handicapped Children In the School.* Springfield, Ill.: Charles C. Thomas, 1960.

Cruickshank, W. M., F. Bentzen, F. Ratzeberg and M. Tannhouser. *A Method of Teaching Brain-Injured and Hyperactive Children.* Syracuse, New York: Syracuse University Press, 1961.

Dupont, Henry (ed.). *Educating Emotionally Disturbed Children.* New York: Holt, Rinehart and Winston, 1969.

Hellmuth, J. (ed.). *Educational Therapy.* Seattle, Wash.: Special Child Publications, 1966.

Kaelbling R., R. M. Patterson. *Eclectic Psychiatry.* Springfield, Ill.: Charles C. Thomas, 1966.

Long, N. J., W. C. Morse and R. G. Newman (eds.). *Conflict In the Classroom: The Education of the Emotionally Disturbed Child.* Belmont, California: Wadsworth Publishing Co., 1965.

Morehouse, Ruth (ed.). *Transitional Programs In Psychiatric Occupational Therapy.* Dubuque, Iowa: William C. Brown, 1968.

Newman, R. G. *Psychological Consultation In the Schools.* New York: Basic Books, 1967.

Sattely, Cecilia (ed.). *Approaches To the Treatment of Patients With Neuromuscular Dysfunction.* Dubuque, Iowa: William C. Brown, 1962.

Schwartz, Herman S. *The Art of Relaxation.* Elmhurst, New York: Sessions Publishers, 1954.

Schwartz, Herman S. *Home Care for the Emotionally Ill.* Elmhurst, New York: Sessions Publishers, 1957.

White, Mary Alice and Myron W. Harris. *The School Psychologist.* New York: Harpers, 1961.

White, Robert W. *The Abnormal Personality.* New York: Ronald Press, 1948.

PART II

THE NATURE AND DIAGNOSIS OF MENTAL ILLNESS

CHAPTER

CHAPTER 4

THE DESCRIPTION OF MENTAL ILLNESS

COLTER RULE, M.D.

"PSYCHIATRY SUFFERS from words. Look at some of the words: schizophrenia, hypochondriacal, hebephrenia, masochism, pathergasias, psychoneurotic, manic-depressive, psychoanalysis, dissociative dysmnesic disorders, narcissistic. These are beautiful words and, once you have mastered them, you can lead them around like pets. They serve much the same purpose as a vicious looking bulldog. They prevent the intrusion of strangers into your private domain and they give you a feeling of security. I may know exactly what my terms mean, but, unfortunately, when I use them, even among the fully initiated members of my own lodge, I can never be sure that the fellow members recognize them as meaning just what I think they mean. When I use them outside the lodge, they make me seem mysterious and it is mystery which has done psychiatry harm in its contact with the general public." Preston, (1940)

This statement made by a psychiatrist nearly a third of a century ago becomes increasingly relevant with the passing years. It is evident that disturbances of behavior, emotions and thought processes are well-nigh universal and that they are not the province of any professional group, cult or sect, rather they should be the concern of every member of society to the extent of his curiosity, intelligence and interest. As matters of public concern, complex and abstruse classifications and diagnoses following medical and surgical models can interfere with public interest and understanding, a most regrettable situation. The very attempt to set up diagnostic categories has been challenged by some professionals Szasz (1961).

In the course of any doctor's practice it is, of course, not surprising that the patient who appears for treatment will complain of suffering from a physical illness when exhaustive examinations and tests fail to reveal any physical cause. Such problems have been designated as "mental." Estimates of the number of such patients attended by other than psychiatrists range from 10% to 70% of all patients. This high figure is backed by other studies, the Cornell study of ten years ago revealed that 80% of the population suffered from a "mental" or psychological disorder of sufficient severity to interfere with full function for living. That one of every two hospital beds in the country is occupied by a "mental" patient should provide final proof of the extent of "mental" disturbances and an idea of immeasurable cost, not only in dollars, but in suffering which afflicts our society.

THE SEARCH FOR DIAGNOSTIC CATEGORIES

Any student of mental abnormalities is struck by the wide range of behaviors, mood disturbances and irrational thought processes which occur. From this welter of confusion a succession of theories, dating back to the dawn of history, has been postulated to account for the abnormalities. Primitive man thought of the victim as one possessed by evil spirits. Hippocrates, the father of medicine, is credited with asserting that such a view was incorrect, and that mental conditions, like physical diseases had a specific cause, and ran a specified course, differing from the previous views that they were the result of the operation of evil spirits, or the mischief or punishment of the gods. This rational explanation was, of course, substantiated by the observable fact that delirium followed fever, that behavioral abnormalities followed head injuries by accident or weapons. While the Hippocratic roots of rationality continued to be held through the centuries, his views were overshadowed by the general view that diseases of all kinds represented the punishment for sins, and —during the Middle Ages—the accepted cause lay in the explanations of demonology, i.e., "possession" by demons. Thousands of the emotionally troubled were put to death because of the view that they were possessed of the devil, or practiced witchcraft spreading evil throughout society. This theory was rejected only after centuries, is documented in the Salem witchcraft trials within the history of our own nation, and still persists among primitive peoples.

Modern attempts to explain and classify mental illness following the medical model of clearly defined syndromes began in the nineteenth century. While the benefits of this effort are obvious and set the background for a rational approach it carried with it a blindness to the social and developmental roots of mental illness and the necessity of investigating and changing the social causes responsible. Before describing recent trends a brief review of two major contributions of the last century, those of Kraepelin and Freud should be noted.

At the beginning of the nineteenth century, several physicians noticed that there were certain patients in the mental hospitals who had fairly similar symptoms. These patients often had poor memory, defective speech, and difficulty in walking or doing skilled movements and yet, at the same time, maintained that they were capable of the greatest deeds. Invariably, these patients got worse and eventually died in the hospital.

During the course of the next 60 years it was gradually learned that more men than women were affected, that the onset of symptoms was usually during middle age, and that certain reflexes were abnormal. It becomes increasingly evident that this complex of symptoms had a typical onset, a typical course, and a typical outcome. By the end of the nineteenth century it had been fairly well established that this disease, later called paresis, was caused by damage to the spinal cord and brain due to syphilitic infection. Once this was known, various methods of prevention and treatment were instituted.

During the latter part of the nineteenth century, a German psychiatrist named Emil Kraepelin began to study large numbers of case histories in the mental hospitals. His aim was to establish various groupings of symptoms that were associated by virtue of a common onset, common course, and common outcome; just as had been done previously for general paresis. Kraepelin eventually classified mental diseases into two major groupings which he called the manic-depressive psychosis and dementia praecox (or schizophrenia). Within each major grouping he proposed several subgroups.

This system, with relatively few changes, has been in use by psychiatrists up to the present time. It is used as a basis for the legal determination of insanity, the establishment of wards for custody, the screening of military personnel, the preparation of census data, the estimation of prognosis, and the treatment of patients. Experimental research with patient populations usually uses these categories as the descriptive basis for selection of subjects and evaluation of results. Here again, description and classification precede experimentation.

While Kraepelin was achieving renown for his systematic classification of mental hospital patients, Sigmund Freud was beginning his studies of hysteria. Hysteria, a puzzling malady, recognized many centuries before, is characterized by a large assortment of symptoms which could include blindness, deafness, paralysis, anesthesia of parts of the body, and convulsions. For a long time it had been believed that hysteria was due to a disorder of the nervous system, but Freud and others introduced surprising observations.

It was discovered that most of the symptoms of hysteria could be produced by hypnotic suggestions and then eliminated by further suggestions. It was shown that in some actual cases of hysteria the symptoms could be removed by hypnosis. Other peculiar facts were the existence of anatomically meaningless signs and symptoms, e.g. paralysis of body parts unexplainable by any anatomical lesion, and disappearance of these signs when the patient went to sleep.

In an effort to clarify these issues, Freud published an essay in 1893 which described the differences between paralyses due to organic lesions and those due to hysteria. After giving a detailed description of these differences between organic and hysterical paralyses, Freud noted that the particular symptoms that develop seem to depend on common, popular ideas about the organs and parts of the body. He then predicted that no one would find hysterical symptoms in patients that mimic certain well-known effects of brain or nerve injury (e.g., certain visual field defects, or certain kinds of partial facial paralyses) because the symptoms seem strange to the unscientific mind. Finally, Freud concluded that in all cases of hysterical paralysis there is a strong subconscious emotional feeling associated with the organ whose function is lost, and that cure requires the elimination of the connection between the emotion and the organ.

Freud's writing, as is well known, provided the basis for many of the descriptive and explanatory terms still used by psychiatrists. However, there has never been complete agreement and several attempts have been made to provide a consistent nomenclature.

One of the first attempts to create an organized classification of "mental diseases" was made at Bellevue Hospital in New York City in 1903 and then revised in 1911 and 1922. An alternative classification was proposed by the forerunner of the American Psychiatric Association in 1918. Although an attempt was made to develop a single classification system in 1933, the American Psychiatric Association and the American Neurological Association could not compromise their diagnostic differences so that similar or identical diagnoses were differently coded.

World War II had an important impact on psychiatric thinking because it either produced or uncovered a large number of psychiatric problems. This in turn led to extensive revisions in nomenclature. In 1952, the American Psychiatric Association noted in retrospect: "By 1948 the situation in psychiatric nomenclature had deteriorated almost to the point of confusion which existed throughout medical nomenclature in the twenties." One of the major shortcomings concerned the classification of mental disorders associated with organic brain disease.

The World Health Organization in 1948 and again in 1955 tried to develop an internationally acceptable nomenclature. The result, however, was to increase the diffuseness of the definitions. In 1966, the World Health Organization and the American Psychiatric Association jointly approved a new revised diagnostic nomenclature and it is this schema which is now in current use. Basically, the committee which made the recommendations tried to determine what well-informed psychiatrists generally agreed upon. However, it "tried to avoid terms which carry with them implications regarding either the nature of a disorder or its causes and has been explicit about causal assumptions when they are integral to a diagnostic concept." The report of the committee points out that it was impossible for the members to agree on just what schizophrenia, the most widely studied of the mental diseases, is; they "could only agree on what to call it."

Despite the desire of the committee to avoid inconsistent or ambiguous terminology the final result which was achieved used a variety of approaches. Some of the diagnostic categories are purely descriptive (e.g. hysterical personality type), some are of mixed type in terms of description plus presumed etiology (e.g. involutional melancholia), and some are primarily etiological (e.g. psychophysiologic disorder). It is also possible for a person to show symptoms that are considered to be diagnostic of several different states (e.g. depression).

The result of these complex factors is that precise diagnosis is often difficult, and it is not uncommon for experts to disagree with one another. As previously noted, there has been a recent movement whose advocates prefer to describe mental illness as a myth (Szasz, 1961), and who try to emphasize its non-medical, social aspects. In the absence of definitive, etiological information about mental illness, any diagnostic scheme used by psychiatrists is not highly reliable or fully satisfactory (Klein and Davis, 1969).

One of the major reasons that diagnostic nomenclature is unreliable is that signs of mental illness can be produced by so many different factors. It has been established that mental abnormalities can be produced by bacterial infections such as tuberculosis, meningitis, whooping cough and syphilis. In the 19th century one of the important bases for mental hospitalization was syphilitic infection. Mental abnormalities can also be produced by viral infections such as measles and encephalitis, as well as certain parasitic diseases. Prolonged exposures to toxins such as carbon monoxide, insecticides, lead, and carbon tetrachloride can also produce mental symptoms. In addition, in the current age of experimentation with drugs, there are many mental symptoms which have been produced by drugs such as LSD, psilocybin, amphetamines, barbiturates, and the like.

Vitamin deficiencies are another established source of mental abnormality. Insufficient vitamins B or C can produce both physical illness and mental symptoms, but because the brain is generally more sensitive to the effects of deprivation than other organs, mental symptoms will often appear before other biological diagnostic signs. The Nobel prize winner Linus Pauling (1967) has pointed out that enzyme abnormalities could probably underlie many signs of psychosis, just as the malfunctioning of an enzyme system is the basis for one form of mental retardation, phenylketonuria. In the 1930's many patients in mental hospitals in the southern United States were there because of vitamin B deficiencies related to the ingestion of bleached white flour. After this was discovered a change in diet alone produced remission of symptoms in many individual cases. All these examples which have been cited emphasize the multiplicity of factors which influence the appearance of aberrant mental symptoms. It is no wonder that the problems of diagnosis and determination of etiology are so difficult.

SOME MAJOR SYNDROMES

Any attempt to exhaustively describe all the syndromes of mental illness would require a text book. As an alternative, a brief description will be given here of the types of mental aberration that are most commonly seen in mental hospitals. Three types of patients will be described: the paranoid schizophrenic, the depressed, and the manic or agitated patient.

Paranoid Schizophrenia: Patients who most commonly develop paranoid schizophrenia are in their late teens or early twenties. It is found in all social classes and in people with a wide range of intelligence. Quite often, the patient who develops this illness reports an adolescent period during which he was relatively withdrawn and solitary. He tended to develop sexually relatively late, usually did not become involved in contact sports such as football or basketball and was not considered a behavior problem either at home or in school. Pupils who sit quietly in the back of the room are usually overlooked by teachers.

The constellation of symptoms associated with this illness is a progressive withdrawal from people, a feeling of depression and the development of certain bizarre signs. For example, the adolescent may lock himself in his room and refuse to go into the street or he might keep the lights on all night and be heard to pace restlessly around his room. Sometimes he may begin to cry or show a sudden temper outburst. He may talk strangely about sexual matters or about particular individuals who are trying to harm him. Quite frequently such patients will use individuals or organizations who are currently in the news as a basis for their delusion. For example, ten or fifteen years ago, a paranoid schizophrenic might have the belief that communists or the FBI were constantly watching him. Today he might identify his watchers as CIA agents or Black Panthers. Sometimes the patient will report hearing voices talking to him which tell him bad things. The voices might, for example, tell him that he was no good, that he was a homosexual or that he should kill himself. It is important to note that hallucinations are not necessarily a part of the psychosis.

Usually, the way a patient gets into a hospital is because some crisis occurs in the family and the family members then take the patient to an emergency room. The usual treatment is Thorazine, one of the major tranquillizers and in most cases the more florid symptoms decrease or disappear within a month or two. Quite often, however, patients of this type have a recurrence of symptoms and have a series of hospitalizations over the years.

Depression. Depression is probably the most common psychiatric symptom in America today. It has been estimated that more than 10 million people suffer from various degrees of depression and that more psychotropic drugs are sold for the alleviation of depression than for any other symptom.

Depressions may occur in people of any age and are often related to real life situations associated with important experiences of loss. Death of a family member, or loss of a job or girlfriend may precipitate a depression. However, depressions often occur without good reasons or unconnected with any disturbing life event. Some women have mild depressions that are clearly related to their menstrual cycle. Occasionally women have severe post-partum depressions associated with the birth of a child. Certain drugs taken to deal with medical conditions will induce depressions in a small number of cases. Many women who go through the menopause experience varying depths of depression. Certain diseases of the pituitary gland and the adrenal gland will induce depressions. It is clear that a large variety of possible causes exist for any case of depression.

The personal experience of depression in terms of symptoms also varies a good deal. Most such patients report feelings of emptiness, worthlessness, sadness and hopelessness. They feel unable to do their normal work be it housework, factory work, or administration. They find it difficult to concentrate and feel unable to make normal decisions. They withdraw from social contacts, stop telephoning, often eat less, lie around passively during the day, but sleep poorly at night. Interest in sexual activity decreases or disappears. Often a feeling of irritability develops.

Sometimes the patient becomes very passive as these changes develop, but at other times the patient might become quite active and agitated. In most cases, the patient's thinking remains relatively normal in the sense of making appropriate responses to questions or requests. However, in some smaller proportion of the cases a thought disorder occurs along with the depression. In such cases, the patient may have bizarre thoughts, or delusions or highly irrational thinking. The psychiatrist then distinguishes between psychotic depression and neurotic depression.

Most depressions are of relatively short duration, lasting from a few weeks to a few months. Though the use of antidepressant drugs (many chemical varieties are available), most patients show a favorable response, and long-term depressions lasting more than a few months are now the exception rather than the rule. In the case of recurrent depressive illness, it has been shown that the average duration of depressions, even without treatment of any kind, is about three to four months. Depressions are dangerous and must be taken seriously because the probability of self-inflicted injury or suicide increases. It is important to remember that people who make suicidal threats are more apt to carry them out than those who don't. Appropriate referrals are often necessary.

Manic or Agitated Behavior. The term manic in relation to mental illness usually refers to the type of illness called manic-depressive. Manic depressive patients typically show a pattern of behavior which is marked by recurrent episodes of mania, depression or both. However, since this form of illness is relatively uncommon and accounts for only a small proportion of mental hospital patients it will not be considered further. Instead the term manic will be used as roughly synonymous with agitated behavior and although this is an over-simplified usage it includes many more patients actually seen in hospitals.

The manic or agitated patient begins to show the following kinds of symptoms to a gradually increasingly degree. He feels as if he has boundless energy and reports that he can work as much as 20 hours a day. His need for sleep decreases and when he does sleep he sleeps restlessly. He begins to feel like being with people more and often increases the number of activities in which he is involved. He reports that he can not sit still and that he has been working faster than usual. At the same time feelings of anger and irritation increase and he becomes less tolerant of frustration. If he has money, he spends the money freely and sometimes irrationally and quite often there is an increase in sexual drive.

This kind of manic state can occur at all ages. Quite often people who show this pattern of behavior have some similarity to it even in their normal pre-psychotic state. They typically have a strong craving for attention and they are often found in the forefront of things. They are gregarious, lively and popular both in their normal state and when they are patients.

Quite often such patients find that they cannot stop talking and not uncommonly may be brought to the hospital at the point of exhaustion. Sometimes, but not always, they show bizarre thinking; but even when this is not the case they show a strong tendency to jump from subject to subject in some disconnected fashion and are often difficult to follow. When such a patient enters a hospital he is usually given phenathiazine derivatives which act to reduce the agitation and over-activity and the more overt signs usually disappear in a month or two. Recently lithium carbonate has been used fairly effectively to calm these patients without necessarily sedating them.

The Neurosis. The preceding descriptions have dealt with the more typical symptom complexes which are seen in mental hospitals or which usually require some degree of hospitalization. Now we will present a brief discussion concerning the neuroses.

There is at present no unanimous agreement on just what a neurosis is or what causes it. In the last century the term was applied to certain symptoms which interfered with normal life but which were not considered as bizarre. For example, people with unusual compulsions such as constant hand washing were considered to be neurotic. People with unusual fears or phobias were also so classified. Some patients who were classified as hysteric showed peculiar lapses of memory or loss of sensation from a particular body part or showed an apparent paralysis of some muscles.

As time went on the definition of neurosis was gradually expanded to include a variety of things. For example, it included people with depression and people who acted-out in some aggressive way. Some psychiatrists wanted to include delinquents and criminals under this rubric. About the only thing that these many different states have in common is that the individual feels as if he has an inner compulsion to behave in some way which is not necessarily satisfying to him and is often not socially useful. This sense of being controlled by inner forces which are beyond one's own control seems to be a key element in the definition of neurosis. Although some psychiatrists insist that anxiety is a necessary correlate of neurosis, others have pointed out that in many cases of depression or psychopathy (delinquent acting-out) there are very few signs of unusual anxiety. Some observers have tried to show that so-called normal individuals show a pattern of behavior which is a kind of golden mean between sets of extremes. In one study (Plutchik, 1961) in which neurotic children at a child guidance clinic were compared with delinquent or psychopathic children who were engaged in criminal behavior, a series of differences between them were noticed on seven major dimensions. This is shown in Table 1. In every case the normal child could be conceptualized as falling mid-way between the neurotic and the psychopathic child on the different personality dimensions.

Since the behavior of the neurotic is less troublesome than that of the psychopath, both for himself and for society, there has been less attention directed to the precise measurement of change that can be brought about by treatment. A large variety of treatment procedures have been used in dealing with the signs of neurosis including: suggestion, hypnosis, psychodrama, persuasion, education, non-directive therapy, other types of psychotherapies as well as all kinds of drugs. Every one of these methods has undoubtedly been successful to some degree in helping to alleviate the symptoms of neurosis. In fact, a study by Eysenck (1958) has reported that neurotics who went to general practitioners showed as much improvement as those who went to psychiatrists. A study by Levitt (1963) showed that children who were treated for a year in a Child Guidance Clinic showed no more improvement after a two year follow-up than a comparable group of children who were not treated. These findings and many others of a similar sort all suggest that there is a great deal that we do not know about psychiatric problems and how to treat them. It is certainly evident that we are still in the pioneering stage of understanding the multiple causes and courses of psychological disorders and that new understanding and new theories will be part of Man's increasing understanding of himself in relation to the world and the society in which he lives (Rule, 1967). Meanwhile, there exists unlimited opportunity for all mental health workers, professional and paraprofessional, to make significant contributions to the understanding and treatment of "mental illness" in any of its many forms.

PSYCHOSOMATIC MEDICINE

During the past 30 years or so a new branch of psychophysiological stress under the name of psychosomatics has developed, which has attempted an integration of psychiatry with internal medicine. The view has gradually evolved that certain physical illnesses are brought about as a result of certain types of emotional stresses, and that existing illnesses are exacerbated by emotional stress. These views are based upon observations which have often been reported by physicians and others, but it is only relatively recently that any systematic attention has been directed to these issues.

Physicians who have been involved in this field point out that our language is filled with expressions that suggest a connection between emotions and physical changes in the body. For example, we get "butterflies in our stomach" when we are frightened, or our "stomach becomes tied up in knots," or we get "scared stiff" or "scared shitless." People who are angry may "bust a gut," or become "livid with rage." Feelings of "disgust may make our skin crawl" or give us "goose pimples." The assumption is made that long-lasting states of fear, anger, disgust, or depression may bring about changes in the stomach, lungs or heart and blood vessels, skin and other organs which can be pathological and which will eventually become real physical illness at some point. Thus, it is claimed that certain emotional states may bring about an actual ulcer in the stomach, or an inflammation of the bowel (colitis). Some psychiatrists have gone on to suggest that even such diseases as coronary thrombosis, uticaria, various skin conditions and even cancer can be brought about by emotional stresses of various kinds.

Another aspect of psychosomatic theorizing refers to the kind of person who develops a particular illness. The question arises: "Why did this particular *person* develop this particular *illness,* at this particular *time* in his life." To talk only of emotional stress ignores the special character structure of the person who is under stress. Different people, even in concentration camps and prisoner of war camps, respond differently to the same general circumstances. This leads to the idea that certain personality traits and abnormal structure may *predispose* an individual to react with a certain emotional pattern to a given situation.

For example, it has been claimed that people who develop ulcers are usually driving, highly ambitious persons, who, at the same time, have a strong need to be dependent. The conflict between the dependency and the ambitious strivings leads to frequent feelings of disappointment and resentment, which in turn become expressed in the stomach lesion we call an ulcer. Similar speculations have been made about other types of illnesses.

There are thus three elements to the general psychosomatic framework: the personality trait pattern, the particular constellation of emotional stresses, and the persistence of these over a long period of time. Those views seem plausible at the very least, and a number of attempts have been made to confirm or justify them. Unfortunately many of the attempts at confirmation have simply been case histories reported by enthusiastic therapists. Although such case histories are often fascinating to read they cannot provide convincing evidence of any of the tenets of psychosomatic medicine. There is no way to control the many variables which impinge on an individual's life. There is no way to take into account the many emotional stresses an individual experienced without having a physical illness. After all, therapist typically sees the patient only after an illness has developed and he then has to reason backwards, so to speak, to arrive at possible causal factors.

Also unsatisfactory are many of the studies which are of a more research nature in which groups of patients are considered. Different investigators have often reported different personality traits associated with a particular illness (e.g. ulcers) or have disagreed on causal factors. For example, it was noted during World War II that some business men who had ulcers and were put in concentration camps by the Nazis, lost their ulcers despite the terribly stressful conditions of the camps. As another example, although several studies have shown that physical illness often occurs shortly after a severe personal loss (e.g. death in a family), there has been no consistent connection established between the loss and any one specific illness. Severe depressions apparently weaken body defenses in some ways that enable diseases to occur more readily. But this is far from establishing a precise connection between a particular personality interacting with a certain stress to produce one unique illness.

In conclusion, although research has shown that widespread bodily

Table I

THE PERSONALITY DIFFERENCE BETWEEN NEUROTIC, NORMAL AND DELINQUENT CHILDREN

Personality Dimension	*Neurotic*	*Normal*	*Delinquent*
Expression of Emotions	Shows mostly fears, sadness and anger directed at himself	Can feel and express *all* emotions at appropriate times	Mostly concerned with aggression, courage and manliness
Expression of Action	Tends to be compulsive (and inhibited in action)	Can be spontaneous at times and thoughtful at others	Tends to be impulsive and very quick to "fly off the handle"
Feelings of Empathy	Overly sensitive to feelings of other people, animals and things	Sensitive to feelings of other people but not to excessive degree	Almost insensitive to the feelings of other people
Feelings of Guilt	Guilty about many things; tends to blame himself	Can feel guilty about certain things but goes to neither extreme	Guilty about almost nothing. Will blame other people but rarely himself
Feelings of Insecurity	Tends to feel insecure, inferior or worthless	Is aware of own limitations as well as abilities	Tends to be vain, narcissistic with little apparent insecurity
Feelings of Distrust	Very sensitive to criticism and possible rejection	Exercises some caution but enjoys situations and people	Apparently insensitive to rejection. "Doesn't give a damn."
Social Contacts	Tends to be alone. Has few friends.	Can enjoy being alone as well as group contact	Inability to be alone. Excessive need to be with a group

changes occur during emotional stresses, the assumption that every illness is based upon emotional stress is not warranted, nor is the assumption that each major illness occurs to people of certain limited and definable personality types. Considerably more research must be done before the tenets of psychosomatic medicine can be taken as proved.

REFERENCES

Dunbar, F. *Emotions and Bodily Changes.* New York: Columbia University Press, 1941.

Eysenck, J. H. "The Effects of Psychotherapy," in H. J. Eysenck (ed.), *Handbook of Abnormal Psychology.* New York: Basic Books (1961), pp. 697–725.

Grece, W. J., Wolf, S., and Wolff, H. G. *The Human Colon.* New York: Hoeber, 1951.

Groen, J. *Life Stress and Bodily Disease.* A Research Publication of the Association for Research in Nervous and Mental Diseases. Baltimore: Williams & Wilkins (1950), pp. 16–17.

Haugen, G. B., Dixon, H. H. and Dickel, H. A. *A Therapy for Anxiety Tension Reactions.* New York: The Macmillan Co., 1958.

Klein, D. F. and Davis, J. M. *Diagnosis and Drug Treatment of Psychiatric Disorders.* Baltimore: Williams & Wilkins, 1969.

Pauling, Linus. "Orthomolecular Psychiatry," *Science* (1968), pp. 160 and 265–271.

Plunkett, R. J. and Gordon, J. E. *Epidemiology & Mental Illness.* New York: Basic Books, 1960.

Plutchik, R. "Implications of a Neurosis-Delinquency Continuum," *J. Assoc. Psychiatric Treatment of Offenders* (1959), pp. 3, and 4–5.

Preston, George H. *Psychiatry for the Curious.* New York: Rinehart & Co., Inc. (1940), p. 3.

Rule, Colter. "A Theory of Human Behavior Based on Studies of Non-Human Primates," *Perspectives in Biology and Medicine.* University of Chicago (1967), 10 (2).

Selye, H. *The Stress of Life.* New York: McGraw-Hill, 1956.

Szasz, T. S. *The Myth of Mental Illness.* New York: Norton, 1961.

Wolff, H. G. *Life Stress and Bodily Disease.* Baltimore: Williams & Wilkins, 1950.

CHAPTER 5

THE INTERVIEW PROCESS*

LEONARD HOCHMAN, PH.D.

IT HAS BECOME APPARENT in the process of treating people that the patient's presenting problem is most often related to events which took place prior to the acute onset of the discomfort. Although the patient may report some particular accident or strain which explains the present difficulty, further examination may reveal that there is a historical basis for the maladaption. The patient's history may reveal either a chronic weakness in that area, chronic tension affecting the area or a pattern of reaction to stress which manifests itself in an attack on the weakened portion of the body.

If the practitioner keeps in mind that the patient facing him across the desk brings with him a long history of reaction to stress, prior injuries, familial patterns, and a rich and complex life style, the history taking may be as important in determining the course and outcome of treatment as is the treatment itself. If one wishes to uncover reaction patterns one must be able to lead the patient on a voyage of discovery through his own history. Often the discovery of these patterns and the identification of their origins leads to solutions which interrupt the further development of the symptom. A program of care must, we believe, be designed so that the patient does not experience recurrent episodes of the same complaint.

The general practitioner cannot justify the beginning of a course of treatment without first determining the patient's overall situation. It is as important to identify the function of the symptom in terms of its object as it is to determine the consequences. Freud in the development of the idea of "secondary gain" very clearly stated that every chronic symptom has for the patient some positive value. It is often difficult to see the value but from the point of view of the "private logic" of the patient it is real. One must determine the nature of the gain * if one is to treat successfully.

It is often the opening of the door to the patient's "private logic" which is the key to treatment. The taking of a careful history provides the greatest insights into the person's private system of thought. Dreikurs has suggested that on a test of functional versus organic causes for distress we simply ask the patient how his life would change if the symptoms were relieved. If no

* For an explanation of the possible "secondary gains" see page 167. Ed.

clear change can be arrived at, he suggests that the symptom is clearly organic in nature. However if relief of the symptom would bring about dramatic change in the person's life, particularly as it effects significant behavior changes toward others in the environment, the complaint is most likely functional.

The method of history taking depends to a great extent on the person and the establishment of the doctor-patient relationship. The practitioner should keep in mind that he is questioning for a specific purpose. He is attempting to both understand the person and the nature of the complaint and work out an acceptable solution. If one is to understand the functional meaning of an ailment for a particular person one must first understand the person. If one is to change the direction of the person one must understand what makes him move. History taking cannot and should not be done solely during the first visit. As the course of treatment proceeds, additional information can be obtained. As the patient develops confidence in the practitioner he may be more and more willing to reveal facets of his life.

Taking full records at an early stage may save time with the garrulous patient who wishes to cover the same ground over and over. He can be told tactfully that it is already in the record. Records also serve to point up the improvements that have taken place, for the neurotic's deficient perspective makes him prone to forget his earlier difficulties and dwell on the remaining symptoms. The fact that the practitioner is sufficiently interested in keeping good records often convinces the patient of his deep interest. The information thus obtained by the practitioner plays a major role in determining a remedial program not based upon guesswork or hasty conclusions. The thorough examination is often the means by which the initial rapport so vital to constructive personal relations takes place. Many patients are thereby impressed with the efficiency, thoroughness, and interest of the practitioner.

Because of this larger meaning attached to whatever the practitioner does, he should never become careless, impatient, or feel this process is a waste of time. He must execute the examination in an orderly and effective manner. Nevertheless, the entire procedure of history-taking should be done quietly and leisurely. The "easy-does-it" attack is most effective. It is actually much simpler in operation than this discussion sounds. The practitioner must show lively interest in the patient, permit him to talk freely, and then make coherent notes of the information obtained.

Useful attitudes in the taking of a patient's history are:

1. *LISTEN:* Too often in the examining room patients are cut off, not allowed to talk, ignored while the practitioner mechanically gathers information.
2. Develop the use of open-ended questions: "How did you injure yourself?" instead of "Did you injure yourself in a fall?" This gives the patient an opportunity to talk and elaborate, which may provide much additional information.

3. Do not press the patient for information he is unwilling to reveal.
4. Continue history taking in subsequent visits.
5. Watch the patient's use of gestures, grimaces, and body movements. To the trained observer this often reveals a great deal about the patient's chronic reactions to stress.
6. It is frequently useful to have the patient write out and bring to the office a detailed description of an average day. Dr. Herbert Nilchin suggests that this often provides information concerning the patient's illness which he may regard as unimportant. He describes a patient he was working with as having brought in the following description: "I get up in the morning, shower, shave, brush my teeth, dress, go down, and have breakfast. Then I go upstairs, vomit, brush my teeth again and leave for work." In the initial history taking the patient had left out the daily vomiting behavior completely. He regarded it as entirely within normal limits and not worth mentioning to the practitioner.
7. Pay careful attention to the patient's response to the first treatment session.
8. Do not question the patient when he is in an agitated state. It is frequently necessary to first help him relax and build trust in the practitioner before he can respond to questions.

Taking and maintaining complete records on every patient is of course essential for a variety of reasons. However, for the person experiencing stress, the practitioner with a pen and pad in hand may represent distance. Notes concerning specific issues should be obtained early, recorded, and put aside for the remainder of the session. The history of a human being unfolds much like a novel. As trust develops, persons other than the patient appear in the story. It is best to complete the record as soon as the patient leaves the office. The practitioner must train himself to listen and record, mentally, important factors and directions for exploration. Careful records often lead to the discovery of distortions and discrepancies in the patient's perception of an event. These are, of course, fruitful avenues for exploration.

It is best to maintain an easy and relaxed approach to the patient. The practitioner must maintain an attitude of interest in and concern for the person he is working with. History taking when done properly is relaxed and natural, following the flow and movement of the patient's ideation. The practitioner must keep in mind that many of the patients who come to him come for the magic of the "cure." They expect something to be done to, or for them. If these expectations are not met, the patient often leaves with a feeling of disappointment. While disavowing the possession of a "magical power," the practitioner must be careful not to destroy the patient's hope in the treatment. He comes for relief. It is important that he finds in the practitioner, sustaining interest and concern. Giving the patient the privilege of telephoning between visits helps to fulfill that need for relief.

Patients frequently come in with complaints which mask the real problems. For example, a patient may come in with a gastrointestinal problem. During the course of the examination, questions are asked concerning dietary and eating habits, sleep patterns, irritability, bowel problems, etc. The patient is encouraged by the nature of the questions to talk freely. He soon begins relating details concerning fears, conflicts, interpersonal relations, compulsive behavior regarding food and so on. The practitioner becomes aware that the nature of the emotional conflict is involved in the gastrointestinal problem. Important data as to the onset of the problem, when it is most acute, under what kind of conditions the pain is most troublesome can be obtained directly from the patient's history. This offers an invaluable source of information as to the management of the problem.

It is essential that the practitioner carefully observe the patient during the questioning period. Changes in facial expression, posture, repeated use of specific gestures, shifts in mood, all are suggestions of underlying difficulties. The practitioner must become aware of the "sore spots" in the personality as well as the "sore spots" in the musculature. In normal social interaction people train themselves to avoid areas for discussion which create conflict in others. In treatment, these are the very areas that should be explored. If the patient shows reluctance in dealing with an area the first time it comes up, the practitioner should return to it in subsequent visits, phrasing the question differently.

Establishing and clarifying the major complaint should always be the starting point. The patient, as Wilhelm Reich suggested, must be educated as to his therapy. He can then help himself to a greater extent. Emotional problems which center around or stem from the major complaint should be explored. The patient's medical history should be inquired into. Exploration of psychic distress associated with earlier illnesses is often revealing in indicating behavioral patterns to which the practitioner should be alerted. It is after the patient leaves that the careful recording of information obtained during the session should be done. Time to reflect on the session and think about the patient all add to the sharpening of one's "clinical intuition."

This brings us to an extremely important aspect of treatment, the doctor-patient relationship. Frequently in examining this aspect of treatment, all of the focus is on the patient. However, the behavior and attitude of the practitioner is crucial. He, by his attitude, will decisively influence the course of treatment. The patient must believe in the practitioner's ability to help, but too much reassurance, given too early in treatment, can often lead to disappointment, frustration, and the patient's loss of belief in the procedure. The difficulties involved, the limits to be expected, and the end results of treatment should be carefully and honestly presented to the patient. Rapport has often been interpreted to mean friendliness; it should really represent concern, confidence, and trust. Empathy, warmth, and honesty are all important aspects of the relationships. Where they are present rapport will develop on its own. When genuineness on the part of the practitioner is not present, all of the jokes, back-slapping, and friendliness will not result in the establishment of rapport appropriate to treatment.

The work of Veyslanck, Greenspoon, Mattarazzo, and others all points out that the posture, facial expressions, and vocalizations of the therapist, including the judicious "aha" and "uhuh" responses, directly influence the behavior of the patient. A worried expression on the practitioner's face can result in increasing the patient's fears surrounding his complaint. Too detailed or tenacious questioning over specific incidents or complaints can create worry and fear in the patient.

In the sessions spent together, the practitioner should attempt to increase his knowledge concerning details of the patient's present life and history which produce worry and tension. Changes in the living situation, changes in the working situation, problems with children, friends, neighbors all can add to the difficulties in treatment. A key issue is the ability of the patient to cope with stress; can he adjust to stress?; can he move in other directions?; is he flexible?; what is his level of maturity? Can the patient establish and articulate goals?; can he delay gratification?; can he wait?; can he accept therapeutic intervention?; does he carry out suggestions? These, again, are crucial in determining the approach to the patient and the eventual outcome.

When dealing with a patient of a low level of maturity, the practitioner can look forward to a long course of treatment. Attention should be paid to determining the major components of the personality. Is the patient dependent, curious, evasive? Is he overly conscientious, ambitious, fearful? Upon these factors, predictions can be made as to his future behavior. One should also watch for physical reactions; blushing, perspiration, trembling, tears, unusual breathing patterns all indicate emotional responses for further exploration.

The most important skill the good interviewer develops is timing. He should be aware of when the patient is ready to deal with a particular issue. Every therapist has had the experience of a patient asking, "How come you never brought that up before?" when he has been asked exactly that question for four or five weeks or perhaps months. This indicates that the patient simply was not ready to reveal the answer, so he didn't hear the question.

The patient must be assured that everything he tells will be in the strictest confidence. He often tests the practitioner before he tells what really troubles him. He will watch the reactions of the practitioner. Expressions of shock, distaste, boredom, annoyance do much to undermine the confidence of the patient. When one becomes aware of the patient's struggle with difficult material, the most useful response is concerned silence. The patient may be encouraged by the practitioner's assuring "it's all right." One should watch for deep sighs, postural shifts, and sudden quietness. They frequently signal the patient's readiness to deal with emotionally charged material.

All therapeutic suggestions given to the patient should be within the ability of the patient to follow. Suggestions like, "Move out of the house," when it is impossible; "get married," when it is impossible, or "change jobs," when jobs are difficult to find all lead to the eventual rejection of the doctor by the patient. Asking the patient to do what is beyond him is destructive in that it increases feelings of inadequacy and worthlessness. Any treatment procedure, no matter what the specialty involved, should result in the patient acquiring a more positive feeling about himself. In the course of treatment the practitioner should continually question the patient in terms of "what also troubles you"; "are there other complaints I might help you with"; "what other changes would you like to make?" "would you be happy if all your symptoms disappeared?" The patient who leaves the office feeling more positive about himself and about his ability to deal effectively with the world he lives in can be considered a therapeutic success.

REFERENCES

Adler, Alfred. *Individual Psychology*. New York: Basic Books (Heinz Ansbacher and Lowena Ansbacher), 1956.

Aldrich, C. Knight. *Psychiatry for the Family Physician*. New York: McGraw-Hill Book Company (The Blakiston Division), 1955.

Freud, Sigmund. *Collected Papers*. New York: Basic Books (translation by Joan Riviere), 1959.

Greenspoon, J. "The Effect of Verbal and Non-Verbal Stimuli in the Frequency of Members of Two Verbal Response Classes." Doct. Dissertation, University of Indiana, 1950.

Kaelbling, Rudolf and Patterson, Ralph M. *Eclectic Psychiatry*. Springfield, Illinois: C. C. Thomas, 1966.

Nechin. *Personal Communication*.

Reich, Wilhelm. *Character Analysis*. New York: Noonday Press (translated by Theodore Wolfe), 1949.

Veyslanck, W. S. "The Control of the Content of a Conversation: reinforcement of statement of opinion," *J. of Abnormal and Social Psychology* (1955), pp. 5, and 668–676.

Wolberg, Lewis R. *The Technique of Psychotherapy*. New York: Grune and Stratton, 1954.

Ziskind, Eugene. *Psychophysiological Medicine*. Philadelphia: Lea and Lebiger, 1954.

CHAPTER 6

THE DIAGNOSIS OF PERSONALITY FROM THE BODY*

Bioenergetic Analysis

ALEXANDER LOWEN, M.D.

INTRODUCTORY COMMENTS

Dr. Alexander Lowen presents bio-energetic analysis *as "a psychotherapy devoted to the analytic study of the form and movement of the body." Many features of this system can be of particular interest and value to the doctor who is concerned with a more comprehensive understanding of the patient and the effectiveness of his work. Here, the reader will find valuable information that can challenge as well as heighten his perception in evaluating the patient's past and present organismic stress as it reveals itself through the body surface.*

Although the author deals largely with the schizoid personality, the basic information he presents, as to what expressions and bodily features to look for, can apply to every patient, irrespective of the diagnostic label that has been placed upon his disorder. To understand the patient in emotional distress, we must utilize all the known diagnostic procedures. The taking of a fairly extensive case history is always indicated, but basically we must learn to observe the impact of the patient's stress upon his body. When the D.C. uses his visual, audial and tactile senses, he can determine with additional certainty the cause or causes of the malady, and decide what procedure to use and whether or not to seek a consultation or make a referral. Dr. Lowen says, "No words are as clear as the language of the body expression once one has learned to read it."

In the many seminars that he conducts, he gives unstintingly of all his studies and long years of successful experiences in practice. Most frequently, the large lecture room in New York where some of his seminars and work shops are conducted, is overflowing with behavioral scientists. Many are seated on the floor; all watch in amazement at what the body reveals to this specialist's keen observation and insight.

Dr. Lowen looks at patients as though with a third eye, just as Theodore

* Reprinted by permission of the author and publisher—The Macmillan Co., N.Y., 1967. From *The Betrayal of the Body*.

Reick listened as though with a third ear. In effect this means seeing and hearing without the blinders or stoppers that most people put on in their contacts with one another.

Through his methods, it is possible to detect the patient's stress as it reveals itself through the structure and function of different parts of the body. He has developed this art and science to a great degree. Those who are body-conscious appreciate his methods most. Those who have been blind to the body's expressions are fascinated by his analysis. When the patient starts to tell his story, it verifies Dr. Lowen's observations.

The nervous system, the vertebral column, and the muscles of the body receive the brunt of the social, environmental and ego stresses throughout life. The reactions to these stresses are reflected in the somatic and structural body.

From the material that the author so generously gave us permission to use, we allowed ourselves to only extract a few of his observations on body analysis. As far as his techniques are concerned, how to release the patient's muscular armour, we are of the opinion that this cannot be learned through reading; it must be studied under individualized expert teaching and demonstrations.

In diagnosis, the use of modern scientific tests and instrumentation cannot be overlooked, but it seems that a first step is to observe the features and expressions of the body, and the body structure. That often tells a fundamental story: the life style, the life history of the person. We can learn that story through the use of our most valuable instrument—our sense of observation. This chapter will be an eye-opener to the student and practitioner alike.

H.S.S.

* * *

PSYCHOANALYSIS had its origin in Freud's attempt to comprehend a somatic disturbance (hysterical symptom) in terms of a psychic conflict. The next big problem to command Freud's attention was the distinction between the anxiety neurosis and neuresthenia. Throughout its development psychoanalysis has never been able to dissociate itself from the physical manifestations of emotional conflicts. Yet with respect to the physical function of the organism the psychoanalytic attitude has been to approach it from its psychic reflection. One can proceed in the reverse direction with greater effectiveness, that is, from the physical problem to its psychic representation.

Ferenczi supplemented the traditional method with techniques which sought to involve the body more directly in the analytic procedure. Reich placed even more emphasis upon the somatic functions, especially upon the relation of respiration to the problem of emotional control. In addition, Reich introduced the concept of a physical energy as a counterpart to Freud's concept of a mental energy.

There is no neurotic problem which does not manifest itself in every aspect of the individual's function. This follows logically from the gestalt concept of the organism as a unity. Because we express our personalities or character in every action and in every attitude it becomes possible to determine character traits from such diverse expressions as handwriting, the walk of the person, etc. The bioenergetic analyst, like any other therapist, does not depend on any one manifestation. The history, the appearance, the manner of speech and even psychological tests are used to arrive at a correct diagnosis of the character structure. Most important, however, is the patient's physical appearance at rest and in movement. No words are as clear as the language of body expression, once one has learned to read it.

Reading the language of the body is not a mechanical process. Body expression is not a static or fixed phenomenon like printed words on a page. It is constantly changing. The observer must, therefore, be alert to these changing nuances of meaning if he wishes to understand the individual. He must be sensitive to quick impressions and sufficiently in touch with his own responses to understand their significance. And he must be able to relate one expression to another for no single bodily sign has meaning except in relation to the total personality and to the immediate situation of the individual.

Despite the subtleties and nuances of body expression there are many body signs which are clear and unchanging. In fact the absence of subtlety is itself a sign that something is amiss. Where the healthy body is constantly moving and changing, the disturbed body shows a relative fixity of attitude and expression. These fixed bodily attitudes and postures tell us much about the nature of the disturbance. A fixed smile, for example, informs the observer that it is a defensive maneuver not a genuine expression of feeling. Similarly when we see an overall pattern of bodily rigidity or flaccidity we derive its meaning from its chronic character, for normally healthy people may also go rigid or become limp in appropriate situations.

Generally the most important single feature of a person's body which strikes the observer is the look of his eyes. The eyes have often been described as mirrors of the soul yet this aspect of their function is ignored in medical practice. Some people's eyes are bright and shining, others are sad or angry. Quite often, however, we see eyes that lack expression; they look lifeless and seem to stare at us or through us or past us. This is especially true in schizoid and schizophrenic individuals. The eyes of these individuals have been described as "off," "blank," "vacant" or "out of touch." This lack of expression in the eyes is so characteristic of these disorders that it alone may be used to diagnose the presence of these disturbances.

The common denominator in all schizoid persons is the inability of the individual to focus his eyes with feeling upon another person. His eyes may be wide with terror but he does not look at one with terror nor does he feel the terror. In the same way his eyes may occasionally show an expression of rage but it is not directed and not perceived. The schizoid is not conscious of his eyes because feeling has been withdrawn from them. This is particularly true of a person in a catatonic state whose eyes have a glassy quality indicating his withdrawal of feeling from and his break of contact with the external world.

The meaning of eye contact is revealed by Ortega y Gasset in a delightful essay entitled "Point of View in the Arts." He writes, "Proximate vision has a tactile quality. What mysterious resonance of touch is preserved by sight when it converges on a nearby object? We shall not violate this mystery. It is enough to recognize this quasi-tactile density possessed by the ocular ray, and which permits it, in effect, to embrace, to touch the earthen jar. As the object is withdrawn, sight loses its tactile power and gradually becomes pure vision."

We can draw a distinction between seeing and looking based on Ortega's analysis. Seeing is pure vision, looking is vision that has a quasi-tactile component. The words, themselves, imply another distinction. To look is to direct one's vision according to the dictionary definition of this term. Looking is, therefore, an active or conscious process, seeing is passive. The ego is involved in the function of looking whereas it is not required for seeing. Generally speaking, the schizoid individual sees but doesn't look. He doesn't come into contact with the world through his eyes and on this level he is out of touch with the world and necessarily with himself.

We must look at people's eyes to learn what they feel or to sense their response to us. Their eyes will tell us if they are glad or sad, angry or amused, frightened or relaxed. Because the schizoid's eyes tell no story, we know that he has suppressed his feelings. In treating my patients I pay very close attention to their eyes. I look at their eyes and into them. When I reach them emotionally, that is, when they respond to me with feeling their eyes light up and come into focus. This also happens spontaneously when a patient gains more feeling in his body as a result of breathing and moving. The color of the patient's eyes become more vivid, they look more alive and they focus with feeling upon you. The responsiveness or lack of it in the eyes of a patient gives me a clearer indication of what is going on with him than any verbal communication. More than any other single sign, the expression in the eyes of a person indicates to what extent he is in touch with the world around him and, therefore, with himself. It tells me the degree to which he is "in possession of his faculties."

The impression one gets from a person's eyes is not determined by the eyeball itself. The lids, the brows, and the fine lines about the eyes contribute to this impression. Our impressions will be as varied and subtle as the expressions eyes are capable of conveying. I can only discuss a few of the more significant ones. Among these is the fairly common one in which the brows are knitted and lowered while the lids are narrowed. In some people it is seen as a typical expression. In these cases it impresses me as an attempt to maintain focus against a force acting in the contrary direction. The person looks as if he is trying to penetrate a veil behind which he senses a threat. If one presses with two thumbs on the underside of the brow alongside the nose, the expression will often change into one of bewilderment. The knitted brow can be interpreted, therefore, as a defense against an underlying feeling of bewilderment. Both the feeling and the defense can be traced analytically to early experiences in childhood in which the child fought against being bewildered by parental behavior that he could not understand. Knitting the brow somehow protects the child's vulnerable ego against the disintegrating effects of confusion. In this connection it is interesting to note that Schilder places the ego in the region of the glabella which is the area between the brows.

When one looks from the eyes to the total expression of the face, other signs of personality disturbance become evident. Since we instinctively know that the face is that aspect of the personality which we present to the world, we all look at faces and their expression to tell us what each person is feeling. Often, however, we look but fail to see. We do not allow the vision to register its meaning in our consciousness. I recall a professor I had whose brow was so raised that lines of astonishment and surprise were engraved on his forehead. No one else in the class paid the slightest attention to this expression, least of all the professor. Yet if one duplicates this expression voluntarily, the feeling of surprise and astonishment is so strong as to be disturbing. When an expression becomes engraved in the features, one loses consciousness of it. Like our old clothes these expressions become so much a part of us that we become aware of them only by their absence.

Not infrequently two conflicting expressions are shown on the face at the same time. For example, one often sees a rigid jaw set in an expression of defiance together with eyes that have a vacant or frightened look. The rigidity of the jaw is maintained by chronically tight and contracted jaw muscles. The tension in these jaw muscles blocks off or prevents any feeling from becoming manifest in the eyes. If one releases this tension, one can elicit an expression of fear or terror in the eyes. The rigid jaw may be seen, therefore, as a defense against the terror. In effect, this person is saying, "I won't be afraid." But he is saying this more to himself than to others, and while such a bodily maneuver may serve to keep his courage up, it is done at the expense of his eyes; that is, by reducing their capacity to look and see the danger. Another very common split expression on the face is the fixed smile about the mouth and cheeks which contradicts the evident sadness in the eyes. I need not elaborate the meaning of this contradiction since we are all taught that no one wants to see our sadness. And so we attempt to mask it from others and also from ourselves.

Most people wear a mask over their face to hide their feelings. It is most manifest in the schizoid personality where it covers all feeling and where one can hardly see the normal play of expression that makes a healthy face look so alive. The mask takes several forms: it may show the bewilderment of the clown, the knowing look of the sophisticate, the haughtiness of the aristocrat, or the innocent look of the naive. Each mask is associated with a fixed smile the characteristics of which are 1) its unvarying quality, 2) its lack of appropriateness, and 3) its unrelatedness to a feeling of pleasure. In fact the smile frequently appears when the individual is in a state of tension or pain. It can be understood as an attempt to relieve the tension of the mask when feelings arise which the individual cannot express or communicate. It is really part of the mask which hides and denies the existence of a negative response.

Masks are not removable at will. They represent facial attitudes which have become fixed or frozen by fear. Mothers are always afraid that children's expressions may become permanent aspects of the child's countenance and often warn their children "not to look that way." We must know that in the case of the schizoid individual the mask enables him to appear before the world without causing the shock that a cadaverous expression or look of terror would otherwise provoke. Harvey Cleckly refers to the schizoid expression as a "mask of sanity." To remove the mask the frozen condition of the face must be thawed out, the fear and terror must be made conscious and their grip upon the personality relaxed.

The schizoid condition develops from the suppression of feeling due to fear. These suppressed feelings are locked up in the body where they form a volcanic nucleus that is always liable to explode. When feeling erupts it is not an ego symbolic phenomena. The schizoid person is out of control and his ego is overwhelmed by the feeling. In these circumstances his facial expression becomes so distorted that it looks inhuman. If a feeling of anger arises, for example, the face takes on a demonic aspect. The eyes become dark and the brows knit as if a storm was brewing. Instead of anger one sees a frightening black rage which is, often, quite destructive. This rage is the reverse of terror and its intensity is directly proportional to the fear that spawned it. If it is crying that breaks through, the mask collapses and one sees an expression of despair.

The key tension in all individuals, schizoid or neurotic, is found in the muscles of the jaw. By setting the jaw one can control the expression of feeling and to some extent the feeling itself. I mentioned earlier that a defiant jaw can block out the look or the feeling of fear. A determined jaw can hold back one's tears and prevent one from sobbing. A retracted jaw limits one's self-assertion. Tension in the jaw muscles is responsible for bruxism, the tendency of people to grind their teeth while asleep. And because a set jaw inhibits the expression of feeling it markedly affects a person's respiration. We have found in bioenergetic analysis that it is impossible for a person to breathe freely and deeply unless his jaw is relaxed.

The jaw occupies a key role in personality disturbances through its involvement in the oral activities of the organism. Frustrations of the sucking and biting impulses in the baby and young child, together with the fear that the expression of these impulses will evoke a hostile response from the parents, act to partially immobilize the jaw. A jaw that has a defiant expression also says "I don't need you." A retracted jaw clearly denotes an inhibition of biting impulses. It also indicates that the individual is afraid to get a good bite on life or to sink his teeth into life. This limitation on oral aggression later extends to the whole personality. And while it may be compensated by the use of other aggressive modalities, the eyes and the arms, still constitutes a weakness in the individual's total pattern of reaching out and taking in.

Muscular tensions are not isolated phenomena. They are parts of meaningful patterns. Thus we find that tension in the muscles of the jaw is associated with tension in the nuchal muscles at the base of the skull. These tensions at the base of the skull also serve to hold back reaching and biting impulses. This holding pattern is most evident in the schizoid personality where it is so strong that it immobilizes the upper half of the head. We can appreciate this fact if we realize that biting is a function of the upper teeth which bite down upon the object. The lower teeth serve to hold the object against the bite. Immobilization of the upper part of the head is related to the schizoid sense of terror.

The severe contraction of the nuchal muscles at the base of the skull is the root, I believe, of the tension headaches that plague so many people. They exert a pull on the muscles and aponeuroses that cover the top of the head and forehead. It is surprising how quickly such headaches can disappear if one loosens these tensions. Holding the person's forehead in my left hand, I use the fingers of my right hand to knead the muscles at the base of the skull. Then I place both my hands around the crown of the head and relax the scalp. This procedure may take no more than two minutes but the feeling of relief is almost immediate. In my opinion tension headaches are related to the holding back of feelings of anger. The holding back is related to the fear described above.

Anger and fear are opposite directions of movement. In anger one strikes out, in fear one pulls back. These movements, towards a foe in anger or away from the foe in fear, occur within the body as well as in space. The emotions of fear and anger, like those of love and hate, refer to movements within the body of the person. An e-motion is a movement from the center of the body to the periphery where it appears as an expression. The individual experiences this movement as a feeling, that is, he feels the e-motion. The observer senses the movement through its expression and knows the e-motion manifested in the expression. Terror and rage are intensified emotions qualitatively similar to fear and anger but carrying a much stronger affective charge.

The head and face offer many other diagnostic clues to the personality of an individual. In fact, so many that it is impossible to comment on all of them in this review. Some have found their way into our language. For example, we speak of a person as being long-faced or having a long face. One dictionary defines it as "an expression of solemn concern" but I have seen many people with long faces. Their expression struck me as a mixture of disappointment and sadness with a sullen quality. We speak of people as being "down in the mouth" and we see these expressions on their faces. The head and face may have a gaunt look which indicates a lack of joy in the personality. If the head is small as compared with the rest of the body, it indicates, to my thinking, a weakness in the ego functions. I regard the face as the flower of the personality.

The neck serves to connect the head with the trunk. Necks may be long and thin, or short and thick. These differences have meaning. We find the long, thin neck in asthenic bodies associated with the schizoid personality. In these personalities the functions of the head are often dissociated from those of the body, this means that there is a dissociation between thinking and feeling, between perceiving and acting. The long neck places a distance between the two sets of functions and creates the impression that those related to the head have little to do with those related to the body. In some individuals the head is carried in such a way that it looks as if the person were saying, "I (my head and ego) am above all this body business." One may detect a note of haughtiness in this person's bearing. The short, thick neck has the opposite connotations. The thick neck gives a person a bull-like appearance. These individuals tend to be chargers or pushers. They drive themselves and others. Since the thickness of the neck is, in general, due to a contraction and holding in the neck muscles one can suspect strong tendencies to stubbornness and spitefulness in these people. In most cases these suspicions are verified as one gets to know the person.

A stiff neck has long been associated with pride—a stiff-necked pride. The stiff neck prevents the head from bowing down or "giving in." The metaphor is, of course, literally true. The stiffness is due to tension and spasticity in the muscles at the back of the neck where it can be easily palpated. Chronic muscular tensions such as these are responsible in some cases for arthritic changes in the joints which often show up in x-rays of necks. Massage of these tight neck muscles along the back and sides of the cervical vertebrae together with a pressure exerted through the fingers upon the tight areas while the person is breathing often loosens the neck. The head drops lower and the person feels a sense of release as he finds himself more able to let go of his head. Occasionally one sees people who seem to have no neck at all. The head is held close to the shoulders, an attitude which strongly suggests that the person has pulled his head in, as a turtle does, in a protective maneuver. In one of his plays, Tennessee Williams describes these individuals as "no-neck monsters." Pulling the head in is the opposite of sticking the head out and indicates that a person who carries his head this way would have great difficulty in self-assertion.

When we look at a person's body from the neck down, we try to evaluate its overall quality before studying it in detail. Is the body over-developed muscularly or under-developed? An excessive muscular development transforms the body into a fortress. If I get this impression from a person's body, I know that his massive musculature is a defensive device to protect a sensitive inner self. This inner self is often perceived by the patient as a small child who guards his vulnerability by a formidable exterior. On the other hand, the person whose body is under-developed muscularly suffers from a lack of aggressive capability. Aggression, in its primary sense, means to "move towards." Movement is a function of the musculature which is obviously limited when the musculature is weak or rigid.

Bodies also show varying degrees of rigidity or flaccidity. Some are so rigid that the person can hardly bend backward or forward while others are too flexible bending like reeds. I like to think of the human body as the shaft of a bow. It functions on the principle of a bow in many situations as when one bends backward to throw a ball or strike a blow. If the body is too rigid, this bowing action cannot occur. The same thing is true, however, when the body is too flexible for then the bow has no tensile strength to send the arrow winging.

The posture of the individual is also significant in this connection. Does he stand straight or is he hunched forward? How many people have you seen who walk and stand as if they were carrying the weight of the world on their shoulders and backs? An excessive bodily rigidity represents structural strength at the expense of motility. It is found, for example, in persons who hold themselves out as the "pillars of society." Analysis of their personalities shows that they have dedicated themselves to upholding certain principles about which they are rigid and unyielding. When flaccidity dominates the picture, one has the impression that the individual cannot hold himself up and that he collapses easily. In these persons one also senses a decreased vitality or a diminished level of energy. The collapse is seen in the way the upper half of the body folds and rests upon the lower half. This is what happens physically when a person "folds up."

We think of the backbone as the important structural element in the body. It is not the bones that constitute the strength or weakness of the backbone, but the muscles that support and move the bone structure. Any weakness in the functioning of these muscles has serious consequences for the personality. Thus when we say that an individual lacks backbone it means that these muscles do not function to sustain his position or his aggression. Our language reflects these functions. A person can "back up" his position or "back down" from it. He can hold back when necessary or back off. If the musculature of the back is either too rigid or too flaccid, these functions are handicapped. These deficiencies can be overcome by mobilizing these muscles through appropriate movements.

Rigidity in the muscles of the back is also mainly responsible for the very large incidence of lower back pain in people. I have treated many patients with lower back problems. In all these cases I found that the back "goes out," that is, the lower back develops a severe spasm when the person is under stress and stiffens instead of collapsing. Stiffening is this person's typical response to stress even in situations where giving or collapse would be the healthier reaction. In each case reduction of the tension in the lumbosacral muscles, mobilization of pelvic motility, analysis of the underlying emotional conflict with a resolution of the problem of the inhibited impulse results in the disappearance of the symptom and a strengthening of the lower back. The rigidity of the backbone is evident not only in the loss of flexibility but also in the palpable tension of the lumbar musculature.

We shall now continue our analysis of the body in a segmental way starting from the shoulders down. The position and motility of the shoulders are as significant to the ego functions as the legs and pelvis are to the sexual functions. Several attitudes are easily discerned. Retracted shoulders represent repressed anger, a holding back of the impulse to strike; raised shoulders are related to fear; square shoulders express the manly attitude of shouldering one's responsibilities; bowed shoulders convey the sense of burden, the weight of a heavy hand. The shoulders play an important role in the motility of the chest since the shoulder girdle extends from the spine in back via the rhomboids to the sternum in front via the pectoral muscles. Disturbance in the shoulder girdle will, therefore, affect the respiratory function. Since the basic function of the arms in the primates is to reach out to take or give, to seize or strike, the extent and quality of the reaching out is a measure of the ego.

In neurotic structures the arms and body form a unity which is subject to the limitations of the character structure. The oral character complains of feelings of weakness and impotence in his arms. In his body structure we observe that the muscles which hold the scapula to the body and control its movements are overdeveloped and chronically contracted. The most visible ones are the pectoral muscles in front and the trapezius behind. Par contra, the muscles which hold the arms in the sockets are weak and underdeveloped. This accounts for the difficulty the oral character has in reaching out to take or give.

There is an antithesis between the upper and lower halves of the body. It is not uncommon to see a broad-shouldered man with narrow hips and thin weak-looking legs. It is as if all the energy were concentrated in the upper half leaving the bottom half impotent. We find in practice that as the legs strengthen and as sexual potency increases the shoulders drop, the chest becomes smaller and the center of gravity drops appreciably. The distribution of the musculature in the human body is such that the greater part is concentrated in hips and legs. This gives man support for his need to maintain the upright position. The muscles of the upper half of the body have been spared the function of supporting or moving the body. They should be soft, relaxed and available for quick, sensitive movements.

Another aspect of the body that is significantly revealing is dysplasia, the presence of features which belong to the opposite sex. It is characteristic of the schizoid body. Android features such as narrow hips, slender thighs, and a male distribution of pubic hair are frequently found in the female. In the male, gynecoid tendencies are present in the form of a full, rounded pelvis, an incipient mons veneris (a mound of fatty tissue over the pubic bone in the female), and a feminine distribution of pubic hair in the form of an inverted triangle.

Since all of my patients suffer from some degree of lack of aggression, the physical passivity enjoined by the prone position or the sitting position in therapy constitutes some handicap. If we think of "aggression" in terms of its dictionary meaning, to move to, the standard analytic position imposes a limit upon aggression and movement. I do not mean to imply that simply putting a patient on his feet could overcome such serious problems as depression and the inability to work. Much more is involved than this. But working from a standing position illustrates the literal significance of such expressions as "to stand on your own two feet," to be "on your toes," "to hold your ground," etc. Sometimes, very rarely, the patient is spontaneously aware of the immediate connection between his emotional problem and the somatic disturbance. When this happens the therapeutic endeavor is greatly facilitated.

The legs and feet are the foundation and support of the body and the ego structure, but they have other functions. It is through our legs and our feet that we keep contact with the one invariable reality in our lives, the earth or the ground. An individual who feels that he has no control over his legs usually feels he doesn't know where he is going. Tall persons frequently complain of loss of contact with their legs or with the ground. Sometimes one gets the impression of a patient that they are up in the clouds. The technical problem is how to bring the patient down to earth and how to anchor him there. The sense of belonging, or having roots, must be directly related to the feeling of intimate contact between the feet and the ground.

The problem of emotional security cannot be divorced from the question of the physical security of one's footing. While the problem can be tackled on the verbal level, it yields more quickly and more completely to a therapy which combines analysis "from above" with direct work on the physical disturbance below. Bioenergetic therapy aims to bring the patient into contact with his feet and with the ground and at the same time to make the patient aware of the relationship between his emotional problem and its physical counterpart. The therapy proceeds on two fronts simultaneously, although at any one time the analytic work may predominate while at another time the emphasis shifts to the physical side.

When one examines the legs from a dynamic point of view, one becomes aware how weak the foundations are which support some seemingly strong ego structures. A robust person with a round face and a full body who has a pair of thin, spindly legs, narrow hips and is suffering from hypertension can be seen as compensating for the weakness of the lower half of his body by the seeming security and strength of the upper half. The functions of the upper half of the body which are essentially oral in nature dominate his personality. These have to do with taking in or charging up. The relative underdevelopment of the lower half indicates that the functions of energy discharge are severely restricted while the discharge of energy in movement and sex is greatly reduced. Bioenergetically one could interpret the hypertension as the result of a preponderance of energy charge over energy discharge.

The lack of contact with the feet and the ground can be related to the common experience of falling anxiety. This symptom is manifested in dreams of falling, in fear of heights, and in the fear of falling in love. Where there is a basic insecurity in the lower half of the body, the individual compensates by holding on with arms and eyes to objective reality. In addition to the functions of support, balance, and rooting, the legs are the most important structures in the function of body movement. Where the function of support is weak, we may also expect a disturbance in motility. One can gauge the motility in the legs by the ability of the individual to freely swing his pelvis without using any part of the trunk in the movement. This is very close to the motion demanded by such dances as the samba, the mambo, and the rhumba. These dance movements require a relaxed, flexible knee joint, a looseness of the pelvis on the trunk, and relaxation of all the leg muscles. I have found that there are three conditions which impair this basic motility: weakness, massiveness, and rigidity of the leg musculature. The legs may be weak, they may be abnormally heavy or they may be rigid. Frequently the legs will show a mixture of these elements. In the analysis of structure, attention is paid to each component as well as to the total aspect. The feet may be narrow or broad, the toes pinched together or spread apart, the arch collapsed, relaxed or tightly contracted. The calf muscles may be shapeless or knotted. The position of the feet in the person's natural stance may be straight and parallel, turned outward as a result of spastic gluteal muscles, or pigeon-toed. Each disturbance is interpreted in terms of its effect on the functions of support and movement.

An approach to personality through the interpretation of bodily expression depends upon the ability of the doctor to relate the physical characteristics of an individual to his attitude and behavior. All people unconsciously interpret personality from physical expression. The analyst has to make these interpretations consciously. He has to know the significance of the physical distortions that a patient's body presents.

Only the total picture enables one to make the diagnosis of the schizoid personality or of any other psychiatric personality. The details may vary, because each person is an individual with a unique life experience, which is reflected in his body. The look in the eyes, the expression of the face, the carriage of the head, the posture of the body, the color of the skin, the tone of the muscles, the timbre of the voice, the stance of the legs, the motility of the pelvis, the spontaneity of gesture—these, and many more indices add up to the total picture we are seeking. When this total picture is one of unity, integration, and self-command we regard the person as being "all there," in possession of his faculties and emotionally healthy. The schizoid body lacks these qualities. The schizoid picture is that of a forsaken body from which the psyche has fled in terror.

Analytical therapists are confronted daily with individuals whose structure and personality are defective to the point of being inadequate to handle the pressures of reality. In their struggle to survive such individuals develop compensating mechanisms to overcome their weaknesses. Adler's theories about organ inferiority and the striving for power and superiority derive from such clinical observations. Unfortunately, compensating mechanisms never correct the fault of weakness. Bioenergetic analytic therapy attacks the basic disturbance as it manifests itself in the adult pattern of behavior, thereby diminishing the need for compensations and adjustments.

REFERENCES

Cleckly, H. *The Mask of Sanity*. St. Louis: C. V. Mosby (1955), pp. 423–25.

Ferenczi, Sandor. "The Further Development of an Active Therapy in Psychoanalysis." *The Theory and Technique of Psychoanalysis II*. New York: Basic Books, 1953.

Ortega y Gasset, "Point of View in the Arts," in *The Dehumanization of Art, and Other Writings, on Art and Culture*. Garden City: Doubleday (1956), p. 103.

Reich, W. *Character Analysis* (3rd ed.). New York: Orgone Institute Press (1949), p. 481.

Schilder, Paul. *The Image and Appearance of the Human Body*. New York: International Universities Press, 1950.

Sheldon, W. H. *The Varieties of Human Physique*. New York: Harper & Bros., 1940.

Sheldon, W. H. *The Varieties of Temperament*. New York: Harper & Bros., 1942.

CHAPTER 7

THE ROLE OF MUSCULAR TENSION IN MALADJUSTMENT*

ROBERT PLUTCHIK, PH.D.

A. INTRODUCTION

The term personality may be said to refer to the relatively permanent and idiosyncratic aspects of an individual's behavior. This is in no sense an atypical usage of the term. Gardner Murphy has written, for example, that "personality (is) something that enters into and persists through every situational adjustment." Thus any form of behavior which is relatively enduring may be considered part of one's personality. From this point of view an individual's posture, typical gestures, or characteristic facial expressions are aspects of personality. This has long been recognized. Yet there have been few systematic studies of the formation and significance of persisting muscular patterns of behavior, and of their effect on health and adjustment. This review is an attempt to draw together in a systematic way the various lines of evidence which bear on the relation between muscular tension, personality formation, and maladjustment. This evidence, drawn from both experimental and clinical sources, will be presented in four parts; first, muscular activity as a form of personality expression; secondly, the processes which lead to the production of tension; and thirdly, the effects of persistent muscular tension. The paper will conclude with some implications for psychotherapy.

B. MUSCULAR ACTIVITY AS A FORM OF PERSONALITY EXPRESSION

The various studies of the judgment of personality through expressive movements such as posture, gait, and gesture are unanimous in showing, first, that these muscular modes of activity do reveal such character attitudes as dominance, apathy, or inhibition, and secondly, that expressive movements are fairly stable characteristics of the individual and relatively independent of mood or situation.

In his experiment concerning the analysis of spontaneous facial expressions during experimentally induced emotion, Landis found that although

* Reprinted by permission of the author and the publisher—*The Journal of General Psychology,* 1954, 50, 45–62.

facial postures were not characteristic of emotions, they were characteristic of individuals. Similarly, Davis, in a study of the relation of muscle action potentials to frustration induced experimentally, reported that "individual consistencies in muscular activity are pronounced." In two early studies of muscular tension as related to emotional tendencies, Duffy found that subjects showed marked individual differences in muscular tension. High tension individuals rated lower on stability and degree of adjustment to the environment and tended to show a greater degree of reaction in the experimental situation. In a more recent experiment, Duffy had subjects perform eight different tasks at different times, while muscle tension measurements were taken. By the use of factor analysis she found that a general tension factor operates which is more or less independent of the task, of the mode of tension measurement, and of the time at which the measurement is made. She concludes that tension level is a more or less persistent characteristic of the individual, and is, in this sense, an aspect of personality. Freeman similarly has found that there is a basal level of postural tension which varies from individual to individual which is characteristic of a given person.

Many clinical observations concerning the relation between muscular tension and personality have been reported. Freud was probably the first to systematically call attention to the emotional significance of seemingly meaningless acts and to emphasize their usefulness in the study of personality. Restless muscular movements of the body, face, fingers, and arms, he considered to be motor discharges of psychic tension and attempts to overcome anxiety. Ferenczi found regular parallelisms between motor acts and psychic functioning. He noted that many patients in states of resistance display an exaggerated stiffness of their limbs. In the progress of analysis, the physical tensions sometimes disappeared with the resolution of mental ones. A similar observation has been made by Fenichel. Frequently, a patient in psychoanalysis who can no longer avoid seeing that an interpretation is correct, but nevertheless tries to, shows a cramping of his entire muscular system or parts of it. Many patients, according to Karl Abraham, spontaneously speak of a "tension" in the body as well as a state of mental "tension." Reich has observed that in the compulsive character, all muscles of the body, but particularly those of the pelvis and pelvic floor, of the shoulders and the face are in a state of chronic hypertonia. Dunbar has stated that muscle tension is of fundamental importance as an expression of the personality's habitual defenses and that these defenses are revealed in postural attitudes, voice, and in fact, any persistently contracted muscles. Similar conclusions have come out of studies at the Johns Hopkins' hospital. Ascher found that changes of motor behavior of hospitalized patients was the most reliable factor in evaluating their therapeutic progress. The patients were often unaware of showing certain attitudes through their motor behavior, such attitudes, for example, as dependency, hostility, ambivalence, withdrawal, etc.

One of the most conclusive studies showing the relationship between personality and tensional behavior is reported by Deutsch. He systematically recorded basic postures and changes in postural behavior of patients under analytic treatment. A characteristic posture appears, Deutsch noted, immediately or soon after the analysis is begun. As psychological changes occur during treatment, the postural pattern becomes transitorily or permanently altered. He found that verbal expression of memories and feelings correlates with postural expression, and that in states of conflict, the defenses and the repressed emotions are readily reflected in bodily behavior. He reached the conclusion that posture is expressive of attitudes, and that movements seem to aim at the release of tension and are repeated until the tension tends to be discharged.

To answer the possible objection that these persistent postural tensions are easily modifiable by conscious control, an experiment by Jacobson should be noted. In a carefully controlled study he found that daily rest alone without special training in relaxation has little or no effect on the level of muscular tension of an individual.

The evidence which has been presented appears to justify the following conclusions: (a) Persistent muscular tensions are an aspect of personality; they vary from individual to individual. (b) Certain attitudes are associated with certain characteristic muscular tension patterns; (c) Personality changes that take place in the course of psychotherapy will parallel fairly enduring changes in the condition of tonus of the body musculature. Clinical observations further suggest that these tensions have meanings, e.g., the expression of certain attitudes toward the environment, the attempt to reduce anxiety, or possibly both.

This problem will be clarified by a discussion of how persistent muscular tensions originate. In the following section, the view will be developed that tensions result from frustrations or conflicts, and that persisting tensions are an index of persisting conflicts. Frustration differs from conflict in that the latter involves mutually exclusive demands on the behavior of the individual while frustration may consist in neglecting to bring any of the primary body functions into action.

Before proceeding, it should be stated that there are a great many different techniques which have been used to measure muscle tension. Davis classifies them into six major groups: (a) those applying external forces mechanically and recording resistance to movement offered by limb or muscle; (b) those recording slight movement of parts of the body; (c) those eliciting reflex responses; (d) those requiring the subject to perform some voluntary response; (e) those recording electrical properties of the skin; and (f) those recording the electrical properties of muscles. Although Davis considers the recordings of action potentials from the muscles as the most adequate measure, all the devices mentioned have been used.

C. HOW MUSCLES BECOME CHRONICALLY TENSE

In everyday life one recognizes a connection between inhibited emotional expression and the making rigid or fixed of a particular muscular pattern. Witness such comments in ordinary conversation as "keep a stiff upper lip" to keep from crying, or "keep your chin up" as a way of hiding or overcoming one's sadness. Someone who shows no emotion is a "dead pan"; a snobbish or arrogant person might be "stiff-necked"; and the statement that "discipline steels one's character" may be more than figurative.

The concept that "holding back" (as a result of frustration or conflict) leads to chronic tension, is not new. In *The Problem of Anxiety,* Freud writes that in the infant "increase of tension (arises) from non-gratification of its needs." Luria has observed that "the active inhibition of the affective symptoms always produces tension."

These observations are understandable on the view that conflict or frustration produces emotional reactions which are actually extensive muscular preparations for action. In his study of anger, Gates found that the most frequent impulses in anger were to make a verbal retort; to injure the offender physically; to injure inanimate objects; to run away or leave the room; to cry, scream, or swear. These actions obviously involve tremendous muscular preparation and activity. If such activity is blocked, impeded, or prevented adequate expression, the preparatory tensions will not be released and will remain in a residual form primarily in those muscles which were principally involved in the anticipated action. Relevant to this latter point are the two following studies. Jacobson, investigating the effects of an imagined contraction, found that it is impossible to conceive an activity without causing fine contractions in all those muscles which produce that activity in reality. Katzell has recorded muscle action patterns from different muscle groups before and during task performance. His results indicated, that when the tasks were within the performance capacity of the subjects, the patterns of preparatory tension were approximately diminished, covert duplicates of the patterns occurring during subsequent overt performance. In general, it may be expected that those individuals who express their feeling most directly and adequately for the situation will possess least residual tension. In partial confirmation, Zander has noted that subjects who responded most aggressively to experimentally induced frustration, were also more relaxed and friendly outside the experimental situation, and seemed better adjusted.

Frustration or conflict not only leads to anger but under certain conditions, to the production of muscular tensions as well, which may persist over long periods of time. Many experiments confirm the view that frustration is the basis for the development of persistent muscular tension. Using 25 nursery school children as subjects, Williams found that with an increase in the strength of a barrier (e.g., tower-building, tapping, and guessing tasks) there is a concomitant increase in general tension as determined by an index of respiratory activity. In summarizing the relation between muscular tension and performance, F. A. Courts points out that the increased muscle tension which accompanies a novel environmental situation may be considered a symptom of the maladjustment of the organism to the environment. "In frustration, where the readjustive response is prevented by the difficulty of the required behavior or by other factors, muscle tension would be expected to persist on a higher level longer than it does when readjustment is comparatively more easily obtained."

G. L. Freeman has found that internal stimulation, such as increased bladder pressure, heightens the general level of postural tension in an individual; the increased tension persists until relieved by an appropriate act. Further, a conflict-situation or the frustration of any goal-oriented activity heightens the level of postural tension and the heightened tension from conflict or frustration persists until some adjustment can be made.

Several clinical investigations bear on this same problem. The results of one of the experimental studies on headache carried out at the Cornell Medical Center justified the conclusion that "noxious stimulation of the head or emotional tension lead to sustained contraction of the scalp and neck muscles." The case is reported of a man with "anxiety and emotional tension," periodic headaches, pain in the neck and shoulders, stomach trouble, and some loss of memory. Electrical records showed marked muscle contractions although the patient was completely unaware of them. Following psychotherapy and chemotherapy, the patient was symptom free and "feeling like a new man." His myogram showed no muscle potentials.

Weiss has reported that a person with strong hostile feelings which are unexpressed is unable to relax and that the rebellion takes the form of constant muscle tension. The explanation he offers is that the muscles serve as means of defense and attack in the struggle for existence, and internal tension is most easily released by muscular action. Hence, if the external expression of aggressiveness in the form of muscular action is inhibited by repressing forces operative in the individual, muscular tension may result which is felt by the individual as pain and limitation of movement. Sustained tensions in one group of muscles have been found to spread gradient fashion to the other muscles in the body.

In the light of these facts and studies which have been presented, the conclusion may be drawn that the existence in any individual of persistent muscular tension is an index of the fact that an equally persistent conflict exists, or that the individual has experienced frustration which is in some sense still unresolved. Chronic muscular tensions, therefore, can be conceived as a continuous state of readiness, indicating present day conflicts or frustrations. The tensions reflect attitudes which are usually verbally unexpressed.

These conclusions lead immediately to a preduction. Those people who are known to have definite conflicts, such as neurotics and psychotics, should therefore have larger than normal amounts of residual and persisting tension. The next section will review those investigations which demostrate the truth of this proposition and will discuss some of the harmful effects on the organism of chronically contracted muscles.

D. THE EFFECT OF PERSISTENT MUSCULAR TENSION

Several authors have developed the concept of a biological energy equilibrium. Freud's hypotheses of the libido is such a concept. Kurt Goldstein has presented a similar notion. G. L. Freeman has attempted to justify the view that "all total behavior is homeostatic-regulatory." Darrow and others have presented evidence in support of this view.

In the light of this concept of a neuromuscular homeostasis—and the theory is in many respects well established—the existence of chronically contracted muscles can be seen to provide a continuous source of internal stimulation. The energy of the neural impulses, set up by chronic muscular activity must be handled in some way or other, and will be expressed either by bodily restlessness, stereotyped movements, tics, increasing tension in other muscles, such as the heart and capillary system, or increased activity in the glandular and secretory systems. The problem of which of these particular forms the discharge will take is a very difficult problem, and will depend on such factors as the nature of the frustrating influences in an individual's life, his constitutional makeup, and probably other factors. In any event, it should be possible to compare such symptoms of tension in various diagnostically defined groups. Several such comparisons are available.

Using hand tremor and general bodily movement as measures of tension, Sherman and Jost found an increase in muscular tension during frustration in both normal and neurotic children, but more so in neurotic children. The neurotic children also showed greater tension during the rest and attention periods than normal. Weiss studied 40 patients with so-called psychogenic rheumatism encountered in a larger study of 200 patients with chronic fatigue. He observed that this group of patients complain of aches and pains in the muscles and joints, in addition to chronic fatigue, and often have slight elevation in temperature. Psychosomatic study showed that these patients had significant emotional conflicts and that marital maladjustment was a frequent underlying problem. Chronic resentment, of which the patient was usually totally unaware, produced a state of tension which was reflected in the musculo-skeletal system, causing so-called muscular rheumatism. Similarly, Boland and Corr found psychogenic rheumatism to be the most frequent cause of disability in 450 consecutive cases diagnosed as arthritis or allied organic conditions in an Army general hospital. The majority of the patients had definite psychoneurotic manifestations before entry into military service. Ellman, Savage and others examined 50 patients diagnosed as long standing cases of fibrositis (i.e., inflammation of fibrous tissues, such as muscle). All patients had minor degrees of stiffness and pain, and half had definite limitations of movement. Thirty-five of the patients showed decided psychoneurotic features. Another striking finding has come out of the observation of two thousand cases of neurosis in a military hospital in England. The mean blood pressure of the neurotics who did not have an organic disease (3.4 per cent) was found to be higher than the accepted normal. These studies are very strong evidence for the belief that individuals with persistent conflicts (neurotics) have equally persistent muscle tension in various forms.

More evidence for this view has come out of investigations of the startle reaction in normal and maladjusted persons. Jacobson performed an experiment in which the subjects were instructed to sustain, voluntarily, three degrees of tension: high, medium, and complete relaxation. A startle stimulus was suddenly introduced and kymograph records were taken of upward and backward movements as a measure of startle, and it was found that the start or response was greatest under high tension and least or zero when the subjects were relaxed. The studies of Landis and Hunt on the startle reaction to a pistol shot, as recorded by high speed camera, found that the startle response was intensified in schizophrenics, particularly in the patients of the catatonic subgroup, and somewhat intensified in the manic-depressive and involutional groups. Paretics and encephalitics responded normally. In consideration of Jacobson's findings, these results can best be explained as indicating that psychotics possess greater muscular tension than normals. In further confirmation of this hypothesis, Darrow mentions that excessive fast EEG activity of the cortex is more or less typical of conditions of anxiety or tension, and that in anxious and schizophrenic persons such self-maintained activity (and low potential EEG's) may persist to the point of exhaustion. With regard to neurotic subjects, Luria reports that their motor reaction to a startle stimulus is much more marked in intensity than the normal reaction and differs in form. He notes that "patients with functional neuroses exhibited a picture of intense motor conflicts."

Further evidence for the thesis that maladjusted persons possess large amounts of residual tension is obtained from studies of reaction to pain. Under controlled experimental conditions, Jacobson produced pain in subjects by means of an electric current. When the only noteworthy variable was the degree of tension in the muscles being stimulated, he found that the intensity of the sensation as reported by the subjects varied accordingly, the degree of pain being least when the muscles were most relaxed. He suggests that a tense or spastic organ tends ipso facto to be hypersensitive. In agreement with this, Wolff and Wolf found that when the stomach was stretched by glass rods, the pressure needed to produce pain was 100 grams per square centimeter when the contractile state of the stomach was average. However, when the stomach wall was strongly contracted, pressure of 50 grams per square centimeter or half that originally applied was found sufficient to produce pain. On the other hand, when the stomach was relatively relaxed, 150 grams per square centimeter were necessary to induce pain. A finding which can be interpreted in this light was obtained by Chapman, Cohen, and Cobb using the Hardy-Wolff radiation apparatus. They investigated the level of perception and reaction to painful heat stimulation in 94 neurotic patients and 44 healthy individuals. They found that the level at which the neurotics (anxiety neurotics and asthenics) react (i.e., wince, pull away) is lower than for the control subjects. Chapman, Finesinger, et al. compared the heat sensitivity of 50 psychoneurotic patients with that of 56 normal subjects. These studies also indicated that the patients had an essentially normal threshold of pain perception but an increased tendency to reactions of motor avoidance.

Thus these two lines of investigation—of the startle response and reaction to pain of normal and maladjusted people—lead to essentially the same conclusion: Those individuals with severe conflicts and maladjustments, also have more or less of their body musculature in chronic contraction.

What is the effect on the body economy of chronic muscle tension? In a review of the work on pain, Wolff and Wolf write: "Noxious stimulation of the ureter has been shown to result in contraction of abdominal muscles which when sustained, may become a source of fresh noxious impulses. At length the pain from the contracted muscles may overshadow that from the ureter. Such secondarily contracted muscles may also give rise to local rigidity and tenderness." In this same work, the authors point out that a large proportion of headaches, especially those accompanied by stiffness or tenderness in the neck and occipital region, find their origin in unduly sustained increase of the contractile state of underlying head muscles; and, that it is likely that a similar mechanism explains many backaches. Studying sciatica, Elliott has observed localized muscle spasms, which he considers to be the source of the pain and tenderness. Electrical activity due to muscle spasm has also been recorded in "fibrositis" and various rheumatic disturbances. Travell, Rinzler *et al.* treated 58 cases exhibiting pain in the shoulder region and arm by intramuscular infiltration with procaine hydrochloride. They obtained 62 per cent complete remission of pain, 31 per cent improvement, and 7 per cent no relief. Procaine is known to relax the localized muscle spasm. These doctors conclude that "the pain is the consequence of a sustained spasm of the skeletal musculature." They also note that all the varied procedures which relieve pain in the upper extremity (such as procaine, ethyl chloride, local anaesthesia, mechanical pressure, etc.) have in common the effect of relaxing muscle.

The evidence that has been presented above strongly implies the belief that abnormality is associated with increased muscular tension, and that ability to relax can be considered as at least one of the diagnostic signs of adjustment. But it is not muscular tension per se, but its chronicity and degree that constitutes abnormality.

E. IMPLICATIONS FOR THERAPY

This paper has tried to show: first, that patterns of muscle tension and overt activity are valid indices of attitudes and personality, and that changes in tension patterns are adequate indicators of the progress of therapy; second, that frustrations of various sorts or the interruption of strongly motivated goal-directed activities are the "reason for being" of persistent tensions, and that these tensions reflect a continuous state of readiness of which an individual may often be unaware. Freud has pointed out that "the true aim of repression is to suppress the development of affect," and that "repression demands a constant expenditure of energy." From the point of view development in this paper, repression is indicated by the existence of chronic muscle tension; and a constant supply of energy is needed to maintain this condition. Thirdly, continued muscular preparation acts as a continuous source of internal stimulation, the energy of which is handled by some sort of an "overflow" mechanism.

Besides chronic muscle tension being causally related to many physical illnesses, it has also been found to be associated both with neuroses and psychoses. A new definition of normality might be proposed: freedom from chronic muscular tension.

R. W. White has stated that neuroses take their start when the defenses against a condition of threat are "frozen" and that therapy involves the "unfreezing" of these defenses. This is another way of stating that a person's mode of reaction to a condition of frustration becomes chronic. Recent psychological approaches to therapy have emphasized changing the patient's perception of a threatening situation. If, however, the views advanced above are at all correct, this is only a partial solution. Muscles which have been persistently tense over a period of many years will not relax simply because the patient perceives a situation differently. In experiments with typists and with children in competitive situations, the results indicate that subjects who discharge relatively more of their aroused energies through the motor channel specifically appropriate to the experimental displacement also tend to recover equilibrium quickly, and to be left with only small amounts of residual tension. Since tensions have arisen precisely because adequate motor responses were not made in earlier frustrating situations, it would seem clear that the course therapy should take is to allow the uncompleted responses reflected in bodily attitudes to be completed under more favorable circumstances than would be possible outside of the therapeutic situation. The patient should be helped made aware, at the same time, of the meaning of his actions. This, of course, is the statement of a therapeutic ideal, not the statement of a specific technique. It is based on the postulate that one is healthier without persistent muscular tensions than with them, a fact which this paper has attempted to demonstrate.

F. SUMMARY

The experimental and clinical evidence, which has been presented concerning the formation, significance, and effect of chronically contracted muscles, is considered to be adequate justification for the following conclusions:

1. Patterns of movement, posture, and facial expressions are consistent aspects of personality and have been found in many instances to be more revealing indices of changes in personality than verbal reports.
2. Chronic tensions arise because adequate motor responses to conditions of conflict or frustration are impeded or blocked. Tensions reflect a continuous state of readiness of which an individual may often be unaware.
3. Besides chronic muscle tension being casually related to many physical complaints, it has also been found to be associated both with neuroses and psychoses.
4. In the light of these facts and conclusions, it is suggested that a universal criterion of normality might be: freedom from chronic muscular tension. Some considerations relevant to therapy were also presented.

REFERENCES

Abraham, K. "A constitutional basis of locomotor anxiety" (1913), in: *Selected Papers of Karl Abraham.* London: Hogarth Press (1927), p. 527.

Allport, G. W., & Vernon, P. E. *Studies in Expressive Movement.* New York: Macmillan (1933), p. 269.

Arnold, M. B. "A study of tension in relation to breakdown," *J. Gen. Psychol.* (1942), 26:315–341.

Ascher, E. "Motor attitudes and psychotherapy," *Psychosomat. Med.* (1949), 4:228–235.

Balken, E. R. & Masserman, J. H. "The language of phantasy: III," *J. of Psychol.* (1940), 10:75–86.

Boland, E. W., & Corr, W. P. "Psychogenic rheumatism," *J. Amer. Med. Assoc.* (1943), 123:805–809.

Cason, H. "Common annoyances: A psychological study of everyday aversions and irritations," *Psychol. Monog.* (1930), 40 (2).

Chapman, W. P. "Measurement of pain sensitivity in normal control subjects and psychoneurotic patients," *Psychosomat. Med.* (1944), 6:252–257.

Chapman, W. P., *et al.* "Measurements related to pain in neurocirculatory asthenia, anxiety neurosis, or effort syndrome," *J. Clin. Investigation* (1946), 25:890–896.

———. "Measurements of pain sensitivity of patients with psychoneurosis," *Arch. Neurol. & Psychiat.* (1947), 57:321–331.

Clites, M. S. "Certain somatic activities in relation to successful and unsuccessful problem solving," *J. Exp. Psychol.* (1935), 18:708–724.

———. "Certain somatic activities in relation to successful problem solving: Part II and III," *J. Exp. Psychol.* (1936), 19:106–115, and 172–192.

Courts, F. A. "Muscular tension and performance," *Psychol. Bull.* (1942), 39:347–367.

Darrow, C. W. "Psychological and psychophysiological significance of the electroencephalogram," *Psychol. Rev.* (1947), 54:157–168.

Davis, R. C. "The relation of certain muscle action potentials to 'mental work,'" *Ind. Univ. Publ., Sci. Ser.* (1937), 5.

———. "The relation of muscle action potentials to difficulty and frustration," *J. Exp. Psychol.* (1938), 23:141–158.

———. "Methods of measuring tension," *Psychol. Bull.* (1942), 39:329–346.

Davis, A., & Havighurst, R. J. "Social class and color differences in child rearing," in Kluckhohn, C. and Murray, H., *Personality in Nature, Society, and Culture.* New York: Knopf (1948), p. 561.

Denslow, J. S., & Graham-Service, D. M. "The spread of muscle action potentials from active to inactive areas," *Fed. Proc.* (1948), 7:27.

Deutsch, F. "Analysis of postural behavior," *Psychoanal. Quart.* (1947), 16:195–211.

Duffy, E. "Tensions and emotional factors in reaction," *Genet. Psych. Monog.* (1930), 7:1–79.

———. "The measurement of muscular tension as a technique for the study of emotional tendencies," *Amer. J. Psychol.* (1932), 44:146–162.

———. "Level of muscle tension as an aspect of personality," *J. Gen. Psychol.* (1946), 35:161–171.

Dunbar, F. "Character and symptom formation," *Psychoanal. Quart.* (1939), 8:18–47.

———. *Emotions and Bodily Changes* (3rd ed.). New York: Columbia Univ. Press (1946), p. 604.

Eisenberg, P. "Expressive movements related to feeling of dominance," *Arch. of Psychol.* (1937), 3 (211).

Eisenberg, P., & Reichline, P. B. "Judging expressive movement: II. Judgments of dominance-feeling from motion pictures of gaits," *J. Soc. Psychol.* (1939), 10:345–357.

Elliott, F. A. "Tender muscles in sciatica," *Lancet.* (1944), 246:47–49.

Ellman, P., Savage, O. A., Wittkower, E. & Rodger, T. F. "Fibrositis," *Ann. Rheumatic Dis.* (1942), 3:56–75.

Estes, S. G. "Judging personality from expressive behavior," *J. Abn. & Soc. Psychol.* (1938), 33:217–236.

Fenichel, O. *Outline of Clinical Psychoanalysis.* New York: Norton, 1934.

Flugel, J. C. "A quantitative study of feelings and emotion in everyday life," *British J. Psychol., Gen. Sect.* (1924–25), 15:318–355.

Freeman, G. L. "Postural tensions and the conflict situation," *Psychol. Rev.* (1939), 46:226–240.

———. "Dr. Hollingworth on chewing as a technique of relaxation," *Psychol. Rev.* (1940), 47:491–493.

Freeman, G. L. & Haggard, E. A. "Reactions of children to experimentally induced frustrations," *Psychol. Bull.* (1941), 38:581.

Freeman, G. L. & Pathman, J. H. "Effect of voluntary and involuntary inhibition of motor discharge upon physiological recovery from experimentally induced displacement." (In press) Cited in Freeman, G. L., *The Energetics of Human Behavior*. Ithaca: Cornell Univ. Press (1948), p. 344.

———. "The relation of overt muscular discharge to displacing stimuli," *J. Exp. Psychol.* (1942), 30:161–174.

Freeman, G. L. *The Energetics of Human Behavior.* Ithaca: Cornell Univ. Press (1948), p. 344.

Freud, S. "The unconscious" (1915), in: *Collected papers of Sigmund Freud,* Vol. 4. London: International Psychoanalytic Press (1925), p. 508.

———. *Repression* (1915), in: *Collected papers of Sigmund Freud,* Vol. 4. London: International Psychoanalytic Press (1925), p. 508.

———. *The Problem of Anxiety.* New York: Psychoanalytic Press (1936), p. 127.

———. "The Psychopathology of Everyday Life," in: *The Basic Writing of Sigmund Freud.* New York: Modern Library, 1938.

Fromm-Reichmann, F. "Transference problems in schizophrenia," *Psychoanal. Quart.* (1939), 8:412–426.

Gates, G. S. "An observational study of anger," *J. Exp. Psychol.* (1926), 9:325–336.

Gerard, M. "The psychogenic tic in ego development," in *The Psychoanalytic Study of the Child,* Vol. II. New York: International Univ. Press (1946), p. 424.

Goldstein, K. *The Organism.* New York: American Book (1939), p. 533.

Grinstead, A. D. "Bodily movement accompanying problem solving activity (abstract)," *Psychol. Bull.* (1939), 36:620.

Halverson, H. M. "Infant sucking and tensional behavior," *J. Genet. Psychol.* (1938), 53:365–430.

Hollingworth, H. L. "Chewing as a technique of relaxation," *Science* (1939), 90:385–387.

———. "Psychodynamics of chewing," *Arch. of Psychol.* (1939), 34 (239).

Howell, W. H. *A Textbook of Physiology* (11th ed.). Philadelphia: Saunders (1930), p. 1099.

Jacobson, E. "Response to a sudden unexpected stimulus," *J. Exp. Psychol.* (1927), 10:19–25.

———. *Progressive Relaxation.* Univ. Chicago Press (1938), p. 493.

———. "The effect of daily rest without training to relax on muscular tonus," *Amer. J. Psychol.* (1942), 55:248–254.

James, W. T. "A study of the expression of bodily posture," *J. Gen. Psychol.* (1932), 7:405–436.

Jost, H. "Some physiological changes during frustration," *Child Devel.* (1941), 12:9–15.

Jost, H. & Sontag, L. W. "The genetic factor in automatic nervous function," *Psychosomat. Med.* (1944), 6:308–310.

Katzell, R. A. "Relations between the activity of muscles during preparatory set and subsequent overt performance." *J. of Psychol.* (1948), 26:407–436.

Krout, M. H. "Autistic gestures: an experimental study in symbolic movement," *Psychol. Rev. Monog.* (1935), no. 208.

———. "The social and psychological significance of gestures," *J. Genet. Psychol.* (1935), 47:385–411.

———. "Further studies on the relation of personality and gestures: A nosological analysis of autistic gestures," *J. Exp. Psychol.* (1937), 20:279–287.

Landis, C. "Studies of emotional reactions: II. General behavior and facial expressions," *J. Comp. Psychol.* (1924), 4:447–509.

Landis, C., & Hunt, W. A. *The Startle Pattern.* New York: Farrar & Rhinehart (1939), p. 168.

Landis, C., & Bolles, M. *Personality and Sexuality of the Physically Handicapped Woman.* New York: Hoeber (1942), p. 171.

Lashley, K. S. "Physiological analysis of the libido," *Psychol. Rev.* (1924), 31: 192–202.

Levy, D. M. "On the problem of movement restraint," *Amer. J. Orthopsychiat.* (1944), 14:664–671.

Levy, D. M. In: *Encyclopedia of Psychology* (Ed. by P. L. Harriman). New York: Philosophical Library (1946), p. 897.

Luria, A. R. *The Nature of Human Conflicts.* New York: Liveright (1932), p. 431.

Marquis, D. P. "A study of frustration in newborn infants," *J. Exp. Psychol.* (1943), 32:123–138.

McGregor, H. G. "The physical examination of two thousand cases of Neuroses," *J. Neur. & Psychiat.* (1944), 7:21–27.

Murphy, L. "Childhood Experience in Relation to Personality Development," ch. 21 in *Personality and the Behavior Disorders* (Ed. by J. McV. Hunt), Vol. II. New York: Ronald Press (1944), p. 1242.

Murphy, G. *Personality*. New York: Harper (1947), p. 999.

Reich, W. *Character-Analysis* (2nd ed.). New York: Orgone Institute Press (1945), p. 328.

Ribble, M. A. "Infantile experience in relation to personality development," ch. 20 in *Personality and the Behavior Disorders* (Ed. by J. McV. Hunt) Vol. II. New York: Ronald Press (1944), p. 1242.

Sherman, M., & Jost, H. "Frustration reactions of normal and neurotic persons," *J. of Psychol.* (1942), 13:3–19.

Simons, D. J., *et al.* "Experimental studies on headache: muscles of the scalp and neck as sources of pain," *Proc. Ass. Res. Nerv. & Ment. Dis.* (1943), 23: 228–244.

Taylor, J. H. "Innate emotional response in infants," *Ohio State Univ. Stud. Contrib. Psychol.* (1934), no. 12:69–81.

Travell, J., Rinzler, S., & Herman, M. "Pain and disability of the shoulder and arm," *J. Amer. Med. Assoc.* (1942), 120:417–422.

Van Alstyne, D. "Relaxation and some related factors," *Child Devel.* (1935), 6:310–321.

Watson, J. B., & Morgan, J. J. B. "Emotional reactions and psychological experimentation," *Amer. J. Psychol.* (1917), 28:310–321.

Weiss, E. "Psychogenic rheumatism," *Ann. Int. Med.* (1947), 26:890–900.

Wenger, M. A. "Some relationships between muscular processes and personality and their factorial analysis," *Child Devel.* (1938), 9:261–276.

White, R. W. *The Abnormal Personality*. New York: Ronald Press (1948), p. 613.

Whitehorn, J. C. "Guide to interviewing and clinical personality study," *Arch. Neur. & Psychiat.* (1944), 52:197–216.

Williams, M. F. "Tension and respiratory pattern in young children," *J. Genet. Psychol.* (1942), 60:71–84.

Wolff, H. G., & Wolf, S. *Pain*. Springfield, Ill.: Thomas (1948), p. 90.

Wolff, W. "Involuntary self-expression in gait and other movements," *Char. & Personal.* (1933), 2:328–344.

———. *The Expression of Personality*. New York: Harper (1943), p. 334.

Zander, A. F. "A study of experimental frustration," *Psychol. Monog.* (1944), 56, (256).

PART III

THE STRUCTURAL AND NEUROPHYSIOLOGICAL PREMISE

CHAPTER

CHAPTER 8

CHIROPRACTIC ANALYSIS*

MORTIMER LEVINE, D.C.

INTRODUCTION

J. Lamoine De Rusha, D.C.

The behavioral scientific community today is becoming more cognizant of the influence of the neuro-musculo-skeletal system in evaluating the aberrations of function, as well as the attendant sequellae which may arise from anatomical disrelationship of the aforementioned systems.

Dr. Levine helps one to realize that the biologic union between structure and function has always been an integral part of chiropractic. In addition to contemporary diagnostic and laboratory procedures, the chiropractic discipline emphasizes this relationship. Chiropractic analysis, as Dr. Levine postulates, is the building of a ratio between structural disrelationship (histological or gross) and the functional disturbances resulting therefrom via the neurological bed. The ensuing cellular pathology further makes the organism receptive to bacterial invasion, viruses, chemical insult, and micro-trauma: physical, emotional, and ideational.

Levine discusses some of the chiropractic tenets: "The Spinal Subluxation," "The Principle of Basic and Compensatory Distortion," "Myotonic Variance," and other features of chiropractic analysis. All these help one to appreciate that musculo-skeletal and neural integrative functions and controls are of cardinal significance in chiropractic concepts of etiology, diagnosis, therapeutic adjustive procedures, and prognosis.

These principles today are buttressed and substantiated by concepts such as the stress and adaptation syndromes of Selye (1950–1954), the homeostatis of Cannon (1939), and the cybernetic control systems based on engineering principles (Norbett Wiener, 1953). Kelly (1948) speaks of a nidus of irritation arising from any area of the sensory portion of the nervous system, irradiating outward to excite both the "internuncial pool" of the central nervous system, and the "self re-exciting neuronal circuits" in the neural communicating system of the total body. This irradiation of stimulus may discharge into

* Reprinted by permission of the author and the publisher—The Comet Press, N.Y., 1964. From *The Structural Approach to Chiropractic.*

ascending projection systems and the alpha fiber systems and be responsible for disturbances of cortical function, or it may spill over into the lateral horn of the spinal cord and be responsible for varied autonomic "concomitants."

The Biologic Law of chiropractic, (Carver, 1910), states that the radiation of nerve stimulus over its organized channels the C.N.S. and the peripheral nervous system causes all animation or life. It is substantiated by Cannon (1932), who considers the autonomic nervous system to be the chief regulator of homeostasis. Chiropractic biomechanics, embracing myotonic variance and skeletal disrelationship mentioned in this chapter, are augmented by Yamamoto and Brebeck (1965). Those familiar with the contemporary references should find it easy to relate to chiropractic concepts as laid out by Levine.

The author has done well to point up chiropractic analysis, as formulated by Carver (1910). It is supported by contemporary thinking of structural psychotherapists, such as Lowen (1958 and 1967), Rolf (1962), Alexander (1941), and others. Chiropractic analysis parallels the central theme of much present knowledge, namely, that structure and function are interdependent, cannot be divorced one from the other, and that they comprise the "togetherness" of body unity. Hippocrates, Sherrington, MacKensie, and Bernard were harbingers of these concepts years ago. The trite adage, "A Sound Mind in a Sound Body," and the reverse, might be a manifestation of this "togetherness."

* * *

IN THE BROADEST SENSE all healing arts are based on the study of man, how he is constructed, how he functions and how he acts and reacts to his environment, to his fellow man and to his inner stresses. The proposition that a living organism is the result of molecular activities and biologic forces which man is utterly incapable of designing or creating is not subject to dispute. However, one does not have to have transcendental views or believe in a particular cosmic scheme of things to acknowledge that the restoration of health depends more on the correct organization of inner processes than it does upon any outside efforts thought to be therapeutic.

Chiropractic is based upon the premise that the body is self-stabilizing and self-regulating. Biologic processes are not static, living tissues are always being repaired and rebuilt to serve their intended function. Nature has a remarkable power of self-restoration which no outside agency is completely capable of supervising. The concept that nature is smarter than man is not novel. Nor did it originate with chiropractic. It is a very old idea, but perhaps more relevant today than ever before. Although we live in an age of moon trips, laser beams and heart transplants, the psycho-biological functions that go on in a living human organism are so complex that no man or group of men understand more than a fragment of this complex.

CHIROPRACTIC ANALYSIS

Chiropractic analysis is the determination of the equation between the body's structural distortion and the functional abnormality resulting from that distortion. This equation holds, even though it is often difficult to recognize a concomitant relationship between structure and function in a given case of pathology. The difficulty in equating the degree of distortion with the magnitude of symptoms is due to subjective interpretation of symptoms, the patient's relative health conception, and the time and manner in which the distortion was acquired or developed.

Chiropractic views a disease process as the conduct of disrelated anatomy. It postulates that a living organism is healthy if all its parts are in proper position and relation. In order for the gross anatomy to maintain its proper relationships, the microscopic anatomy or morphology of the histologic structures that make up the gross part must be true to form. The integration of structure and function indicates that health or lack of it may be interpreted on architectural and mechanical criteria.

A perfectly normal body structure, one in which each and every part of the assemblage is in proper relation to each and every other part, expresses perfectly normal function. But a body assemblage in which there exists anatomical distortion cannot express normal function. Thus functional change tends to be proportionate to structural change. In short, a chiropractic analysis is the attempt to ascertain how and why a given distortion in a particular person is causing abnormal function in that person. When the chiropractor has made his analysis, he can then devise the adjusting techniques to correct the distortion (if corrigible) relying on the body's endogenous biologic resources to change pathologic processes to physiologic ones.

CHIROPRACTIC DIAGNOSIS

Perhaps the greatest fallacy about chiropractic is that the chiropractic doctor does not diagnose. Nothing could be further from the truth. Chiropractic analysis is an advanced additional dimension to physical diagnosis and is inclusive of all other diagnostic methods. Furthermore every chiropractic college teaches physical examination and diagnostic procedures. Students are taught and tested in physical, neurological, clinical, laboratory, and differential diagnosis. Roentgenology, pediatrics, geriatrics, dermatology, nutrition, and the study of communicable disease processes are all part of the chiropractic curriculum. Before receiving a license to practice chiropractic, candidates are examined in diagnosis either by official State Boards or by the National Board of Chiropractic Examiners or both.

The doctor who has had chiropractic training is well versed in clinical care, patient management, and symptomatology. However, an understanding of chiropractic is impossible by merely memorizing signs and symptoms of disease processes, because no matter how complex symptoms may be, the chiropractic doctor values them only as evidence of a structural or tissue condition. He knows that the bond between structure and function is inseparable and that symptoms are the expression of distorted and disrelated anatomy.

It is important to remember that distortion of a dynamic organism such as the human machine always involves altered relationship rather than a changed place in space, as would apply to a static structure. No molecule, cell, vertebral segment, or organ has a place per se. A cell, bone, or organ has position only in relation to relative tissues. Therefore, a comprehensive overview of the entire organism, plus an intimate and detailed knowledge of the organism's construction, is necessary to determine whether the relationship is normal or whether distortion exists.

One of the basic operational principles on which the practice of chiropractic is founded can be succinctly summed up in the following statement. Any interference with the receipt, transmission, or application of the impulses that travel over the nervous system causes functional abnormality or disease.

WHEN DOES NERVE INTERFERENCE MANIFEST ITSELF?

Interference takes place when tissue displacement, whether cellular, segmental, or organic, is sufficient to change the character, consistence, or relation of nerves so as to alter their ability to conduct and transmit stimuli either on a quantitative or qualitative basis.

Since it is a fact that the nerve system manifests its function only by producing changes in other tissues, interference always exhibits a dual effect. These two phases of nerve interference are: (1) Immediate—interference to the nerve itself, and (2) Remote—interference to the parts ramified. It is not to be construed that these phases take place separately. The moment a nerve is disturbed, the parts it controls are also disturbed. The more important the nerve and the greater the area it governs, the more devastating the effect of interference.

The chiropractic diagnostician understands that interference with nerve stimuli may be a cardinal cause of functional abnormality. Therefore his primary concern is to locate subluxations and their adjacent tissue distortions that interfere with the normal transmission of stimuli. He knows that when he has located and appraised these distortions, he will then know a somatic source of the patient's disorder. He is also aware that proprioceptive input markedly influences the patient's mental state, and that psychosomatics is a two-way street.

THE SUBLUXATION

The subluxation is the unit of distortion and has been the focus of attention and research since the discovery of chiropractic. Although often represented as a simple concept, research has proved the opposite to be true. The mechanics and reactions involved in subluxation are exceedingly complex and can influence every function of the organism.

In order to define the term, subluxation, we must define the word from which it was derived, which is luxation. *Luxation:* A dislocation, specifically a disturbance or derangement of the bones entering into the formation of a joint. *Subluxation:* A subluxation is a partial, minor, or incomplete luxation or, more precisely, a fixation within the range of motion of the involved joint. It is a condition in which a vertebra has come to rest somewhere within its normal scope, but not at its zero point or central resting position. The reciprocal joint facings are in a position of motion when they should be in a position of rest or vice versa. The precise moment when subluxation becomes luxation is when the osseous components of the joints exceed the limits of their physiologic range of motion.

Subluxations can lay the foundation for disease processes, because it reduces the ability of the articulation to perform its designed physiological function. It should be made clear that subluxation can and does occur to any and all joints of the skeletal frame. Naturally, when it occurs in the vertebral column, the pathogenic implications are far more profound.

No discussion of subluxation would be complete without analyzing its effects on the nerves themselves. We know that afferent stimuli are continuously radiating centrally from all body tissues, but they cause reflex action only when the stimuli become adequate to bridge the synaptic gaps between the neurons which receive the stimuli and the neurons which effect response. Noxious stimuli, initiated by a subluxation, lowers the threshold of response of the motor neurons, thereby causing them to fire at a stimulus below that which they would withstand if there were no subluxation. In other words, these nerve circuits become hyperirritable and reach a state wherein a lesser stimulation is more than adequate to generate impulses.

The patient with the acute low back syndrome who reports that all he did was to bend down and tie his shoelace, or some other equally innocuous act, is the perfect example of how prior subluxation is the forerunner to what may appear to be a new condition. The presence of previously acquired subluxations at different levels of the vertebral column clarifies and explains why one man under stress conditions develops headaches, a second man may suffer from gall bladder disturbance, and a third man will have a bout of colitis. Each man had a pre-existing weak point located in a different portion of his spinal column. *Thus, subluxation is not only the source of its own pathology, but may predispose the organism to many other pathogenic factors.* However, time modifies all things and all processes. Subluxation is no exception to this rule. This can account for the fact that the person may acclimate himself to his subluxation and go on functioning—at an impaired level, but adequately to meet his needs.

THE PRINCIPLE OF BASIC AND COMPENSATORY DISTORTION

Carver (1910) formulated this most important canon in chiropractic, *Definition:* When a basic structure moves in relation to the body gravity line, relative and superimposed structures must alter their relation to that line or equilibrium is lost.

The same proposition stated more simply: When a weight-bearing structure is distorted, nature automatically attempts to restore body balance by developing compensatory counter-distortions. Dr. Carver's elucidation of this law of equilibrium was a major breakthrough to a clear and comprehensive understanding of the mechanism of postural change. It now becomes apparent that many of the distortions found in the vertebral column are compensatory in nature, and are the result of the need to redistribute weight because of a basic distortion. No attempt should be made to correct these counterbalancing curves, unless the basic distortion that brought them into being is first corrected.

PELVIC DISTORTIONS

The initial step in postural analysis is to locate and determine the basic distortion. Since the seat of most basic distortions is the pelvis, let us direct our attention to the various types. There are two main classes of pelvic distortions. They are: I. *Distortions of the Pelvis as a Unit.* This class of distortion involves a change of relationships between the pelvis and the trunk above without changing the relationship of the bones that comprise the pelvis. The lumbo-sacral articulation bears the brunt of these stresses and is the prime area of subluxation. There are eight distinct unit pelvic distortions: four in the medial plane, two in the coronal plane, and two in the horizontal plane. The second class of pelvic distortions is:

II. *Distortions in the Pelvis or Sacroiliac Subluxations.* This category consists of a disarrangement of the bones that comprise the pelvis. It always involves subluxation of one or both sacroiliac joints. The sacroiliac mechanism is without a doubt the most complex articulation in the skeletal frame. Therefore, it is not surprising that some differences in the understanding of the mechanics and function of these joints should exist. For years most orthopedists have maintained that the sacrum is immovably wedged between the two ilia, while chiropractic has taught that the sacroiliac articulation is freely movable within a very narrow range. Cineroentgenography (moving picture x-rays) has proved that those articulations are freely movable.

Apart from their complexity, the sacroiliac joints play a vital role in the general health of the individual. A normally functioning sacroiliac mechanism is the sine qua non of normal posture and good body mechanics. The prime function of the sacroiliac joints is shock absorption. These joints are unique in being the only articulations which are not directly activated by muscles. It takes an inertial force such as is provided in walking, running, and jumping to mobilize them. Neural disturbances follow fixation of any articulation which directly or indirectly supports the spinal cord. Loss of the shock absorbing function, due to sacroiliac subluxation, transforms each step into an irritative jar which can shock the delicate nerve tissues.

The two sacroiliac joints do not operate simultaneously, but rather in a reciprocal progressive synchronization as follows: When the right sacroiliac articulation is activated, the left innominate and sacrum move in relation to the right innominate, and vice versa. The pubic joint acts as an accessory joint to the sacroiliac joints and is activated whenever they are activated. All three bones change their positions, but always in a two-to-one ratio with the innominate and sacrum on the side that is not in motion, while maintaining an unchanged relationship to each other. The vast majority of acute sacroiliac subluxations are unilateral. One joint may be fixed in subluxation while the other side can continue to operate. However, with the passage of time, the increased strain on the side still in operation may cause it also to become fixed if the original point is not adjusted.

THE TYPICAL COMPENSATORY, DOUBLE-OPPOSED, ROTATIONAL SCOLIOSIS

As its full name implies, it is a series of four compensatory alternating rotational scoliotic curves. Starting from the bottom and proceeding headward, we find: The *first curve* is a right rotational scoliosis extending from the 5th lumbar to the 2nd lumbar . . . the *second curve* is a left rotational scoliosis ranging from the 2nd lumbar to the 7th dorsal . . . the *third curve* is a right rotational scoliosis stretching from the 7th dorsal to the 7th cervical . . . the *fourth curve* is a left rotational scoliosis extending from the 7th cervical to the occiput.

Thus we have two curves on each side of the body gravity line counterbalancing each other, and all four curves counterbalancing the basic distortion, which is the inherent weakness of the right sacroiliac joint. Carver, who discovered, described, and explained this common human frailty more than sixty years ago, held the opinion that 90% of the human population is afflicted with the typical distortion.

Since the double-opposed, rotational scoliosis seems to be an inherited asymmetry and the practical postural normal of all people, any attempt to correct it would prove fruitless. What then is the significance of studying and knowing the typical distortion? Knowledge of it imparts the following information:

1. *It enables the doctor to recognize all atypical distortion patterns.*

2. *It illustrates the ideal compensation in the coronal and horizontal planes for a one-sided basic distortion.* In this instance we refer to the right side, but the pattern for the left side would be the same except for the reversal of the direction of the curves. The double-opposed, rotational scoliosis is the ideal pattern, because it reestablishes equilibrium with only a slight rearrangement of parts and with the least amount of bilateral imbalance. This means that subluxations and visceral accommodations for framework changes are held to a minimum. The closer the organism approximates its basic ideal design, the better it can cope with stresses and strains, and the more adequately it can equalize daily wear and tear.

3. *It explains the mechanogenesis of rotational scoliosis.* The orientation of the head is a cardinal factor in the ability of the body to maintain balance at the same time that it is accommodating and adapting to other distortions. In the typical distortion, the occiput is found facing directly forward in the horizontal plane and tipped sufficiently feetward on the left in the coronal plane to cause the head to be transversely level.

The mechanics of the atlanto-occipital area provide for the occipital condyles to rock forward and backward on the cradle-like facets of the atlas. However, the dihedral angle formed by the chords of the arcs of the planes of the headward facets of the 1st cervical allows a slight amount of side slip in the coronal plane. Thus the typical double-opposed, rotational scoliosis terminates with the coronal and median planes of the head coincident with the body gravity line. This means that the head has been centered. The equilibrating mechanisms of the body (proprioceptors, semicircular canals, eyes, cerebellar centers, etc.), are again ready to respond best to the constantly shifting demands of dynamic balance.

MYOTONIC VARIANCE

This principle was first elucidated by Dr. H. Lewis Trubenbach. It concerns the various tension states of muscles. Muscles have five states of tone. They are:

1. Tonus: the state of tension in a muscle at rest.
2. Tonic Spasm: the state of tension in a muscle undergoing active movement.
3. Hypertonus: the state of tension in a muscle when it is in fixation and will not relax. This is a pathologic state.
4. Sleep Tone: the state of tension in a muscle when the organism is asleep. In this state the muscle attains maximum physiologic relaxation.
5. Unconscious Tone: the state of tension which is so slight that it is barely existent. This state is always pathologic.

It is self evident that bones do not move themselves. Their movements are accomplished by the pull of the muscles connected to them. In fact, bone position is primarily a reflection of the pull tensions exerted by its attached muscles. Bones that are gripped too tightly or held too loosely cannot function efficiently. It is the unequal tension of opposing fellow muscles that prevents vertebral segments from assuming their normal juxtaposition.

Excessive tension is recognized by psychiatry and other healing disciplines as being responsible for a host of disease processes. High blood pressure, ulcers, angina pectoris, coronary occlusion, colitis, asthma, speech disorders, and even psychosis are only a partial list of disorders that are attributed to excessive tensions.

This recognition of excessive tensions is an awareness of environmental stressors such as personality clashes, injustices, frustrations, unhappy circumstances and other emotional strains. However, not until these tensions become structuralized in the body's tissues does the conduct of the organism become diseased.

Myotonic variance is the correlating and unifying concept which explains bodily behavioral changes regardless of the cause of those changes. Muscle spasm results in faulty bone opposition, which is subluxation and distortion, whether the tension precipitating factors are mechanical, chemical, or emotional. This is a fundamental principle stated by D. D. Palmer in 1905. When we consider that all body movements and functions and the inhibition of movements and functions, take place through the medium of muscles and nerves, it becomes evident that the dichotomy of the psychological and the physiological, mind and body, does not exist. All actions and reactions are psychophysical in nature.

THE CHIROPRACTIC EXAMINATION

The chiropractic examination is primarily, but not exclusively, a spinal and skeletal analysis. It is designed to reveal the patient's static and kinetic postural defects, which are causing or contributing to the patient's faulty functions. It is accomplished via seven steps in the following manner:

1. *Locate the basic distortion.* This means that the doctor must find and determine the primary subluxation which is producing the patient's present postural pattern.

Since the sacrum is the foundation for the normal and abnormal curves of the spinal column, it is the seat of most basic distortions. In judging the position and relation of the sacrum to relative and superimposed structures, the doctor must estimate the following: (a) Has the sacral angle increased or has it decreased? (normal is 38 to 45 degrees). (b) Are the iliac crests equidistant from the floor? If they are not, is the discrepancy due to an anatomical short leg or to a sacroiliac subluxation? (c) Is the pelvis rotated in the horizontal plane in relation to the feet or to the thorax?

2. *Check to see if the compensatory distortion is commensurate with the basic distortion.* Here the doctor must evaluate how well the spinal curves are counterbalancing the basic distortion. (a) Is the spinal distortion in the same plane or planes as the basic distortion? (b) Is the magnitude of the spinal distortion greater or less than the basic distortion?

3. *Consider the ratio of the compensatory curves and decide which is the short radius curve.* In this step the doctor notes whether the counterbalancing distortion is distributed equally throughout the vertebral column. If it is not, which area of the spine is disproportionately distorted?

4. *Link the short radius curve to the symptoms via nerve tracing and reflex zones.* Here we have the key to the structure-function equation and the neuro-mechanical cause or component of the disease process. The short radius curve is made up of the severest subluxations and is therefore the most likely site of nerve interference.

When the symptoms manifested by the patient are in tissues ramified by the nerves which can be traced back to the subluxated area, the genesis of the neuro-dystrophic process is virtually certain.

5. *Check myotonic variance for the time element of the case.* The determination of the state of tension in the muscles and the testing of the range of motion in the involved area will indicate whether you are dealing with an acute or a chronic condition. Hypertonus of muscles and marked restriction of movement of the involved articulations denote an acute condition. Trophic imbalance of muscles and a moderate reduction of range of motion point to a chronic condition.

6. *See if there are any contra-indicative factors to spinal adjusting.* These factors would be pathologic conditions that might preclude the use of the dynamic thrust, such as: fractures, tuberculosis and malignant neoplasms of the spine. X-ray investigation is the best tool to disclose these conditions.

7. *Build a hypothesis of correction and adjust.* At this point, the doctor knows *what* he is going to do, *why* he is going to do it, and *how* he is going to do it.

The spinal and skeletal analysis is now completed. However, the application of chiropractic produces great changes in the patient's condition. This necessitates frequent checking and re-analyzing of the patient in order to know when to stop or change the adjusting procedure.

In conclusion, the words "diseased" and "cure" have become so concrete in our understanding that they shape our very thoughts and beliefs. The tradition of thinking about a disease process of and by itself is so arbitrary and so ingrained in the human mind, that even those doctors who profess that an individual's health is proportionate to his wholeness and that "cure" depends on the correct organization of inner processes are reluctantly influenced to conform to the conventional fragmented understanding.

Yet in real life, we never deal with things in isolation; things and processes are linked together in subtle ways. Body chemistry and the body's neuro-mechanical relationships are inextricably woven together in the living process called metabolism. The chemistry of the body, when not due to hereditary gene abnormality, is the result of controlled coordinated cellular activity. Normal nerve system function means normal body chemistry, as long as the essential nutrients are provided in the optimum kind and amount.

The difficulty lies in our inability to perceive that the difference between what we term a functional disease process and an organic disease process is only a difference of degree. The parenchyma of a liver does not become cirrhosed all at once, articulations do not ankylose overnight, nor does any other lesion become gross before it is histologic, (trauma excepted). Furthermore, nerves, muscles, and articulations are just as much body organs as are viscera. In fact, the whole pathologic panorama is one continuous evolution of intensifying effects. Thus, it is the cumulative effect of short range symptom suppression that makes for long range chronic degenerative disease processes.

All doctors of the healing arts, in appreciating the basic premise that all truths are necessarily an integral part of every other truth, will also look upon the patient as a total entity.

The battle for health will be won by doctors who are predominantly consistent; doctors who can integrate, relate, and reduce to the simplest common denominators the factors which can change pathologic behavior to physiologic behavior. The doctor of chiropractic's constitutional approach teaches that the organism's neuro-mechanical relationship is a decisive factor in the predisposition to, and the maintenance of health.

REFERENCES

Adams, John Crawford. *Outline of Orthopedics.* London: Williams & Wilkins Co., 1961.

Alexander, F. Matthias. *The Universal Constant in Living.* London: Chaterson Ltd., 1947.

Aschner, Bernard. *The Art of the Healer.* New York: Dial Press, 1942.

Beatty, Homer G. *Anatomical Adjustive Technique.* Privately Published, 1939.

Boyd, William. *Text Book of Pathology.* Lee and Ferbiger, 1958.

Burr, Harold Saxton. *The Neural Basis of Human Behavior.* Charles C Thomas, 1960.

Calliet, Rene. *Low Back Pain Syndrome* (1962).

Carver, Willard. *Carver's Chiropractic Analysis* (Two volumes). Oklahoma City: Dunn Printing Co., 1922.

Carver, Willard. *Psycho-Bio-Physiology.* Oklahoma City: Carver Chiropractic College, 1920.

De Jarnette, B. *Sacral-Occipital Technique.* Nebraska City: Privately published, 1940.

Dintenfass, Julius. *Chiropractic.* New York: Pyramid Press, 1966.

Dubos, Rene. *Mirage of Health.* New York: Harper & Bros., 1959.

Gillet, Henry. *Belgian Notes on Fixation.* Brussels, Belgium: Privately printed, 1970.

Goldthwait, Jack E. *Essentials of Body Mechanics.* Philadelphia: J. B. Lippincott Co., 1941.

Homewood, A. E. *The Neurodynamics of the Vertebral Subluxation.* Toronto: Chiropractic Publishers, 1963.

Illi, Fred W. *The Vertebral Column Life Line of the Body.* Chicago: National College of Chiropractic, 1951.

Jackson, Ruth. *The Cervical Syndrome* (1958).

Janse, Joseph. *Chiropractic Principles and Technique.* Chicago: National College of Chiropractic, 1947.

Ligeros, Kleanthes. *How Ancient Healing Governs Modern Therapeutics.* New York: G. P. Putnam's Sons, 1937.

Levine, Mortimer. *The Structural Approach to Chiropractic.* New York: Comet Press, 1964.

Maynard, J. E. *Healing Hands.* Freeport, New York: Jonorne Publishing, 1959.

Mennell, James. *The Science and Art of Joint Manipulation* (Vol. II): *The Spinal Column.* Philadelphia, Pa.: The Blakiston Co., 1952.

Palmer, Daniel David. *The Science, Art, and Philosophy of Chiropractic.* Portland, Oregon: Portland Printing House, 1910.

Pottenger, Francis. *Symptoms of Visceral Disease.* C. V. Mosby Co., 1958.

Schmarl, George and Junghans, Herbert. *The Human Spine in Health and Disease.* New York: Grune and Stratton, 1959.

Sobotta, Johannes. *Atlas of Descriptive Human Anatomy* (Vol. I). Hafner Publishing Co., 1957.

Speransky. *A Basis for the Theory of Medicine.* International Publishers, 1943.

Steindler, Arthur. *Mechanics of Normal and Pathological Locomotion in Man.* Charles Thomas, 1956.

Trubenbach, H. L. and Peterson, Thure C. *The Doctrine of Chiropractic*. New Jersey: Academy of Chiropractic, 1942.

Verner, J. Robinson. *The Science and Logic of Chiropractic*. Privately published, 1941.

Williams, Roger. *You Are Extraordinary*. New York: Random House, 1967.

CHAPTER 9

CHIROPRACTIC AND EMOTIONAL DISORDERS*

A. E. HOMEWOOD, D.C.

THE MODERN DOCTOR of chiropractic, like all other conscientious practitioners of the healing arts, is concerned with research into the various causes for mental and emotional disorders.

D. D. Palmer (1910) emphasized that mechanical, chemical or psychological irritations may cause subluxations, which in turn can lay the foundation for physical as well as emotional illness. Heredity also determines the body type, with its specific areas of structural weakness, causing general basic irritability of the nervous system. Then there are the developmental anomalies and asymmetries which add structural predispositions to distortion.

Furthermore, spinal injuries, faulty posture, occupational or recreational asymmetrical development, etc., are of import in determining the site of subluxations causing somatic or emotional stress. Upon such a background, there is added the reflex irritations from the internal organs.

It has also been noted by D. D. Palmer (1910) and enlarged upon by Harper (1964) and Homewood (1968) that the environmental stresses tend to overcome the normal resistance of the individual and create structural disrelations and dysfunctions of the somatic components of the body. Most of these aberrations are consequences of the response of the nervous system to the irritations of the environment, rather than from the frank, physical trauma to structure.

Emotional factors are then superimposed upon this complex background of mechanical and reflex stress to which the body is subjected. They may therefore be final factors which cause a previously asymptomatic condition to produce various symptoms.

W. Sachs (1936) emphasized that every emotion has its counterpart in the posture assumed. Should an emotion, such as despondency, be persistent, the somatic expression may result in changes of muscular tension with attendant osseous distortion and visceral disrelation. If the emotion persists this may even become more or less permanent. It has also been well established that the emotional state disturbs the function of visceral structures through

* Reprinted in part, modified and updated, from *The Neurodynamics of the Vertebral Subluxation,* by permission of the author and the Chiropractic Publishers, Toronto.

psychovisceral reflexes. Hence, through the mechanism of the visceromotor reflex, the embryologically related vertebral segments may become fixated or subluxated.

THE SPINAL SUBLUXATION AS A PSYCHOSOMATIC DISORDER

There is a growing amount of literature in which the spine and psychic disorders are being related clinically. Brown *et al.* (1954) showed that in a large percentage of cases of low back pain, there was a complicating psychological factor. Levine (1971), in discussing the relationship of depression and back pain, suggests a psychophysiologic mechanism in the pathogenesis of disc protrusion. Scott (1955) demonstrated swelling of intervertebral discs in situations of stress. Depressive patients have been shown to have an upset in mineral metabolism with a significant increase in intracellular sodium. Copper (1969) claims this could be a factor in disc protrusion.

Similarly, many disorders which are commonly attributed to psychic disturbances have been found to have a high incidence of spinal abnormality. One example of this is the research by Kamieth (1958) who reported that, "[in] the majority of patients (with stomach and duodenal ulcers), 86 of 100 had lateral curvature scoliosis of the thoracic portion of the vertebral column. . . . All the scolioses involved the vertebral segments corresponding to the stomach and duodenum, that is T-6 to T-9. . . . Moreover almost 90% of all the patients had pathological changes in the intervertebral disks."

These observations are not to suggest that emotional factors are not involved in visceral pathologies, but rather that causes other than psychic may establish the tissue changes and produce symptoms of many visceral abnormalities. The symptoms which are dependent upon the afferent side of the neural system, to alert the patient of the dysfunction experienced, have their impact upon the emotional centres of the individual. He will then respond in a manner specific to his degree of neural irritability, past experience, and conditioning.

The interference to the normal occupational and recreational functions of the patient are further aspects that will govern the emotional response to the problem. The inability to continue in gainful employment and other productive activities is likely to have a serious emotional impact upon the individual. The emotional turmoil becomes a complicating secondary cause of visceral dysfunction and a much more challenging case to correct. The failure over the years to appreciate the interrelation of the somatic and visceral structures upon mental functions is being slowly corrected.

The brain, spinal cord and nerves are dependent for normal function upon an adequate blood supply via the arteries and venous drainage. In turn, the arteries and even terminal arterioles are under the control of the sympathetic division of the sympathetic nervous system, whose sole outflow of neural impulses is from the first thoracic to third lumbar segments of the spinal cord via preganglionic sympathetics. Therefore, should a spinal subluxation occur in the upper thoracic region, especially from the first to the fourth, an increased neural bombardment of the spinal cord segments from the muscles, tendons, ligaments, joint capsules, intervertebral discs, etc., will cause hyperactivity of the lateral horn cells of the sympathetic system.

Impulses from somatic receptors have been shown to make synaptic connections with the lateral horn sympathetic cells (Coote and Perez-Gonzales, 1970) (Iwamura *et al.*, 1969). Some of these sympathetic neurones send fibres upward through the sympathetic chain to reach the superior cervical sympathetic ganglion before terminating by synaptic connection with the postganglionic neurones. Some of the latter then form a network on the internal carotid and vertebral arteries and their continuingly smaller branches, which finally terminate by the formation of capillary networks that pervade every level of the brain. Hence, overactivation of these sympathetic fibres may well cause vasoconstriction and a degree of ischemia and anoxia with altered irritability of the cells of that portion of the brain.

Subluxations, distortions, muscle tension, and injuries to the soft tissues of the neck may upset the functioning of the sympathetic ganglionated chain or may mechanically and directly disturb the arterial supply and venous drainage of the brain (Kleynhaus, 1970). The vertebral arteries pass headward through foramina in the transverse processes of the cervical vertebrae, and could be directly affected by a severe cervical subluxation. The close approximation of the internal carotid arteries and internal jugular veins to the prevertebral muscles and osseous structures of the neck make the possibility of mechanical interference with optimum blood flow to and from the brain a reality. Again, any dysfunction of the blood supply or venous drainage of the brain alters its function and its ability to respond in an optimum manner to either external or internal environmental changes.

It is well known that much of the reticular formation is concerned with a descending stream of neural influences which can appreciably increase general muscular tone (Birkmeyer and Pilleri, 1966). The muscular tension with its related symptoms is probably due to direct stimulation of the alpha or gamma motor neurones by this system.

Thus, both the cerebral cortex and the general somatic musculature may be influenced by the reticular formation. The increased muscular tension in turn stimulates still other receptors. Additional afferent impulses return in profusion to the central nervous system with consequent influence upon the reticular formation. A positive feedback may thus be established. The cycle apparently continues the perpetuation of both the somatic and emotional tension.

How does the doctor break such a vicious cycle? Certainly not by the "talking it out process" alone or somatic correction alone. Both of these, and more, may be required. There are two primary forms of management of the anxiety afflicted patient. One form is the purely mental approach. The other form is the physical method of releasing tension by restoring the range of articular motion and normalizing the structural integrity through manipulative techniques of chiropractic, and occasionally by the addition of specific relaxation procedures.

Irvin M. Korr (1952) emphasized that, "Manipulation happens to be one of the best therapeutic modalities available today for altering man's patterns of response to noxious and other stimuli in favourable directions and for rendering him less vulnerable." Certainly this position is in harmony with the chiropractic physician's thinking, since it is recognized that the various noxious impulses from subluxations increase the irritability of neural segments, causing an increased erratic response to some additional adverse stimulation. There is no physical symptom in an individual without involvement of the emotions.

THE PSYCHOSOMATIC RESPONSE

Into primitive man was built the simple "fight-flight" mechanism, which demanded adequate expression of fear in musculo-skeletal activity. When the person is unable to fight for his rights, or for his self-preservation, and cannot take flight from it, fright takes possession of him; he freezes in neuromuscular tension, which increases his fear, and lays the foundation for psychophysiological symptoms.

Civilized man is frequently prevented, by the restraints and ethics of society, from responding to the emotion of fear in an adequate muscular manner; nor can an innumerable number of the causes of fear be adequately handled by such a response. (Every physiology textbook explains the alterations in function of this "fight-flight" response.) Unable to express physically his reaction to these emotions, residual tension of somatic muscles and altered function of viscera become the curse of civilized man.

The body's responses to emotion are gross and it is therefore often difficult to demonstrate specific subluxations of the vertebral column as a direct result of emotional trauma. However, psychogenic generalized muscular tension, superimposed upon a weakened area of the spine, can create a localized subluxation in that spinal area.

Teitelbaum (1964) has made the suggestion that spasm of the sternocleidomastoid and trapezius muscles in certain cases of torticollis may be attributed to a psychological problem. He quotes numerous sources in which torticollis patients have found relief through psychotherapy. A spasm of the cervical musculature causing torticollis would seriously affect the vertebral curvature and cause subluxation.

DIAPHRAGM IN PSYCHOSOMATIC DISTRESS

The diaphragm is another revealing source of emotional stress. Sudden diaphragmatic spasm, which can cause dyspnea and chest pain, has been described by Wolf and Goodell (1968). However, diaphragmatic hypertonicity is a found consequence to any unpleasant emotion and the majority of patients demonstrate such tension.

Deep inspiration will reveal diaphragmatic hypertonicity to the experienced observer. If the lower thorax does not lift freely, expand laterally and anteriorly, and the subcostal angle does not become markedly obtuse, there is diaphragmatic tension. Palpation of the sternal, costal and crural origins of the muscle fibres will reveal tenderness and knots of tension. This exploratory palpation may meet with resistance from the muscles of the anterior and lateral abdominal wall, which are very frequently involved, and incapable of relaxing when the individual lies supine. This tension is readily observable since the relaxation of the abdominal muscles should result in a marked depression of the epigastrium, delineating clearly the borders of the subcostal, or substernal angle. The tension in this region of the body is, with few exceptions, a direct reflection of emotional disturbances of an unpleasant nature.

Afferent impulses return to the spinal cord from the diaphragm, entering bilaterally via the posterior nerve roots of the seventh to the twelfth thoracic segments. Intrasegmental synaptic connection may be made with the motor neurones supplying the segmentally associated post-vertebral muscles, since increased tone and bilateral pull upon the posterior arches can be noted.

In accordance with the findings of Joel E. Goldthwait (1941) and the consensus of many anatomists, the diaphragm serves as a "second heart," in that its normal action should materially aid in the venous return from the lower extremities, pelvic and abdominal viscera. No single muscle would seem to be as important to the structural and functional integrity of the human as the diaphragm, and none other is more adversely influenced by the emotional stresses of life.

THE PSYCHO-VISCERO-SOMATIC RESPONSE

A more circuitous route in the production of vertebral subluxations is via the psychovisceral reflex and then, through a viscerosomatic reflex to the paraspinal musculature. Feldenkrais (1949) has established the possibility of emotional stress causing peptic ulcers. Hans Selye (1950) has shown that gastric sites of mucosal erosion are the rule in the "Alarm Reaction" to most stressors, including emotional stress, in those members of society who are aggressive and willing to fight. However, those prone to flight from the unpleasant situations demonstrate a gastric mucosa that is pale and flattened. Once established, the ulcerative condition of the gastric mucosa, as an example, would begin bombarding the sixth to the ninth thoracic neuromeres with noxious impulses, especially to the right halves of neuromeres seven and eight (Rasmussen 1947).

Both Eble (1960) and Downman and McSwiney (1946) have shown that stimulation of the gastric or intestinal wall in a rabbit can lead to somatic muscular contraction. Downman (1955) established that the response was greatest in intercostal nerves on the same embryologic level as the nerve being stimulated, and diminishes as one moves up or down the spinal cord.

Clinically, the somatic reaction, or visceromotor reflex, expresses itself in hypertonicity of the superior portion of the right abdominal musculature and hypertonicity of the postvertebral muscles. Subluxations can be found in this region of the vertebral column and frequently cause gross distortions in the form of scoliosis.

The summation of noxious impulses from a number of sources can become sufficient to produce a degree of postvertebral muscle hypertonicity consistent with the limitation of segmental movement or frank distortion, which may be considered to be a subluxation. This disrelation and disturbance of segmental function become a source of further irritation and either aggravates or perpetuates the patient's problems.

Wilhelm Reich (1949) has explained the tendency of those whose mental and emotional attitudes toward the procreative function have been adversely disturbed to show a retraction of the external genitalia by an anterior nodding of the pelvis. Such abnormality of pelvic relationship to the gravity line necessitates compensatory redistribution of the superimposed body weight around the gravity line. This results in accentuation of the depths of the primary and secondary curves of the vertebral column, which adds stress at the transition areas and the apices of the curvatures. Feldenkrais (1949) and others have stressed that disorders of sexual function, disturbances of breathing and gastro-intestinal function, anxiety and muscular tension are concomitants of the neurotic status.

SOMATOPSYCHIC RESPONSES

Most researchers in psychosomatic medicine have concentrated on the mind as a cause of physical disturbance, but until recently, they have failed to appreciate that disturbances of the body can have a deranging influence upon the mind. It is possible that mechanical or humoral factors may so disturb the neural equilibrium of the individual so that he would be no longer capable of coping with his environmental and emotional stresses.

The mere mechanistic component, the subluxation, may either lay the foundation for psychic aberration or accentuate the psychic abnormality which, in turn, is reflected via the neural system as dysfunction of one or more organs or systems.

The central nervous system receives the information of external and internal change from the total organism, integrates this mass of information and produces the response to the total body or to one or more of its parts. Normally this response is adequate and appropriate to the need and is referred to as health. At other times, the nervous system may cause responses that are adequate to the stimulation but not in the best interest of the total organism. Any organ or system may respond out of phase with the requirements of the total organism. This condition is referred to as disease. Thus, it is apparent that disease can be the body's response to abnormal stimuli, producing functions and tissue changes that are at variance with the best interest of the total organism. This is not to suggest that micro-organisms and other environmental threats are not adequate stimuli to cause the nervous system to produce a set of responses that may be labelled as a disease syndrome.

There is no afferent stimulation from the internal and external environment without involvement of most levels of the nervous system. The term "adequate response" to the stimulus has long been recognized, and the failure of the body to express in action the demanded activity tends to result in one of the many psychic or psychosomatic disorders.

Campion and Smith (1934) stated, "It is a matter of real importance, therefore, that every advance in the powers of sensory perception and discrimination should be brought into relationship with this essential biological need of finding expression in action." If a true adequate response in the form of muscular activity and appropriate action to the stimulus is frustrated, muscular and visceral changes in function will occur which is at variance with the needs of the body. Therefore, the individual is less fit to cope with his changing environment, and as Rene Dubos (1961) stated, "Biological success in all its manifestations is a measure of fitness, and fitness requires never-ending efforts of adaptation to the total environment, which is ever changing."

THE SPINE AS A SOURCE OF ABNORMAL AFFERENT INPUT

". . . The clinician has been so engrossed in the effects of visceral dysfunctions and their outward manifestations, that he neglected the skeletal structures with their disturbance reflected inward on the viscera." (Ussher, 1940.)

Since every muscle, tendon, ligament, facia, joint capsule, intervertebral disc, synovial membrane, periosteum, and blood vessel associated with the vertebral column is richly supplied with receptor nerve endings of various types, there is a continuing stream of afferent impulses from these structures to the spinal cord segment or segments. Stimulation of somatic sensory receptors occurs with resultant alterations in function of the motor pools influenced by the particular segment (Sherrington, 1947). In addition, there is an altered stimulation of the sympathetic cells (Jänig and Schmidt, 1970) which controls the calibre of the blood vessels of both the somatic and visceral tissues. Hence, a disturbance of vertebral structures, as occurs in a subluxation, may affect somatic muscle, blood vessels and viscera.

In recent years attention has been directed to the symptoms associated with myodysneuria, in which a localized segment of a muscle becomes contracted and causes an afferent bombardment which spreads in the spinal cord. The irradiation of neural impulses from the site of myodysneuria, frequently involves the efferent pools of the associated segment or segments with resultant muscular contraction that may produce such conditions as the "frozen shoulder."

Gutstein (1955) has briefly stated that these areas of myodysneuria or "trigger areas" are the result of "Selective involvement of the sympathetics. . . ." He recognizes and discusses the possible reasons for this selective irritability of a few sympathetic fibres which produce a localized vasoconstriction within the muscle, with ischemia of a relatively few muscle fibres, disturbance of the pH, calcium, sodium balance and hypoxia. The noxious impulses arise from the receptors in the area and may spread within the central nervous system to produce many widespread symptoms.

Doctors of chiropractic have been treating these areas of myodysneuria along the vertebral column with considerable success. While not all trigger points occur in the paravertebral musculature, a large number do occur, either as a result or as a cause of the subluxation. The emotional impact from such pain and disability is as potent a disturbing influence as the symptoms of visceral disease. They are dependent, to a significant degree, upon the circumstances, attitude and condition of the patient. It must be appreciated that the vertebral subluxation per se, may well be the factor that disturbs the selected sympathetic pathways. The result is the formation of the trigger point or area of myodysneuria, which shows trophic changes associated with a chronic subluxation.

Skillern (1947) observes that associated with every large plexus there is an "outrigger" or elongated nerve. When stretched or compressed by a spastic muscle through which it passes, or compressed against subjacent bone by a muscle, the nerve becomes irritated and is liable to irritate its plexus. This would give rise to centrifugally radiating pain, and stimulate the somato-sympathetic reflex arc causing spasm of somatic muscles and baneful activity of the sympathetic system. This, in turn, may affect the emotions by bombardment of the sensorium with noxious impulses via the spino-thalamic-cortical tracts. Such symptoms with their disturbing influence upon the psyche are another example of the disrupting effect that afferent neural impulses from somatic structures may have upon the emotions and mind of the patient, whether it's due to be a simple muscle hypertonicity, mechanically irritating a nerve, or the more complex influence of the vertebral subluxation.

Travell and Rinzler (1952) wrote, "Myofascial trigger mechanisms may be initiated by direct trauma to muscle, to joint, chronic muscular strain, chilling of fatigued muscle, acute myositis, arthritis, nerve root injury, visceral ischemia or dyskinesia, and hysteria." As stated above, this overstimulation of sympathetic fibres as a consequence of the afferent bombardment of the appropriate neuromeres may disturb visceral function. The viscera then return afferent impulses to the corresponding neural segments and thereby add to the insult and peculiar somatic response of myodysneuria or "trigger point." The higher brain centers cannot be stimulated by such unpleasant symptoms without drawing emotion into the pattern. The interpretation and significance the patient gives to the symptoms is largely dependent upon past experience, training, temperament and importance in relation to his present status.

Dunn (1952) found that, of 1000 schizophrenic patients studied at the Still-Hildreth Sanatorium, an osteopathic lesion was present at the 5th thoracic vertebral segment in 74.6%, while in 67.6% a lesion was found at the 6th thoracic; in 66% the patients demonstrated axis lesions, and the 4th lumbar was lesioned in 0.7% with the other vertebrae in a variety of intermediate percentages. It should be recalled that the preganglionic sympathetic fibres from the lateral horn cells of the fifth and sixth thoracic neuromeres may ascend in the sympathetic ganglionated chain to synapse in the superior cervical ganglion on each side. From there, the postganglionic fibres carry the neural impulses into the cranial cavity to control the vascular bed of the brain and brain stem (Kobayashi *et al.,* 1971). Neural tissues are very susceptible to alterations in vascular supply, especially if hypoxia from a vasoconstriction occurs. The axis subluxation or lesion may have its detrimental influence either reflexly through the afferent fibres from the multitude of holding elements, or by indirect mechanical involvement of the vertebral arteries. These pass through the foramina transversaria of the axis and atlas, taking a drastic change of direction prior to entering the vertebral canal to pass through the foramen magnum. The vertebral arteries unite to form the basilar artery which is a vital portion and tributary of the Circle of Willis. Abnormalities of mentation should come as no surprise when the somatic structures are such a potent source of possible disturbance to vascularity. Such alterations in irritability of the cerebral structures make them more responsive and even erratic, as they are bombarded by the afferent impulses perpetuated by subluxations, somatic distortions, or visceral dysfunctions, which may have been drawn into the spiral of abnormal function.

Travell and Bigelow (1947) contributed to understanding hysteria in response to "trigger points" or areas of myodysneuria and stated in part, "Thus constriction of the posterior spinal artery or its branches could result in bizarre, glove-and-stocking type of sensory defect by causing ischemia of the afferent tracts in the posterior columns of the spinal cord."

The authors further state, "Such a state of partial ischemia reflexly maintained by somatic trigger mechanisms would also account for the fact that in hysteria, function can be completely destroyed for long periods of time and yet be restored to normal almost at once by the blocking of noxious impulses from somatic trigger areas."

The sensory input from an abnormal spinal stimulus by its ascending and descending collaterals, may draw a considerable number of segments or neuromeres into the functional disturbance (Beacham and Perl, 1966). Further, various afferent fibres from every level of the nervous system have connections in the brain stem which, in turn, send impulses into the appropriate area of the thalamus and cerebral cortex to maintain both wakefulness and direction of conscious attention or awareness (Birkmeyer and Pilleri, 1966). Noxious impulses streaming into the central nervous system from the site of subluxation and other areas of the disturbed spine that may be drawn into the dysfunction are not without influence upon the important reticular activating system.

The importance of the reticular formation and the sensory input to it in the physiology of sleep and arousal has been amply demonstrated (Oswald, 1962). When sleep is desired, every effort is made to minimize the various types of sensory stimuli entering the central nervous system. If a substantial degree of muscular relaxation cannot be attained, the mind may remain active and contribute to the muscular hypertonicity, by way of feedback through the reticular system and the sensory area of the cortex of the cerebrum.

In certain cases, conscious direction of attention to relaxation of the musculature will produce the desired result of sleep. When the mental processes are occupied with less stimulating activity, it will promote the desired relaxation, consequently minimizing the feedback impulses (Schwartz, 1954). Those persons who demonstrate the muscular patterns of anxiety are prone to insomnia. They also suffer from a decreased ability to perform skilled tasks, slurring of words, irritability, hallucination, and even schizophrenic experiences (Oswald, 1962).

Chiropractic has frequently influenced many of these problems when patients initially sought aid for an apparently unrelated symptom. Spinal correction, particularly coupled with muscle relaxing techniques, causes a potent release of tension and is a normalizer of the nervous system. This correction apparently reduces the feedback of afferent impulses, through the reticular system and in this way allows the patient to relax, and induces sleep.

CONCLUSION

This has been a brief and sketchy presentation of some examples of the psychogenic stresses as causative agents in the mechanism of subluxation production. It is hoped that the ideas presented here will act as a stimulus to students and practitioners to delve more deeply into the psychology of the human. The profession should look with renewed respect upon the founder of chiropractic, D. D. Palmer.

It is essential to emphasize again that the majority of subluxations and gross distortions of the vertebral column are the result of summation of a number of causative factors. Perhaps the only subluxations that have a single cause are those resulting from traumatic experiences. Most patients have been subjected to a variety of stress situations.

It is unjustifiable to brand a patient as being neurotic or excuse his symptoms with the convenient diagnosis of "nerves," until the subluxations and other somatic and biochemical distortions have been taken into account and corrected. In the words of Mennell (1962), "Not until every possible physical cause has been explored are we justified in putting 'functional' as a sole diagnosis: cure the physical basis on which the functional element is built up and the neurasthenic element will usually take care of itself and disappear."

Schwartz (1949, 1954, 1958) continues to be a pioneering influence in the chiropractic profession, in postulating the importance of correcting the somatic structure in coping with mental aberrations or environmental stress. Certainly no one in the chiropractic profession has made claims that chiropractic can influence irreversible physical or psychological trauma; nor has any intent been entertained to disparage the need for constructive surgery or psychiatric techniques. Moreover, a plea is made for a cooperative approach in the interest of emotionally disturbed patients, with the assurance that it would demonstrate a higher ratio of results.

The doctor of chiropractic should be acutely cognizant of the importance of structure in every health problem and be astute enough to appreciate when mechanical adjustive ministrations are indicated. If mental stress is the basic cause, structural distortion is a concomitant of it, and is deserving of the doctor's skill and knowledge. If mechanical disrelation has upset the affective mechanism and so disturbed the ability of the mind to cope with emotional stress, then counseling is also indicated.

The correction of structure and normalization of the afferent feedback to the nervous system offers a challenge to the doctor of chiropractic and a hope of success to a great number of patients suffering from the distressing afflictions.

It must be stressed in closing that the patient must be accepted as a holistic entity who has for too long been segmented and compartmentalized for purposes of study, diagnosis and treatment. Only by recognizing and accepting the challenge of the patient as a totality can it be anticipated that his health problems, whether somatic, visceral or emotional, be successfully prevented or treated. There is no single panacea. The answers lie in the willingness of the patient to obey the laws of health and of the doctor to accept the triumvirate of body, mind and environment as an interfunctioning unit.

REFERENCES

Beacham, W. S. and Perl, E. R. "Background and reflex discharge of sympathetic preganglionic neurones in the cat." *J. Physiol.* (1964), 172:400–416.

Birkmayer, W. and Pilleri, G. *The Brainstem Reticular Formation and Its Significance for Autonomic and Affective Behaviour.* Montreal: Hoffman-La Roche Ltd., 1966.

Brown, T.; Nemiah, J. C.; Barr, J. S. and Barry Jr., H. "Psychologic factors in low-back pain," *New England J. Med.* (1954), 251:123–128.

Campion, G. G. and Smith, G. E. *The Neural Basis of Thought.* New York: Harcourt Brace and Co., 1934.

Coote, J. H. and Perez-Gonzales, J. E. "Response of some sympathetic neurons to volley in various afferent nerves," *J. Physiol.* (1970), 208:267.

Coppen, A. "Disorders of mineral metabolism in depressive patients." *Psychiatria, Neurologia, Neurochirurgia* (1969), no. 72, pp. 189–193.

Downman, C. B. B. "Skeletal muscle reflexes of splanchnic and intercostal nerve origin in acute spinal and decerebrate cats," *J. Neurophysiol.* (1955), 18:217.

Downman, C. B. B. and McSwiney, B. C. "Reflexes elicited by visceral stimulation in the acute spinal animal," *J. Physiol.* (1946), 105:80.

Dubos, R. *Mirage of Health.* New York: Doubleday and Co., 1961.

Dunn, F. E. "Altered cervical and thoracic mechanics in psychiatric disorders." *Acad. Applied Osteopathy Year Book,* 1952.

Eble, J. N. "Patterns of response of the paravertebral musculature to visceral stimuli." *Am. J. Physiol.* (1960), 198:429.

Feldenkrais, M. *Body and Mature Behaviour.* New York: International University Press, 1949.

Goldthwait, J. E. *Essentials of Body Mechanics.* J. B. Lippincott Co., 1941.

Gutstein, R. R. "A review of myodysneuria (Fibrositis)." *Am. Practitioner and Digest of Treatment* (1955), 6:570–577.

Harper, W. D. *Anything Can Cause Anything.* Seabrook, Texas: Privately published, 1964.

Homewood, A. E. *The Neurodynamics of the Vertebral Subluxation.* Toronto: Chiropractic Publishers, 1963.

Iwamura, Y.; Uchino, Y.; Kucera, S. and Kudo, N. "Excitatory and inhibitory components of somatosympathetic reflexes." *Br. Res.* (1969), 16:351.

Jänig, W. and Schmidt, R. F. "Single unit responses in the cervical sympathetic trunk upon somatic nerve stimulation." *Pflüg Arch.* (1970), 314:199–216.

Kamieth, H. "Pathogenetic importance of the thoracic portion of the vertebral column." *Postgrad. Med. J.A.M.A.* (November edition), 1958.

Kleynhaus, A. M. "Vascular changes occurring in the cervical musculoskeletal system." *European Chiropractic Union Bulletin* (Oct., 1970).

Kobayashi, S.; Waltz, A. G. and Rhoton, A. L. "Effects of stimulation of cervical sympathetic nerves on cortical blood flow and vascular reactivity." *Neurology* (1971), 21:297–302.

Korr, I. M. "The somatic approach to the disease process." *Acad. Applied Osteopathy Year Book,* 1952.

Levine, M. E. "Depression, Back Pain and Disc Protrusion." *Dis. Nerv. Sys.* (1971), 32:41–45.

Mennell, J. *The Science and Art of Joint Manipulation* (Vol. II), *The Spinal Column.* J. and A. Churchill Ltd., 1962.

Oswald, I. *Sleeping and Wakefulness.* Amsterdam or New York: Elsevier Publishing Co., 1962.

Palmer, D. D. *The Science, Art and Philosophy of Chiropractic.* Portland Printing House Co., 1910.

Rasmussen, A. T. *The Principal Nervous Pathways.* Macmillan Co., 1967.

Reich, W. *The Function of the Orgasm* (Vol. 1). New York: Orgone Institute Press, 1949.

Sachs, W. *The Vegetative Nervous System.* Cassiell & Co., 1936.

Schwartz, H. S. "What is the connection between nerves and nervousness?" *J. National Chiropractic Association* (April edition), 1949.

Schwartz, H. S. "Foundations of Chiropractic Psychosomatics." *JNCA* (June edition), 1949.

Schwartz, H. S. *The Art of Relaxation.* New York: Thomas Y. Crowell Co., 1954.

Schwartz, H. S. *Home Care for the Emotionally Ill.* London: Staples Press, 1958.

Scott, J. C. "Stress factor in the disc syndrome." *J. Bone and Joint Surg.* (1955), 37B.107.

Selye, H. *Stress.* New York: McGraw-Hill Book Co., Inc., 1950.

Sherrington, C. *The Integrative Action of the Nervous System.* London: Cambridge University Press, 1947.

Skillern, P. G. "Clinical observations on (1) Cutaneovisceral (Somato-Sympathetic) reflex arcs; (2) The role of hypermyotonia in bodily aches and pains." *J. Nerv. Ment. Dis.* (1947), pp. 449.

Teitelbaum, H. A. *Psychosomatic Medicine.* New York: Grune & Stratton, 1964.

Travell, J. and Bigelow, N. H. "Role of somatic trigger areas in the patterns of hysteria." *Psychosomatic Medicine* (1947), 9:353–363.

Travell, J. and Rinzler, S. H. "The myofascial genesis of pain." *Postgraduate Medicine,* 1952.

Ussher, N. T. "The viscerospinal syndrome—A new concept of visceromotor and sensory changes in relation to deranged spinal structures." *Annals Int. Med.* (1940), 13:2, 57, and 2090.

Wolf, S. and Goodell, H. *Harold G. Wolff's Stress and Disease.* Springfield, Illinois: Charles C. Thomas, 1968.

CHAPTER 10

PHYSIOLOGICAL PSYCHOLOGY OF CHIROPRACTIC IN MENTAL DISORDERS

W. HEATH QUIGLEY, B.S., D.C.

IT IS THE PURPOSE of this chapter to set forth a rationale, based on sound neurophysiological and psychological principles, to explain how chiropractic may be of psychotherapeutic and/or therapeutic benefit to the patient with a mental disorder. An effort will be made to adhere closely to the principle of parsimony, which states that any hypothesis which fits the known facts and makes the least number of unverifiable assumptions is most likely to be the accurate one.

PSYCHOTHERAPY AND THERAPY

Let us start by defining psychotherapy as the treatment of personality and behavior disorders by psychological means. A preferred definition of successful psychotherapy is the achievement of a corrective emotional experience which makes it possible for a person to perceive his difficulties from a different point of view and to meet his fundamental needs without a sense of fear and uncertainty. Successful psychotherapy in some cases may mean a great deal more, but these listed improved responses represent minimal goals.

There are three ways in which chiropractic may be of value in the treatment of the mental disorders. First, there may be a psychotherapeutic effect. By this it is meant the person will experience a corrective emotional experience. Secondly, a person experiencing a psychophysiologic disorder (e.g. ulcers, asthma, etc.) may obtain relief from these physical dysfunctions, that is, obtain therapeutic benefit. Thirdly, there may be alterations in the biochemical substratum of the patient with a psychogenic mental disorder resulting in recovery. None of these three processes imply an assistance or therapeutic benefit from the doctor-patient relationship in itself, although such an effect is an inseparable part of any constructive communication between doctor and patient.

CHIROPRACTIC AS PSYCHOTHERAPY

To be psychotherapeutic, the corrective emotional experience must enable the person to change his attitude and feeling tone, as well as make a better adjustment to one's life. In the broader sense, it must remove any barriers which prevent him from fully developing his innate potentials. In a simple illustration, if a child becomes inordinately fearful of dogs, an emotional block may occur. Should the parents attempt to persuade the child that there is nothing to fear from dogs, very little change is likely to occur.

However, should the parents wisely buy the child a puppy whose affection is obvious, in due time the child's phobia may change from fear to reciprocal affection, with a generalizing tendency to diminish fear of other dogs. This would constitute a corrective emotional experience. It may seem strange indeed that chiropractic, which is essentially a physical approach could have any such corrective effect. However, it will be seen that this is precisely what it does do in many cases.

There are two basic concepts essential to the understanding of chiropractic as psychotherapeutic. The first concept is conditioning. The second concept is: increased muscular tension leads to increased emotional reactivity.

1. Conditioning

Ivan Pavlov is the best known pioneer in the field of conditioning. Nearly everyone has heard of his experiments with dogs and salivation. Pavlov described conditioning as a process which develops a response to a stimulus which would not otherwise elicit the response. It is widely held today that a vast amount of animal and human learning is brought about by conditioning. According to Wolpe (1958), Ullman and Krasner (1969), and many other adherents to behavioral therapy there is increasing evidence a great many of our phobias have developed on the basis of conditioned responses.

2. Muscular Tension & Emotion

Since neurotic behavior and maladaptive reactions of human beings are not usually present at birth and are not known to be inherited, it may well be that such behavior is learned. The storage of memory and its expression is not limited to the brain, but an extensive portion of the nervous system is involved in the memory process. Consider the spinal cord. It has most frequently been considered merely a bunched network of cells and fibers whose function is to convey impulses to and from the brain. But the spinal cord is a highly complex structure, having millions of neuronal and inter-neuronal connections, forming a vast net-work for retention of learning.

Boycott, Lettvin and Maturana (1965) reported finding a large amount of visual perception organized below the brain. They worked with invertebrates as well as vertebrates. Michael (1969) further enhances this concept by stating that, in certain mammals, complex analysis of sensory information does occur in the retina, before the neural activity moves on to the higher nervous system. Some mammalian retinas, in fact, appear to be capable of a complexity of neural integration that in the cat and monkey is attained only in the visual cortex. In Lettvin's (1965) words, "the eye speaks to the brain in a language already organized and interpreted."

Learning has been demonstrated in reptiles, fish and it even appears in the lowly and primitive flatworm. Horridge (1962) has clearly demonstrated learning can occur in the single nerve ganglion of a cockroach! Thus it appears most likely to occur in the infinitely more neurologically complex spinal cord. Guyton (1966) comments on this possibility when he states, "Most of this storage of information occurs in the cerebral cortex but not all, for even the basal ganglion of the brain and perhaps the spinal cord can store lesser amounts of information." Now it is important to establish that memory, especially of traumatic events, is unconsciously expressed through motor behavior. Thus conscious or unconscious retention of stressful experiences can be disturbing both physiologically and psychologically. Certain forms of disordered functioning in the human body may have been caused by traumatic experiences and may then be perpetuated by conditioning. Dr. W. Horsley Gantt, President of the Pavlovian Society of America, is quoted (1966) as saying that although years may separate an emotional experience from a heart attack, the experience could still cause the attack. The explanation for this phenomenon is that heart beat, blood pressure, and stroke susceptibility are among the most easily conditioned responses of the body. Few have recognized the enduring effect on the blood system of early repressed emotions. Heart rate and blood pressure naturally rise in response to fear. They will also rise in response to something which is completely harmless but associated with fear in the individuals; i.e. a conditioned response. Under normal conditions the cardiovascular system is extremely resistant to change once a reflex has been established. Diven (1937), in a widely quoted experiment, showed that generalization, that is, spreading of anxiety to related situations, occurred even when the subject was unaware of the reasons for his anxiety. In a later repetition of the Diven's experiment by Lacey *et al.* (1955), it was found that generalization spread more widely and intensely when the connection between the stimulus and the conditioned response was perceived only unconsciously.

In brief, although conscious memory of an event may be lost, the cardiovascular system has been trained to react and does react in a highly maladaptive manner. Many similar responses are found in other visceral systems, notably the gastrointestinal system, where conditioning is also notoriously easy to achieve, and difficult to extinguish.

SYNTHESIZING CONDITIONING, MOTOR BEHAVIOR AND CHIROPRACTIC

Turning to the human spinal column, consider a person who has a distinct structural distortion, for example an exaggerated curve as seen from the posterior. On one side of such a spinal column we would find one set of muscles excessively tense, while on the other side of the column we find the opposing set less tense. (See Levine Ch. 8). Guyton (1966) states,

> Certain muscles of the body, primarily the extensor muscles of the legs, hips, and back are specifically adapted for support of the body against

> gravity. These muscles have different characteristics of contraction from the other muscles. Inhibiting much slower contractions and being capable of being contracted for much longer periods of time.

The hypertense muscles (and in some cases irritated visceral tissues) bombard the spinal cord with impulses from the over-active (spastic) muscle. These impulses to the cord are directed across the interneuronal network where the motor neurons in the anterior horn are again stimulated, which in turn keeps the muscle in a continuous state of contraction; a state we may call tension. At the same time the interneuronal pool is excited so that waves of impulses ascend the cord as proprioceptive impulses eventuating in the Reticular Activating System (RAS). The RAS, which has its origin in the brain stem, acts to integrate the higher, middle, and lower levels of brain function, and in addition, acts as a filtering system to dampen down stimuli, and selectively discriminate incoming stimuli from all the sensory receptors. Continuous stimulation of the RAS causes cortical arousal and over-activity of both emotional and cognitive (thinking) functions. Thus, the barrage of proprioceptive impulses from the cord, arising from hypertense muscles results in an excited emotional state, incompatible with healthy emotional adjustment. The very common experience of a night of insomnia in which a person rolls and tosses (motor) and is unable to stop thinking (cognitive and emotional) provides an excellent example of this process.

Returning to the spinal column, when the chiropractic doctor locates the critical point of structural distortion, he corrects the distortion, relieving the spastic state of the muscles. The small but detectable changes in the vertebral relationships (as observed on X-ray film) alter the vectoring of muscle forces, so that relaxation of tension occurs. Significantly such relaxation is not merely a localized response, but represents a generalized relaxation of the body. With the reduction in muscle tension, the cyclic reverberations between the spinal cord and tense muscles is reduced and in turn the RAS is relieved of its excess burden, so that cortical stimulation is similarly reduced. In brief, it is true that a calm body does lead to a calm mind.

NEUROPHYSIOLOGICAL EVIDENCE

What has present day neurophysiology to say about this concept? Wenger *et al.* (1956), say,

> Whenever we experience profound emotion, tension in skeletal muscles also increases . . . suffice it to say that if you become frightened or angry, not only your autonomic nervous system will respond, but also your skeletal musculature. . . . Increases in skeletal muscle tension will facilitate your mental activities to a certain extent, beyond a certain point it contributes to your distraction and will interfere with your efficiency. But such tensions have another influence which you may not realize. They actually contribute to your emotions. In general with increased emotion we are more tense

> muscularly, but also with increased muscle tension we are more emotional. Thus, any factor which increases muscle tension will also increase emotional behavior and other psychosomatic functions. Muscular tension and relaxation are important in human behavior. We have much to learn about their control. Any factor that will exaggerate tension in skeletal muscles will exaggerate psychosomatic problems. Any factor that will decrease tension in skeletal muscles will alleviate psychosomatic problems.

What has just been quoted substantially supports what we have been saying thus far.

THE CORE OF CHIROPRACTIC AS PSYCHOTHERAPY

Edmund Jacobson, (1948) the pioneer investigator of progressive relaxation methods and a number of contemporary psychiatrists, (Haugen, Wolpe, etc.) have shown that a state of anxiety and a state of deep relaxation are incompatible; they cannot co-exist.

We now find ourselves at the core of chiropractic psychotherapy. The chiropractic adjustment applied to the spinal column axiomatically reduces anxiety, because there occurs concomitantly the induction of relaxation. These two events: the adjustment and the reduction of tension, are paired. They provide every element of the classical conditioned response. This conditioned response is of the exact nature as the response we described when the infant learned to respond to a buzzer with suckling. Repetition of the adjustment when required, reinforces the conditioning making it stronger and more durable. Actually, it is more appropriate to refer to this event as counter-conditioning, because we are beginning with an unwanted response and replacing it with a desirable response. The process is identical in principle; the goal is not simply to change behavior, but to change it in a therapeutic manner. With the progressive reduction in anxiety, we must concede that the entire process qualifies it as a first class corrective emotional experience, bringing about a change in attitude, mood, and subsequent behavior. It is therefore successful, as a psychotherapeutic reaction.

Counter-conditioning. For those who may wish to examine the process of conditioning through the chiropractic adjustment more minutely, the following sequence may be helpful in separating each significant element into its proper relationship to the other. Taking the position that the results are counter-conditioning, then the sequence and elements would appear as follows:

Conditioned Stimulus	Frustration, conflict or pressure
Conditioned Response	Anxiety and resultant tension
Counter-conditioning Stimulus	Chiropractic adjustment
Counter-conditioned Response	Relaxation (reduction of tension). *Anti-anxiety*

The response may be strengthened or reinforced by repetition of the chiropractic adjustment when required.

The most common question which is raised by opponents of this explanation is that if what we have just said is true, then in what way does it differ from relaxation induced by massage, heat, or similar modalities?

The application of the chiropractic principle is an art and therefore the techniques vary greatly, but the rationale of any technique of adjusting is basically to correct specific spinal misalignments which are presumably interfering with normal functioning of the nervous system. It is not necessary to make gross changes in the vertebral position to bring about significant changes in function; small changes are often followed by significant effects.

The difference, therefore, between the chiropractic adjustment and that of massage and related modalities of treatment, is that the successful chiropractic adjustment corrects the spinal imbalance and the specific vertebral malposition, not merely inducing relaxation but providing the substratum in which relaxation can be perpetuated. A message may leave one feeling relaxed, but the structural problem remains unaltered.

The larger deeper muscles of the back and hips, the antigravity muscles which maintain posture, are not relaxed by heat or massage but retain their tight grip, holding the spinal column in a misaligned state. The chiropractic doctor often observes a dramatic release of tension and pain following some adjustments. The vast majority of persons with mental disorders suffer from hypertense musculature and it is for these reasons we have observed that chiropractic has a unique service to offer them.

PSYCHOPHYSIOLOGIC DISORDERS

The second major area in which chiropractic can contribute to the alleviation of mental problems is specifically in the field of the psychophysiologic disorders. They are commonly known as psychosomatic disorders, but are more properly defined under the title we have used. *The American Psychiatric Association's Diagnostic and Statistical Manual* (DSM-II 1968) describes these disorders as

> "Characterized by physical symptoms that are caused by emotional factors and involved in a single organ system, usually under autonomic nervous system innervation. The physiological changes involved are those that normally accompany certain emotional states, but in these disorders the changes are more intense and sustained. The individual may not be consciously aware of his emotional state."

Fight or Flight Theory. Cannon (1932) found that when an animal was confronted with any situation which evoked pain, rage, or fear, it responded with a set of emotions to "fight" the danger or to take "flight" from it. He believed these reactions were mobilized by the secretion of adrenin when the cerebral cortex perceived a situation as threatening. A stimulus was sent out over the sympathetic nervous system to the adrenal medulla which then secreted the hormone, adrenin. He wrote:

> "Respiration deepens; the heart beats more rapidly; the arterial pressure rises; the blood is shifted away from the stomach and intestines to the heart and central nervous system and muscles; the processes in the alimentary canal cease; sugar is freed from the reserves in the liver, the spleen contracts and discharges its content of concentrated corpuscles and adrenin is secreted from the adrenal medulla. The key to these marvelous transformations in the body is found in relating them to the natural accompaniments of fear and rage, i.e. running away in order to escape from danger and attacking in order to be dominant. Which ever the action, a life or death struggle may ensue.
>
> In short, all these changes are directly serviceable in rendering the organs more effective in the violent display of energy which fear or rage may involve."

MODERNIZATION OF CANNON'S VIEW

It is widely believed today that after cortical perception of threat, the associational fibers activate the hypothalamus in the limbic area, which in turn triggers the autonomic nervous system (ANS) which primarily activates the changes in the viscera enumerated above, as well as many others. The adrenal medulla is also affected, but is not the primary exciting agent. Since adrenin is sympathomimetic, it supports and acts much as the sympathetic nervous system does, in arousal.

Gellhorn (1943) has demonstrated that the two divisions of the ANS act with greater unity. During the arousal of strong emotion in animals, there is an extensive discharge over both divisions, i.e., the sympathetic and the parasympathetic branches. Although the sympathetic dominates during arousal, the parasympathetic is also activated beyond its normal level. It has been shown that to react effectively in a crisis, a burst of sympathetic activity should be closely followed by a parasympathetic discharge. Balance between these two systems is essential, for when the sympathetic system activates the emergency responses, and they are not compensated for by parasympathetic balance, the emergency reactions lead to both physiological and psychological disorganization. Reciprocal action is necessary to maintain an effective bodily state under all conditions.

MODERN MAN'S THREATS

Man no longer faces major physical threats each day of his life, as did his prehistoric ancestors. Today, man faces threats to his ego, his status, his usefulness; he may feel insecure in his job or his marriage. These psychological threats are perceived by the cortex in exactly the same manner as the physical threats. They arouse the same anger, fear, rage, and depressions. The sympathetic nervous system becomes activated; in turn the parasympathetic is overly reactive and anxiety is felt. When this emotional state is either persistent or too intense the physiologic reactions activated by the emotions bring about a more or less continuously disordered function of the viscera.

A very common example of these disorders is spastic mucous colitis. Let us consider this condition from a chiropractic frame of reference. We postulate that an assumed interference to normal balance between the two branches of the ANS exists. Evidence to date suggests it is the sympathetic branch which is interfered with and thus impaired in its function. If the interference to sympathetic function is removed by the chiropractic adjustment, it is likely that a considerable improvement symptomatically will occur. The restoration of reciprocal action between the two systems, places a brake upon the "runaway" parasympathetic branch. Team action or integration of function has been re-established. Return to a more normal bowel function will reappear and mucous secretion will be adequate instead of inundating.

However, it is not the chiropractic contention that this will be the end of the problem. If maladaptive emotions persist, even the strongest adaptation wears out and the symptoms will recur. The very fact the patient "feels better" after equalization of the ANS functioning, can in itself be a positive reinforcer and reduce anxiety prolonging relief. Therefore, it is the admonition of this discipline, that in recurrence, the source of stress must be discovered and psychotherapy should be sought.

Marcus and Kernis (1969) have shown osteopathic manipulation to be of value in normalization of vasomotor tone, compared to three control groups which were not treated. The study was accomplished with the use of the electrical impedance plethamograph. Fichera and Celander (1969) studied the effect of osteopathic manipulation on autonomic tone as evidenced by blood pressure changes and activity of the fibrinolytic systems. They found that osteopathic manipulation produces an increase *"in vivo"* in the content of profibrinolysin activator that converts profibrinolysin into fibrinolysin, thus decreasing the content of profibrinolysin. This particular study is of interest to our discussion because they felt that the fibrinolytic enzyme system and the fibrinogen level are among the most sensitive indicators of subtle changes in autonomic activity. The significant point is that manipulative techniques can alter autonomic nervous system function.

TENSION REDUCTION

It may be observed that fear and tension are reduced by motor activity. The pacing of expectant fathers and nervous habits of anxious students before an examination are classical examples of tension-reducing activity. By reinforcing the sense of relief, considerable alleviation of fear and anxiety may occur with a balancing of ANS function. Being held inactive in the midst of danger is an agonizing experience, for such inaction intensifies visceral effect or symptoms.

In the case of intense and chronic emotional stresses action does not solve the problem because the patient cannot find an effective mode of action. The principal reason for not finding an appropriate action is that the source of anxiety is largely unconscious; the victim does not know what is really bothering him. The visceral response is that of a person's reaction to emergency, a heightening of visceral activity, not compatible with comfort and a sense of security. If this reaction is aggravated by interference to the balanced function of the ANS, then the proper chiropractic adjustment which should reduce the imbalance, is neurologically analogous to the person having taken appropriate action in the first place. It means that relief is found in the release of sympathetic discharge, in very much the same way as if the patient discharged this accumulated tension through fighting or running.

It would be foolish and misleading to contend that all our psychophysiologic and/or emotional problems are responsive to chiropractic care. However, much can be done through chiropractic adjustments to break the cyclic reverberations of ANS imbalance. Nevertheless, continuous stress will wear out the strongest body in time, as Selye (1956) has so clearly shown.

CHIROPRACTIC AND THE PSYCHOSES

The chiropractic profession maintained two major mental hospitals, until the middle fifties and early sixties. One of these was Forest Park Sanitarium and the other Clear View Sanitarium, both located in Davenport, Iowa. Forest Park was opened in 1922 and Clear View in 1926. Much of what is to be said concerning psychotic disorders, of necessity, is limited to a considerable extent to my experiences as staff member of Clear View for 21 years and the Director from 1951 to 1961, at which time Clear View was closed.

Observed Results. It is not credible merely to state that I have seen large numbers of psychotics emerge from psychoses into normal living. Anyone reading these pages deserves more evidence than one man's observation which could be extremely biased. However, I will attempt to present some evidence, but at the same time point out the extreme difficulty of providing statistical proof.

When I first joined the staff of Clear View Sanitarium in 1940, I held strongly to the view that mental disorders were primarily of emotional origin. I frequently saw agitated schizophrenics, dangerous to themselves and others, arrive at Clear View in straight jackets, completely out of contact with the world of reality. They were not responsive to words, care, or any type of ministration. However, after chiropractic adjustments a dramatic change occurred, in which the patient began to orient himself by asking questions as to who we were, where he was, what had happened to him. Soon he was released from restraints, had freedom of the ward and was eventually released from the Sanitarium. At first I felt this represented those persons who will make spontaneous recovery with or without care. When this type of experience was observed in patients who had been under psychiatric hospitalization for years, the change was difficult to reconcile with a psychological rationale alone. For the most part, the major recovery occurred before one could perform any significant therapy. Certainly, the patient did not have an opportunity to develop "insight", but it was clearly evident that he was perceiving the world from a much different and healthier frame of reference. These recoveries were not limited to schizophrenic types but also to psychotic depressions. What appeared to be arteriosclerosis, evidently represented other neurophysiological changes, in that although complete recovery of the older patient was not observed, social recovery, that is return to the home environment, was possible about one-third of the time. After becoming Director of Clear View in 1951, I attempted to evaluate results obtained through a longitudinal study. I sought the assistance of statisticians in biology, but we were plagued by the inability to have a control population for study, as well as adequate follow-up methods. I did, however, attempt a seven year follow-up, in which each year after release, the patient's family was asked to complete a form relating to the present mental health of the patient. It is clearly evident that the condition of the patient as he leaves a mental hospital is not as important as how long he can remain in society in useful performance. When the Sanitarium was closed, workmen inadvertently destroyed a large number of our records, including much of the material compiled for this survey. I can only comment on some of the earlier material gathered which I happened to have in my own possession. It is neither my intent to present this material as proof, nor as having a great deal of validity. The design of the study was as valid as circumstances would allow, but the loss of the core materials damages the authenticity of these findings. To withhold them completely does not seem justified, so justification for their presentation is only to urge that a closer examination of chiropractic and the mental disorders is warranted.

TOTAL ADMISSIONS FOR YEAR 1972

	Admitted	*Released & Socially Restored*
Schizophrenic	80%	70%
Affective Disorders	8%	33%
Brain Syndromes	8%	33%
Other	4%	6%

Total admissions for year: 72
Total Releases: 39

Documentation of many cases from Clear View has been published by Quigley (1954), (1958). Unfortunately, a statistical design was not feasible, but again an unbiased mind may find it is worthwhile looking at the possibilities. We do have a possible, well developed hypothesis to explain our findings with regard to psychotic patients. However, substantiative evidence is missing.

The only area in which some supporting evidence seems to be found is in the theory of non-specific biological stress as enunciated by Selye (1956).

SUMMARY

Using modern neurophysiology and psychology provides a rationale for the use of chiropractic to provide a psychotherapeutic benefit. By synthesizing the principles of conditioning with those of excessive proprioceptive feedback deriving from immediate or older patterned circuits in the nervous system, insight into neurotic as well as psychophysiologic disorders can be understood from a neurophysiologic framework.

The chiropractic adjustment, which is designed to restore integrity to nervous system function as well as to correct the structural distortion, induces relaxation. This type of relaxation is highly significant because the underlying correction often provides a physical substratum in which deeper relaxation can be perpetuated. The pairing of the chiropractic adjustment with its response of relaxation, provides a counter-conditioned response to anxiety and tension, because relaxation is antithetical to anxiety and its related states. Reduction of proprioceptive feedback from muscles to the spinal cord, and to the reticular activating system, reduces cortical excitation which in turn responds by diminishing the barrage of efferent impulses to the muscles and viscera. Organization and integration of cognitive and conative function is restored and a corrective emotional experience takes place.

The importance of reciprocal innervation of viscera by the autonomic nervous system has been pointed out. The chiropractic subluxation effecting the sympathetic branch(s) is the most likely possibility to provide a vulnerable system in which psychophysiologic disorders may develop. The imbalance between sympathetic and parasympathetic systems leads to dysfunction and pathology. The removal of this interference by chiropractic adjustment may either relieve or diminish the symptomatic intensity of the problem.

Reference was made to chiropractic care in psychotic disorders. Mears (1965) has shown a postural relationship between institutionalized patients and the degree of postural defect. Since the essential nature of psychoses is unknown, a chiropractic rationale has not been proposed. Clinical observation and a longitudinal study, hampered by statistical and distance barriers do weaken the study, but it does represent the only longitudinal information we possess.

CONCLUSION

Although there are many gaps in our information, nevertheless, the preponderance of evidence warrants an unbiased study of chiropractic as a therapy for mental disorders. Not only has it provided the internal conditions favorable for recovery in a long list of documented cases, but there is nothing in chiropractic that is intrinsically incompatible with other therapies. Certainly, psychotherapy of any type can proceed simultaneously with chiropractic methods. Fortunately, many patients benefit from a combination of chiropractic and counseling. Some persons are critical of chiropractic treatment in mental disorders because it is not specifically directed against any symptom or symptom-complex. However, the same is true of many forms of treatment. Shock therapy, ataractic drugs, antidepressant drugs, all represent a wide-band approach without specificity. Further, generality is not a valid criticism against any therapy because anxiety itself tends to generalize; that is, with time, fear and uncertainty tend to spread out and touch many previously healthy areas of the patient's life. Therefore, the lack of specificity may be a highly defensible procedure in many cases.

All in all, clinical experience indicates that chiropractic is a worthwhile therapy in the mental disorders. It is not seen as the only treatment or even the treatment of choice in all cases, but it justifies the most serious consideration. In some instances chiropractic may provide the corrective influence, while in others it may be relatively ineffectual. But there are literally millions who would probably benefit from chiropractic care combined with hospitalization, counseling, and other therapeutic approaches.

REFERENCES

Boycott, B. B., Lettvin, Maturana, H. R., Wall, P. D. "Octopus Optic Responses," *Exper. Meor.* (1965), p. 12, 247, 256, and 247–256.

Cannon, W. *The Wisdom of the Body*. W. W. Norton, and Co., 1932.

Diagnostic and Statistical Manual of Mental Disorder, 1968. Second Edition (DSM-II), *American Psychiatric Association.* Washington, D.C.

Diven, K., "Certain Determinants in the Conditioning of Anxiety Reactions," *Journal of Psychology* (1937), III:298–300.

Feshera, A. and Celander, D. "Effects of Osteopathic Manipulative Therapy on Autonomic Tone as Evidenced by Blood Pressure Changes and Activity of the Fibrolytic Systems," *Abstracts from American Osteopathic Association Journal* (July 1969).

Gantt, H. "Blood Flow Conditioned," *Science News Letter* (Feb. 26, 1966), no. 89135.

Gellhorn, E. "Autonomic Regulations: Tjier Significance for Psychology and Neuropsychiatry," *Interscience Pub.* New York: 1943, XIV and XV:18.

Guyton, A. *Textbook of Medical Physiology* (3rd ed.). Philadelphia and London: W. B. Saunders Co. (1966), pp. 653, 775, 889–903.

Haugen G., Dixon, H., Dickel, H. *A Therapy for Anxiety Tension Reactions.* New York: Macmillan Co. (1960), pp. 21–23, 34.

Horridge, G. A. "Learning leg position by the ventral nerve cord in headless insects," *Proc. Roy. Soc. Series B* (1962), 83:33–52.

Jacobson, Edmund. Revised Edition, *Progressive Relaxation.* Chicago, Ill.: University of Chicago Press (1948), p. 218.

Lacey, J., Smith, R., and Green, A. "Use of Conditioned Autonomic Responses in the Study of Anxiety," *Psychosomatic Medicine* (1955), XVII. (Later reprinted in 1958).

Mears, D., "Mental Diseases and Cervical Spine Distortion," *American Chiropractic Association Journal* (Sept. 1965), 2 (9).

Michael, C. R. "Retinal Processing of Visual Images," *Scientific American* (1969), 220 (5): 104–114.

Quigley, W. *Case Histories of Mental Illness under Chiropractic Care.* Clear View Sanitarium, Davenport, Iowa (1954 and 1968).

Selye, H. *The Stress of Life.* New York: McGraw-Hill (1956), pp. 65–66.

Ullman, L. P. & Krasner, K. *Case Histories in Behavior Modification.* New York: Holt, Rinehart and Winston, 1965.

Wenger, M. Jones. *Physiological Psychology.* Holt, Rinehart and Winston (1956), pp. 372–375.

Wolpe, J. *Psychotherapy by Reciprocal Inhibition.* Stanford, Calif.: Stanford University Press (Holt, Rinehart and Winston), (1958), pp. 37–70.

CHAPTER 11

THE RELEASE FROM ABNORMAL MUSCULOSKELETAL SENSORY ACTIVITY
A Mechanism to Explain Chiropractic Results in Psychological Disorders

SCOTT HALDEMAN, D.C., PH.D.

THERE IS a growing interest in psychotherapeutic literature pertaining to muscular, structural, and relaxation techniques in the treatment of mental and emotional disorders.

Schwartz (1949) conducted a survey of 350 persons suffering from nervous and mental disorders and found that an overwhelming percentage showed improvement under chiropractic care. It was interesting to note that, although all the cases surveyed exhibited subluxations, there was no correspondence between a patient's pattern of vertebral distortion and the peculiar emotional disorder he exhibited.

At the same time, Dunn (1948, 1950) found that patients suffering from psychological disorders, especially those who manifested tension and anxiety, responded to osteopathic manipulation. He also suggested that, apart from the obvious psychological benefits of manual contact and professional care, there is a breaking up of abnormal somatovisceral pathways and relieving of muscular tension.

The role of muscular tension in emotional or psychological disorders has received a great deal of attention by the medical and psychological professions. Plutchik (1954) reviewed the literature on this topic and came to the conclusion that muscular tension patterns are associated with certain personality attitudes. He stated that people who are known to have definite conflicts have larger than normal amounts of residual and persistent tension. (Plutchik also documents that the most prominent psychiatrists and psychoanalysts are cognizant of the concomitant factor of muscle tension with emotional distress.) The advantages of relieving tension in the treatment of these disorders is now well recognized by Haugen *et al.* (1960), Yorkston and Sergeant (1965), and by many psychotherapists.

Although muscular tension is generally considered to be a result rather than a cause of anxiety and emotional states, relief of these tensions has a profoundly beneficial effect. Jacobson (1970) quotes numerous cases of psychotic and psychosomatic illness which responded to his relaxation exercises. Favorable results for emotional and mental disorders were reported in the history of chiropractic, and verified by the Quigley and Schwartz reports of the work done in the Clear View Sanatorium (see Ch. 16 and Ch. 10). It is well known that muscular tension and joint fixation are closely associated with spinal subluxations and that correction of the subluxation leads to a reduction of these two factors, Gillet and Lickens (1970).

During the last twenty years a number of chiropractic theoreticians (Verner, 1950; Harper, 1966; Homewood, 1963) have discussed the possibility of an abnormal sensory input from spinal structures as being involved in certain functional disorders. The theory being invoked states that a spinal subluxation or injury will cause stimulation of the sensory nerve endings in the spinal or paraspinal tissues. These afferent impulses are then considered to travel to the spinal cord where they influence the various spinal neurons to cause abnormal motor impulses to both somatic and visceral structures. Similarly these abnormal impulses have been used to explain chiropractic results on higher brain functions by continually bombarding the reticular, thalamic and cortical nerve cells in such a manner as to adversely affect their function.

The theory being used to explain results in certain psychic disorders have depended on an abnormal afferent discharge from spinal structures. This theory states that the chiropractic adjustment reduces muscular tension and causes mental and physical relaxation (Schwartz, 1949b). In turn, it reduces the input from spinal structures and causes a decreased bombardment of central neurons. This reduces the effectiveness of inputs to centers responsible for psychosomatic disorders. Reduction of the sensory input to the reticular activating system could also prevent one cause of insomnia with its concomitant psychic problems, Homewood (1971).

There has, however, been no review of the current literature to determine the sensory structures which exist in the paraspinal and spinal tissues and which could be irritated by a subluxation. Also, it remains to be documented as to whether or not afferent impulses from these receptors travel along neurons which make contact with the systems involved in the above functions. This chapter will be an attempt to fill this gap and in this way perhaps enlarge the current understanding of these mechanisms.

THE SOMATIC RECEPTORS

A. Muscle Receptors

Since the original discovery of muscle afferents by Ruffini in 1898 there has been a great deal of work done to isolate the various sensory receptors in muscle and to investigate their functional significance. Four different receptors have now been described, each having its own specific stimulus and sending impulses to the central nervous system. A number of these receptors are used in the servo system to control muscular contraction and reflexes while others are primarily for conveying impressions to higher levels for conscious or unconscious sensation. These receptors include:

1. The muscle spindle: The muscle spindles lie between and parallel to striated muscle fibres. A typical spindle has two types of intrafusal muscle fibres, the larger and longer "nuclear bag" fibres, and the smaller "nuclear chain" fibres, Boyd (1961). Each muscle spindle contains approximately four or five intrafusal muscle fibres of which two are nuclear bag fibres and the remainder nuclear chain fibres. The primary spindle receptors are coiled around both nuclear bag and nuclear chain muscle fibres and send their impulses along fast conducting, large diameter (Group I) nerve fibres. The secondary sensory endings arise almost exclusively from nuclear chain muscle fibres, round which they appear to be coiled, or scattered in the classical "flower-spray" endings, Buller (1963); Boyd (1959). These endings give rise to slower conducting afferent fibres (Group II) with smaller diameters. Both primary and secondary receptors in the muscle spindle are stimulated by stretch. This stretch can be brought about by a mechanical lengthening of the muscle or by stimulation of the gamma motor neurons which cause the intrafusal muscles to contract, thus increasing the tension on the receptors. The most marked difference in the behavior of primary and secondary endings is in their phasic responses, Harvey and Matthews (1961). The primary endings are more sensitive to changes in stretch than the secondary endings. During dynamic stretch or relaxation, the primary fibres respond much quicker than the secondary endings. Since there now appears to be separate gamma motor control for the nuclear bag and nuclear chain fibres (Boyd, 1961) it has been postulated (Buller, 1963) that the responses of the spindle afferents to the rate of stretching (dynamic response) and to the degree of stretching (static response) are under separate control. It is suggested that the degree of activation of the nuclear chain fibres determines the static sensitivity, and the relative activation of the nuclear bag and nuclear chain fibres determines the dynamic sensitivity of the spindle.

2. The Golgi tendon apparatus: This receptor was first described by Camillo Golgi in 1880. It is formed around a bundle of small tendon fascicles generally in that part of the bundle that is immediately adjacent to the musculotendinous junction, Merrillees (1962). The receptor is enclosed in a very delicate capsule which is a continuation of the sheath of Henle of the afferent nerve. At each end, the capsule blends with connective tissue of the muscle or tendon. The nerve supply to this receptor is a single large medullated afferent fibre from the intramuscular nerve. This nerve branches on reaching the tendon into short sprays of unmyelinated terminals which are attached to the tendon fascicles. It is, presumably, the distortion of these terminals which fire the receptor. The afferent nerve is a Group I fibre with a slightly lower velocity of conduction than the afferent fibres from the primary muscle spindle. The Golgi tendon organs are primarily stretch receptors

which are affected either by contraction of attached muscle fibres or passive stretch of the muscle tendon, Fulton and Pi-Suñer (1928). Although their sensitivity and threshold for stretch is slightly less than for the primary muscle spindle receptors, the tendon receptors do not decrease their firing rate as the muscles shorten. On the contrary, there is a striking relationship between the amount of muscle force and the frequency of firing of the nerve supplying the tendon organ.

3. Pressure receptors: The most familiar pressure receptor in and around muscles is the Pacinian corpuscle, Paintal (1962). The Pacinian corpuscle for the most part is located in the fascia covering the muscle although the occasional corpuscle is seen within the muscle, Barker (1962). It consists of a number of concentric lamellae with a central unmyelinated nerve ending in the middle. According to Hunt (1961), these receptors are particularly sensitive to rapid mechanical stimuli or vibration but not to stretch of the muscle.

There are, however, not sufficient Pacinian corpuscles in the muscle to account for the number of pressure sensitive Group III nerves which supply muscles. Paintal (1962) states that the muscle pressure receptors are not sensitive to vibration. The vast majority of Group III fibres seem to be distributed within the muscle as free nerve endings, Stacey (1969). Paintal (1960) found that the majority of the Group III fibres could be stimulated by pressure. The threshold of these receptors appears to vary considerably and they adapt rapidly to the stimulus. These receptors have also been considered responsible for the sensation of muscle pain produced by squeezing the muscle or injecting 6% NaCl locally. However, they are not apparently responsible for the pain of muscle ischaemia.

In an attempt to discover the muscle receptors responsible for cardiovascular responses to exercise, Hnik *et al.* (1969) has suggested that certain of the Group III muscle afferents with free nerve endings may be involved. These myelinated nerves can be stimulated by raising the KCl concentration in muscles to values which can be found during muscle contraction. He suggests that the K^+ released by muscle action may be the stimulus for chemoreceptors in the muscle which in turn bring about the cardiovascular responses.

4. Unmyelinated pain receptors: Apart from the slower myelinated fibres which are sensitive to pressure-pain there are numerous unmyelinated fibres which respond to other noxious stimuli. The receptors involved are the free branching unmyelinated terminals of the perivascular nerves (Lim *et al.*, 1962). Iggo (1961) showed that these fibres could be stimulated by ischaemia as well as pressure, 5% NaCl and changes in temperature. They seemed to respond in a non-specific manner.

B. Joint Receptors

As is the case with muscles there are a number of different sensory receptors located in the joints. For the most part these receptors are located in the ligaments and capsule surrounding the joint. Although the majority of the research into joint receptors has been done on peripheral joints, Gardner (1969) feels that sufficient evidence is available to suggest that the vertebral column joints have the same basic system of receptors. These receptors include:

1. The Vater-Pacinian corpuscle: These endings are very similar to the Pacinian corpuscle found in other areas of the body in that they are lamellar endings. These receptors are relatively scarce in most joints and are not found in the synovial membrane. Gardner (1950) feels that they are not the predominant ending in joints. They are stimulated by movements which distort the lamellae. They are also fast adapting receptors (Boyd, 1954) and relatively sensitive to distortion.

2. The complex nerve endings: Gardner (1950, 1969) reviews the literature on the so-called spray or Ruffini-type endings. These endings are non-encapsulated and have been consistently found within the joint capsule as well as the ligaments surrounding the joint. They are supplied by larger myelinated fibres in the joint nerves and fall into, what in muscle nerves would be classified as Group II and III fibres. The occasional Golgi receptor has also been described in the ligaments surrounding the joint as well as a simple coiled end organ in association with the adventitia of blood vessels. The spray endings and the Golgi type of endings are sensitive to the stretch induced by movement or tension or by an increase in intra-articular pressure. The spray endings have been shown to have a characteristic discharge frequency for particular positions and rates of movement, Boyd and Roberts (1953). They are therefore, accurate indicators of movement. When a joint is at rest, certain spray endings continue to discharge for long periods of time. Hence, they are accurate indicators of position as well as movement.

3. Free nerve endings: These endings have been demonstrated in the articular capsule, the external parts of collateral ligaments, surrounding blood vessels, and even in the synovial membrane, Gardner (1950). There is, however, some debate as to the abundance of these endings within the synovial membrane. They are supplied primarily by unmyelinated and small myelinated nerve fibres and are primarily responsible for pain impulses (Gardner, 1969).

In the spinal structures the sinu-vertebral nerve has been found to give sensory fibres to fascia, ligaments, periosteum and intervertebral joints (Pedersen *et al.,* 1956) and to the intervertebral disc, Burke (1964). Burke goes to great lengths to suggest that the intervertebral disc is supplied with free nerve endings responsible for pain impulses. There appears, however, to be considerable debate of whether or not these fibres are of any significance.

A vertebral subluxation with its associated muscle spasm and joint fixation would be expected to stimulate a number of these receptors. The increase in muscle tension would stimulate primary and secondary spindle endings as well as the Golgi tendon organ. Since these receptors adapt very slowly, a very large number of these sensory impulses would be entering the central nervous system. The prolonged muscle action could also be expected to cause release of K^+ and ischaemia which in turn would cause stimulation of the smaller Group III fibres as well as pain receptors. Joint fixation would cause an abnormal continuous stimulation of one set of complex nerve endings and spray endings while not stimulating the other sets. Stimulation of pain receptors in the joints and ligaments as well as those in the disc, meninges and nerve roots would all add to the input to the central nervous system much of which is constant and cannot be released by sleep or sedation. The general psychological effects of conscious pain and discomfort is known, however, it would not be surprising to find that the unconscious proprioceptive input could also affect the psyche. This would depend to a large extent on their central connections.

SPINAL CORD CONNECTIONS

The cell bodies of the afferent nerves from the somatic receptors are located within the dorsal root ganglia and enter the spinal cord through the dorsal root. Once in the spinal cord these fibres can make direct connection with spinal cord neurons or ascend to higher levels to connect with neurons within the central nervous system. The connections an afferent nerve will make is dependent largely on the type of receptor it is connected to.

The muscle spindle and Golgi tendon afferents make extensive monosynaptic and polysynaptic reflex connections in the spinal cord. The physiology of these connections have been well described by Eccles (1962) and many others. Although of importance in normal function it is unlikely that these connections have any effect on the psyche.

The discovery that somatic stimulation could cause visceral responses has lead to a great deal of research being conducted into the spinal interactions between the visceral and somatic nervous system, Haldeman (1971). Coote *et al.* (1969) compared white ramus responses from splanchnic nerve and intercostal nerve stimulation. They showed that the splanchnic nerve evoked responses were smaller but of longer duration than intercostal nerve evoked reflexes of the same segment. The central delay of sympathetic reflexes indicated that the responses were polysynaptic. Sato *et al.* (1969) showed that Group I fibre stimulation did not cause a sympathetic response whereas Group II and III fibre stimulation did have a significant sympathetic response. Fedina *et al.* (1966) showed that the responses had different characteristics. The A fibres elicited a reflex discharge with a subsequent inhibition, while the C fibres caused an overall increase in sympathetic activity. These pathways could explain the augmentation of psychosomatic disorders resulting from spinal receptor activation.

Apart from synapses on local interneurons, most afferent nerves synapse with neurons which ascend to higher brain centres. Eccles (1962) describes monosynaptic connections of Group Ia, Ib and II fibres from muscles onto spinocerebellar tract fibres. According to McIntyre (1962) the only muscle afferents which travel to the cerebral cortex along the dorsal column-lemniscal system are those from Group II and III fibres. Oscarsson (1966) has, however, indicated that certain Group I fibres do ascend in the dorsal funiculus. The dorsal funiculus-medial lemniscal pathway is the primary pathway for proprioceptive impulses from joint and tendon receptors (Gardner, 1969) as well as certain complex modalities such as vibration. Gardner, however, states that even after cutting the dorsal columns, signals from joints and muscles still reach the cerebral cortex. He gives evidence to suggest that the main pathway these impulses follow is the spinocervicothalamic system which ascends in the dorsal part of the lateral funiculus to the lateral cervical nucleus. There it synapses with neurons which cross over and ascend in the dorsal part of the lateral funiculus to the lateral cervical nucleus. Then it synapses with neurons which cross over and ascend to higher levels.

The lateral spinothalamic pathway is the primary pathway for pain impulses from all areas of the body. Gardner (1969) suggests that myelinated fibres in this system in monkeys and man probably carry impulses concerned with touch, pressure, and position sense. However, relatively few of these fibres ever reach the thalamus, most of them terminating in lower reticular formation nuclei.

LOWER BRAINSTEM CONNECTIONS

A number of the lower brainstem nuclei, such as the cuneate and gracile, act primarily as relay stations in the afferent pathways. Most afferent fibres appear to give off collaterals as they ascend and these collaterals have been shown to activate other cells or nuclei in the brainstem. An example of this can be seen in the experiments of Burton *et al.* (1971) who showed direct excitation of lateral reticular nucleus cells following stimulation of the dorsal spinocerebellar tract and muscle nerves. Similarly Pompeiano and Barnes (1971) were able to record potentials in the various vestibular nuclei following muscle vibration and Golgi organ stimulation. Cassinari and Pagni (1969) in their review of the pathways followed by pain impulses have quoted literature to show that the spinothalamic tract fibres give off extensive collaterals to a great number of reticular nuclei in the bulb, pons and midbrain as well as to thalamic nuclei.

A great number of brain stem functions can be shown to be influenced by this system. For example, stimulation of muscle or mixed hindlimb nerves in cats, by Schomburg and Schiemann (1971), caused a change in both the inspiration and expiration phases of respiration as well as an excitation of lumbar fusimotor responses. They contribute these changes to increased excitability of the reticular formation. Similarly numerous changes in the blood vascular system have been noted following muscular contractions (Green, 1941) which presumably occur on a brainstem level. The possibility that inputs to the cerebellum may be influenced by collaterals to the reticular nuclei has also been suggested by Pompeiano and Barnes (1971). It is therefore obvious that spinal muscle tension (the subluxation) could have extensive effects on the visceral centers in the lower brainstem.

THALAMUS AND CEREBRAL CORTEX CONNECTIONS

Practically all afferent impulses synapse with thalamic neurons and eventually reach the cerebral cortex for conscious and unconscious interpretation. The multiple pathways from joint and cutaneous receptors relay in the ventrobasal complex and adjacent nuclei of the thalamus, Gardner (1969). Recordings have been made from thalamic neurons which respond to rotation of joints, distortion of muscle-fascial relations, pressure or heat, Perl and Whitlock (1961). Cassinari and Pagni quote researchers who claim that not all sensory fibres which reach the thalamus end in the specific sensory nuclei. Certain fibres have apparently been found to end in midline thalamic nuclei as well as in the centrum medianum and lamina medullaris nuclei. It is possible that impulses might reach these areas through the reticular formation of the brainstem.

There is a great deal of interconnection between systems in the upper brain stem region. For example, although stimulation of Group II, III and IV afferents have widespread influences on visceral function in decerebrate animals (Haldeman, 1971), it is impossible to get any response in these animals from stimulation of Group I afferents. In the decorticate animal, however, stimulation of these Group I afferents can cause sham rage as well as visceral reactions, such as blood pressure increases and pupillary dilation, Malliani *et al.* (1968). Through this pathway, therefore, even primary muscle afferent stimulation could be involved in somatovisceral and psychosomatic disorders.

From the relay nuclei of the thalamus the afferent impulses are projected to the sensory cortex. Single cell analysis of the somatic sensory cortex in cats have shown that these cells are driven by physiological stimuli such as joint movement, Gardner (1969). Those cells driven by joint movement signal steady position and phasic changes in joint position. There seems to be little doubt that the cortical neurons driven by joint movement are involved in the appreciation of position and motion. Evoked potentials have also been recorded from secondary sensory areas on joint movement and from the motor cortex upon stimulation of deep nerves.

Although the fact that Group III and IV fibres from muscles project to the cerebral cortex is well documented there seems to be some debate as to the projection of the afferent nerves from stretch receptors. Oscarsson (1966), however, has shown that Group I fibres do project to restricted areas of the sensory cortex. These fibres do not seem to be important in the conscious perception of position or movement but instead they seem to represent a feedback mechanism in the integration of movements elicited from the cortex.

DISCUSSION

It is obvious that there are a great many receptors in the paraspinal and spinal structures which send information to the central nervous system. These receptors are sensitive to both static and dynamic situations in the structures and monitor almost any situation or change in situation that can occur. In this brief outline, only the muscle and joint receptors have been discussed, since they are the most important. There are, however, receptors in other spinal tissues such as the meninges, epineurial sheaths and fascia which must also be considered. There can be little doubt that spinal subluxation will cause an increased central input of afferent impulses which can have widespread reflex effects.

Spinal reflex connections can have a positive feedback effect on this abnormal input. The spinal subluxation can cause a severe reflex muscle spasm which in turn could further aggravate the afferent input. For example, one of the common results of irritation of a joint by arthritis is a tonic reflex muscle spasm which is facilitated by the affected joint, Nakamara *et al.* (1966). It is probable that joint fixation would aggravate local muscular spasm which in turn would further fixate the joint. The only way in which such a lack of mobility with its concomitant afferent input could be restored to normal is through specific chiropractic adjustments.

The direct somatovisceral pathways exist to explain a great number of the visceral disorders which accompany spinal subluxations. It is probable that these pathways are also important as augmenting psychovisceral disturbances. Convergence on single spinal neurons of impulses from both somatic and visceral receptors have been shown by Pomeranz *et al.* (1968) and the influence of areas in the brainstem on these reflexes have been well documented, Haldeman (1971). It is possible that a visceral dysfunction resulting from a psychic disturbance would be less severe or even asymptomatic if it was not compounded by abnormal somatovisceral reflex activity resulting from a spinal subluxation or muscle tension.

The interpretation of the effects of spinal structure stimulation on the brain is very difficult at this stage. The pathways exist for the afferent stimulation to affect most functional systems in the brain but whether or not these systems are indeed influenced to any degree remains to be investigated. The influence of somatic stimulation on the reticular activating system seems to be the only well documented effect, Birkmeyer and Pilleri (1966). There is very little doubt that pain and muscle tension can cause insomnia, and this in turn can lead to further problems.

The spinal subluxation causes pain, discomfort, lack of mobility and muscle tension. These factors can cause reflex increase in muscle tension, visceral dysfunction and reticular system activation with insomnia. Correction of the subluxation with the subsequent decrease in afferent input and central reflex activity could, therefore, be at least one of the mechanisms through which the chiropractic adjustment benefits patients with psychological disorders.

REFERENCES

Barker, D. "The structure and distribution of muscle receptors," in *Symposium on Muscle Receptors.* Edited by D. Barker, Hong Kong University Press, 1962.

Birkmayer, W. and Pilleri, G. *The Brainstem reticular formation and its significance for autonomic and affective behaviour.* Montreal: Hoffman-LaRoche Ltd., 1966.

Boyd, I. A. "The histological structure of the receptor in the knee joint of the cat correlated with their physiological response," *J. Physiol.* (1954), 124:476–488.

Boyd, I. A. "Simple and compound mammalian muscle spindles," *J. Physiol.* (1959), 145:55P–56P.

Boyd, I. A. "The motor innervation of mammalian muscle spindles," *J. Physiol.* (1961), 159:7P–9P.

Boyd, I. A. and Roberts, J. D. M. "Proprioceptive discharges from stretch receptors in the knee-joint of the cat," *J. Physiol.* (1953), 122:38–58.

Buller, A. J. "The motor unit in reflex action," in *Recent Advances in Physiology.* 8th Ed. Edited by R. Creese (1963), pp. 122–239.

Burke, G. L. *Backache from occiput to coccyx.* W. E. G. MacDonald, 1964.

Burton, J. E.: Bloedel, J. R. and Gregory, R. S. "Electrophysiological evidence for an input to lateral reticular nucleus from collaterals of dorsal spino-cerebellar and cuneocerebellar fibers," *J. Neurophysiol.* (1971), 34:885–897.

Cassinari, V. and Pagni, C. A. *Central Pain.* Cambridge: Harvard University Press, 1969.

Coote, J. H.; Downman, C. B. B. and Weber, W. V. "Reflex discharges into thoracic white rami elicited by somatic and visceral afferent excitation," *J. Physiol.* (1969), 202:147–159.

Dunn, F. E. "The osteopathic management of psychosomatic problems," *J. Am. Osteop. Ass.* (1948), 48:196–199.

Dunn, F. E. "Osteopathic concepts in psychiatry," *J. Am. Osteop. Ass.* (1950), 49:354–356.

Eccles, J. C. "Central connexions of muscle afferent fibres," in *Symposium on Muscle Receptors.* Edited by D. Barker, Hong Kong University Press (1962), pp. 81–101.

Fedina, L.; Kalunskii, A.; Khayutu, V. M.; and Mitsányi, A. "Responses of renal sympathetic nerves to stimulation of afferent A and C fibres of tibial and mesenterial nerves," *Acta Physiol. Acad. Sc. Hung.* (1966), 29:157–175.

Fulton, J. F. and Pi-Suñer, J. "A note concerning the probable function of various afferent end organs in skeletal muscle," *Amer. J. Physiol.* (1928), 83:554–562.

Gardner, E. "Physiology of movable joints," *Physiol. Rev.* (1950), 30:127–176.

Gardner, E. "Pathways to the cerebral cortex for nerve impulses from joints," *Acta Anat. Supp.* (1969), (56-1 ad 73), pp. 203–216.

Gillet, H. and Liekens, M. *Belgian Chiropractic Research Notes* (8th ed.). Belgium, 1970.

Golgi, C. "Sui nervi dei tendini dell'uomo e di altri vertebrati e di un neuovo organo nervoso terminale musclo-tendineo," in *Opera Omnia* (2nd ed.). Milan: Ulrico Hoepli (1880), 1903 vol., pp. 171–198.

Greene, C. W. "Coronary reflex dilatations accompanying contractions of voluntary muscles." *Am. J. Physiol.* (1941), 132:321–326.

Haldeman, S. "Interactions between the somatic and visceral nervous systems," *J. Amer. Chiro. Assoc.* August Edition (1971).

Haugen, Gerhard B., Dixon, Henry H., Dickel, Herman A. *A Therapy for Anxiety Reactions.* Macmillan Co., 1960.

Harper, W. D. *Anything can cause anything.* Seabrook, Texas: privately published, 1966.

Harvey, R. J. and Matthews, P. B. C. "The response of de-efferented muscle spindle endings in the cats solius to slow extension of the muscle," *J. Physiol.* (1961), 157:370–392.

Hnik, P.; Hudlicka, O.; Kucera, J. and Payne, R. "Activation of muscle afferents by nonproprioceptive stimuli," *Am. J. Physiol.* (1969), 217:1451.

Homewood, A. E. *The neurodynamics of the vertebral subluxation.* Willowdale, Ontario: Chiropractic Publishers, 1963.

Homewood, A. E. *Chiropractic and psychic disorders.* This volume, 1971.

Hunt, C. C. "On the nature of vibration receptors in the hind limb of the cat," *J. Physiol.* (1961), 155:175–186.

Iggo, A. "Non-myelinated afferent fibres from mammalian skeletal muscle," *J. Physiol.* (1961), 155:52P–53P.

Jacobson, E. *Tension in Medicine.* Springfield, Ill.: Charles C. Thomas Publishers, 1970.

Lim, R. K. S.; Guzman, F. and Rodgers, D. W. "Note on the muscle receptors concerned with pain," in *Symposium on Muscle Receptors.* Edited by D. Barker, Hong Kong University Press (1962), pp. 215–219.

Malliani, A.; Carli, G.; Mancia, G. and Zanchetti, A. "Behavioral effects of electrical stimulation of Group 1 muscle afferents in acute thalamic cats," *J. Neurophysiol.* (1968), 31:210–220.

McIntyre, A. K. "Central projections of impulses from receptors activated by muscle stretch," in *Symposium on Muscle Receptors.* Edited by D. Barker, Hong Kong University Press, 1962.

Merrillees, N. C. R. "Some observations on the fine structure of a Golgi Tendon organ of a rat," in *Symposium on Muscle Receptors.* Edited by D. Barker, Hong Kong University Press (1962), pp. 199–206.

Nakamura, R.; Nagano, M. and Doi, M. "The reflex muscle spasm in the chronic arthritis. A factor for determining the joint position," *Electromyography* (1966), 6:55–65.

Oscarsson, O. "The projection of Group I muscle afferents to the cat cerebral cortex," in *Nobel Symposium 1: Muscle afferents and Motor control.* Edited by R. Granit. New York–London: John Wiley and Sons, 1966.

Paintal, A. S. "Functional analysis of Group III afferent fibres of mammalian muscles," *J. Physiol.* (1960), 152:250–270.

Paintal, A. S. "Responses and reflex effects of pressure-pain receptors of mammalian muscles," in *Symposium on Muscle Receptors.* Edited by D. Barker, Hong Kong University Press, 1962.

Pedersen, H. E.; Blunchk, C. F. J. and Gardner, E. "The anatomy of lumbosacral posterior rami and meningeal branches of spinal nerves (sinu-vertebral nerves)," *J. Bone Jt. Surg.* (1956), 38A:377–391.

Perl, E. R. and Whitlock, D. G. "Somatic stimuli exciting spinothalamic projections to thalamic neurons in cat and monkey," *Exp. Neurol.* (1961), 3:256–296.

Plutchik, R. "The role of muscular tension in maladjustment," *J. Gen. Psychology* (1954), 50:45–62.

Pomeranz, B.; Wall, P. D. and Weber, W. V. "Cord cells responding to fine myelinated afferents from viscera, muscle and skin," *J. Physiol.* (1968), 199:511–532.

Pompeiano, O. and Barnes, C. D. "Response of Brain Stem Reticular Neurons to Muscle Vibration in the Decerebrate Cat," *J. Neurophysiol.* (1971), 35:709–724.

Ruffini, A. "Observations on sensory nerve endings in voluntary muscles." *Brain* (1898), 20:368–374.

Sato, A.; Kaufman, A.; Koizumi, K. and Brooks, C. M. "Afferent nerve groups and sympathetic reflex pathways," *Brain Res.* (1969), 14:575.

Schomburg, E. D. and Schiemann, B. "Convertible respiratory and fusimotor reactions to peripheral somatic stimuli in different functional states of the reticular formation in the cat," *Pflug. Arch.* (1971), 327:261–273.

Schwartz, H. S. "Preliminary analysis of 350 mental patients records treated by chiropractors," *J. of National Chiropractic Association* (November 1949), pp. 12–15.

Schwartz, H. S. "What is the connection between nerves and nervousness," *J. National Chiropractic Assoc.,* April, 1949b.

Stacey, M. J. "Free nerve endings in skeletal muscle of the cat." *J. Anat.* (1969), 105:2, and 231–254.

Verner, J. R. *The science and logic of chiropractic.* Englewood, N.J., 1950.

Yorkston, N. J. and Sergeant, H. G. S. "A simple method of relaxation," *Lancet* (1969), pp. 1319–1321.

PART IV

STRUCTURAL PSYCHOTHERAPY

CHAPTER

* deceased

CHAPTER 12

PSYCHOPHYSIOLOGICAL ASPECTS OF THE SUBLUXATION*

EDWIN H. KIMMEL, D.C.

INTRODUCTORY COMMENTS

The force of life expresses itself through the entire organism. When trauma occurs, whatever its nature or cause, its effect is never segmented. At first, it may express itself in minor localized reactions but as it spreads, it may adversely affect the entire organism.

Dr. Kimmel points out some effects of the work of chiropractic which he properly defines as Chiro-kinetics. There are many complex and significant factors involved in the chiropractic management. Its impact on an individual's total health can be far-reaching. He also states that society is beginning to demand that doctors of all schools of healing become involved in the patient's total welfare, which may include a consultive or cooperative effort. The emotional and social ramifications and complexities of a person's sore back affects that person's reactions towards his life, his economics, his loves, his hates, and may sometimes be more important than his locomotive incapacity. The sum total of all healing lore is that treatment shall be given to the whole individual, and any attempt to separate the psyche and soma is not only illogical but impossible.

In this chapter can be found a body of references which graphically and indisputably focuses attention on physical trauma as a definite cause of mental or emotional disturbances. The editor takes this opportunity to acknowledge his debt of gratitude to Dr. Kimmel for his strong support throughout many years in research and the gathering of material for this book.

H.S.S.

* * *

* Presented before the American Academy of Psychotherapists, Twelfth Annual Conference, Warrenton, Virginia, Nov. 1967. Reproduced here with slight changes and additions.

THE QUESTION may arise: How can chiropractic help an emotionally or psychologically disturbed patient? To answer this thoughtful question we posit that chiropractic is a biomechanical and neurological approach to emotional stress.

It has become increasingly evident from the writings of Freud (1938), Reich (1949), Lowen (1958), Feldenkrais (1949), Rolf (1962), and others that the emotions are rooted in the tissues of the body. Thus the biomechanical approach is bound to have an influence upon the total body.

The physical effects of emotional insult remain deep in the tissues. They reveal themselves in the posture and muscular rigidities; they convey a message of distress, which manifests itself in the body's muscular structure (see Lowen, Ch. 6). By the lessening of the neuromuscular-skeletal distortions or irritations, there is release of the residual tensions.

Reich (1949) emphasized the fact that the body's energy flow can be blocked at certain segmental levels, all at right angles to the spine following the path of the spinal nerves. Such muscular rigidities extend from the top of the head (galea apponeuritica) to the sole of the foot (plantar fascia). Unless these muscular armorings are relieved or released, any progress in the emotional growth of the patient is, at best, only temporary.

The individual, living in our rigid society with its multiple stresses, develops muscular tensions and rigidities. They are fed by grief, fear, rage, resentment and anger, which affect his emotional and personality growth. As a result, he unconsciously may develop habits which are potentially negative and self-destructive. His basic wholesome feelings can be blocked by chronic patterns of muscular rigidity, and his behavior can be influenced by these long continued subliminal neurological aberrations.

All body-oriented therapies have, as their goal, the attempted release or dissolution of muscular rigidity. Some of these techniques are gentle and passive (yoga, exercise, Alexander technique, dance therapy, etc.). Other techniques are more rigorous (Reich and neo Reichian, Rolf, Lowen's Bioenergetics).

We postulate that chiropractic is specific and fundamental. As already indicated, there is a sound neurophysiological and neuropsychological basis for such a physical approach to what has been previously designated as purely emotional or psychological aberrations.

In a spirit of inquiry, we here evaluate the potential value of this discipline. We postulate that total health of the organism depends upon a harmonious reciprocal interdependence and integration of psyche and soma via the nervous system. Chiropractic offers a bio-psychological approach to the whole patient by utilizing the kinetics of the body. Many psychopathological reactions can occur as a result of anatomical stress, which disturbs neuro-physiological mechanisms affecting the normal integration of the organism. By lessening or removing anatomical stress, the chiropractor often can play a positive role in affecting mental health. The spinal adjustment procedures of chiropractic have been devised to exert general or specific influence upon the mechanical structures of the body, in an attempt to influence the neuromuscular system, the objective being to re-establish homeostatic balance.

PHYSICAL ETIOLOGY OF EMOTIONAL RESPONSE

Psychotherapeutic literature is replete with convincing evidence that many diseases are of a psychophysiological origin. The 75 year old chiropractic findings indicate that postural and vertebral distortions frequently reveal areas of neuromuscular skeletal stress, which are in turn responsible for many alleged psychosomatic and emotional disorders.

Schutz (1967) stated that "integration of the emotions with the physical structure is required for a more lasting change." He further states that "after many years of being all but ignored, the importance of body-functioning to the emotional states is becoming recognized more widely and applied to growth producing situations, that disturbed body organization and abnormal physiology affect the feelings—a view called somato-psychic." This viewpoint is not new to the doctor of chiropractic. His initial approach to the patient in distress has always been via manipulation of the body structures.

Lowen (1958) looks for the relation between the emotional state and the physical manifestation. He stated that "there is no neurotic problem which does not manifest itself in every aspect of the individual's function. As an important structural element in the body, a weakness in the backbone must be reflected in a serious personality disturbance." Reich (1949) states "Since it is the muscular armoring which causes biopathic restriction of living functioning, this muscular armor has to be dissolved . . . psychic disturbances have their root in the somatic realm." Physical and emotional etiologies and therapy should be considered in their total perspective. In combination they are a holistic approach for psychological disturbances. If we follow the implications of the basic insight, that one great truth does not necessarily negate another, no doctor need ever go astray in this important field.

Chirokinetics concerns itself chiefly with the release of residual muscular tensions associated with recent or latent psychological traumas. Frequently, it will cause long dormant feelings, sensations and memories to surface, as the muscular rigidity associated with that feeling is softened and relaxed.

Often, with only the aid of some minor psychotherapeutic procedures (see Ch.16), in addition to the chiropractic adjustments, the patient may begin to understand how his repressed emotional experiences cause some of his physical distress, and start to cope with them on a more realistic level. For the more severe emotionally disturbed patients, expert psychotherapy is necessary.

PSYCHOSOMATIC DISORDERS

The strong development of "psychosomatics" in the last four decades has not only popularized, but also assembled convincing evidence that with *all* psychic disturbances there is *some* concomitant physical distress; conversely, along with all physical disorder there is some psychological component, whether or not this latter feature is objectively prominent or professionally emphasized in the course of diagnosis and treatment. Since the chiropractic practitioner (like any other straightforward scientific worker) dare not rest content with *partial* truth, but must deal with the TOTAL or WHOLE reality, this elementary psychosomatic principle must control his interpretation of the patient's condition. Specifically, this means that the *release of neuromuscular tension*—a field in which the chiropractor is a genuine specialist—is not only efficacious, but *necessary* in the elimination of emotional stress. Clinical experience with thousands of mild "neurotic" and so-called "borderline" cases demonstrates that people can and do, through chiropractic, become "symptom-free" from established nervous moods and reactions of long duration. The psychosomatic concept is inherent in the very nature of chiropractic. Its elementary principles are based on the sound premise of the complete reciprocal interdependence and integration of the body and the mind (or soma and psyche) via the nervous system.

The natural and logical conclusion to be derived from the very existence of afferent and efferent neural impulses is that every disease condition affects in some way the nervous system and that every chiropractic adjustment can have some influence upon this condition. If we view disease from this apparently novel, but actually quite old, standpoint, it should not be too hard to appreciate why *most diseases can and should be known as diffuse psychosomatic illnesses.* More precisely, diseases are traceable to (1) injuries to the soma, (2) psychic distress, (3) adverse body metabolism, and (4) environmental pressures. D. D. Palmer has stated this essential proposition numerous times in his book published in 1910. It is the chiropractor's normal task to comprehend and react to all these interconnected factors in diagnosing and adjusting any patient brought before him.

He does not conceive of the patient as merely a spine or a disembodied, imperceptible, unfathomable psyche devoid of all corporal roots. The ancient ideal of a sound mind in a healthy or "whole" body can readily be modernized by stressing the converse, viz., *that a healthy body also depends upon a healthy mind*. This interdependence is an A-B-C "natural" for the chiropractor. Since excessive nerve irritation often directly causes much of the discomfort of which the emotionally distressed patient complains, vertebral adjustments definitely make their influence felt in subsequent reports about "feeling better."

Intangible as "thoughts" may be, they are nonetheless *real* things since they are both *effects of certain causes* and in turn produce definitely ascertainable consequences in the experience of the patient.

Chiropractic—the art of restoring disrelated skeletal and/or muscular tissue to its normal design—is psychosomatic per se, because it attempts to correct the faulty structure that may be responsible for the nerve irritations affecting a particular organ, system or gland. Every nerve infringement within the vertebral column or in adjacent or remote tissues is an incipient pathological state involving some concurrent psychic infringement. This initial "malformation" may readily lead to a true psychosomatic condition. Usually the patient superimposes upon this localized neural irritation, additional generalized or widely distributed weight of fear in any one of its protean forms. When initial trauma is increased by a remoter reinforcement from another power area or energy source, the pain is necessarily paralleled by a corresponding growth in fear, worry, and anxiety, and the slow nibbling away of the sufferer's psyche goes on apace.

In this fashion, a minor subluxation can turn into a full-flowered psychic upset if the patient uses his unalleviated discomfort (1) to escape reality, (2) to avoid his obligations to himself and to others, (3) to "get even" with some superior, associate, or family member, (4) as an interpretation of pain, as divine punishment for some offense, etc. If, as is so commonly the case when sedatives are administered, the pain is deadened by medication, then the mental faculties are numbed in some degree. Thus, temporary personality deterioration ensues, normal confidence and poise are destroyed, and childhood fears, frustrations, and feelings of guilt and rejection become prominent to such an extent that the initially uncomplicated "winding base" goes unrecognized by both doctor and patient. In this way a simple fall, blow, or other injury eliciting some anatomical distortion may grow into a full-bodied "neurosis" or "psychosis." Conversely, correcting the distortion brings relief, recovery, and "cure" in enough cases to demonstrate that chiropractic per se is beneficial to the emotionally disturbed, whether used alone or in conjunction with auxiliary, nutritional, or psychological aids.

TIME AND GRAVITY

Man's constant battle against the forces of time and gravity in his effort to maintain his erect posture, and the constant residual muscular tension involved, subjects the human body to a chain of organismic consequences. The strains and stresses upon the joints, ligamentous structures, fasciae, muscles, and unsupported viscera may, like physical disease, affect the ego strength. The asymmetry of the body and the precariously placed center of gravity, which permits utmost agility, does not allow for free and uncomplicated compensation to the forces of gravity which the human has to withstand. The possible emotional effects of "gravitosis"—difficulty in maintaining the erect posture and vertebral joint relationship (Jungmann 1966)—have hitherto been given little recognition as etiological factors. As a pathogen, gravitosis can be analogous to bacterial, ecological, nutritional, and socioeconomic pressures, as well as to other stressors (Selye 1956) to which man is exposed throughout his life. There is ample evidence which substantiates the role of posture in relation to the individual's emotional outlook. Reich (op. cit.) pointed out that what we commonly call "nervousness" is the result of hypersensitivity of highly tensed muscles. The character armor is functionally identical with the muscular armor. Rolf (1963) influenced by Feldenkrais (1949), has also described the psychological manifestations which occur as a result of the physical attitude of the body structure. "In general, every pattern of impulses reaching the CNS from the viscera, muscles, and soma is associated with an emotional state."

The ill effects from the struggle against gravity may not always be acute or sudden. The constant grind and attrition with the concomitant muscular rigidity may often be slow, insidious, and cumulative. We do not usually think of the effects of gravity as an all pervading influence on the total body structure, or on the emotional health of the individual.

Struggling constantly against this ubiquitous and relentless opponent (gravity) subjects the antigravity (extensor) muscles to many dynamic changes daily. The dynamic state of all these muscles concerns the doctor of chiropractic, especially as they relate to the neural bed within the intervertebral foramen, its influence on the autonomic functions, and the effects upon the character structure of the patient.

Feldenkrais (1949) posits that: "To every emotional state corresponds a personal conditioned pattern of muscular contraction without which it has no existence . . . Voluntary directives inhibiting the extensors are observed in all emotionally disturbed persons. In the long run this becomes habitual and remains unnoticed. The whole character is, however, affected. The partially inhibited extensors become weak, the hip joint flexes and the head leans forward."

Postural, occupational, eyestrain, hearing difficulties, or other physical or psychological traumatic stresses produce tension within the muscles and the other supporting elements of the intervertebral joints. As a consequence of such stresses, joint and muscle functions are altered physically. They are no longer able to perform their physiological function. Residual tension begins to build up within the muscles. Biochemical changes also occur due to the narrowing of the blood vessels within the affected parts. Cellular malnutrition and decreased oxygenation may also be responsible for initiating pathological degenerations. Joint fixation and muscular rigidity also occur after accidents especially when structural compensation fails or is inadequate.

Furthermore, we find that reflex hypertonic splintings (fixations) occur in the muscles involved in unsuccessful adaptation to these postural strains. These fixations can become perseverating, self-perpetuating impulses travelling into the posterior (sensory) horn of the spinal cord. They stimulate the anterior (motor) cells of the cord via internuncial neurons, perpetuating a vicious cycle of muscular contraction. There may also be autonomic overtones accompanying this irritating fixation, that is, impulses spilling over into the lateral columns of grey matter of the spinal cord that may be responsible for vaso constriction and trophic changes within the associated viscera by way of the communicating rami of the sympathetic system.

EFFECT OF NEUROLOGICAL STRESS

Rarely is there only one specific area involved in this somato-psycho-visceral complex. Muscular rigidity, regardless of its origin, tends to produce compensatory changes in nearby muscles and fasciae as part of the fundamental adaptive postural mechanism. Neural irritation is likewise plurisegmental. Irritation to the sympathetics at one segmental level tends to produce changes in segmental levels remote from the source of original irritation.

Chronic peripheral changes in the body structure, such as fixed or rigid joints or muscular hypertonus may serve to initiate or maintain increased noxious cerebral activity, by virtue of irritation of the proprioceptor nerve endings. Such irritations may be responsible for a sufficient amount of proprioceptor abuse which can be responsible for abnormal behavioral patterns. Persistent bombardment of excessively strong stimuli from chronic bracing of striated muscles results in the manifestation of symptoms associated with overactivity of the arousal area in the brain. This often culminates in the generation of emotions such as apprehension, fear, anxiety, and other similar phenomena in the cortex (Haugen, Dixon & Dickel, 1958).

The existence of increased muscle tonus, as a manifestation of emotional disturbance, is a matter of clinical observation. The resultant spasticity and painful joints produce local changes which cannot be overlooked and must be treated. Ischemia, edema, inflammation, and degeneration may often remain after the psychogenic factors have been alleviated. These changes may continually perpetuate proprioceptor irritation, thereby maintaining subliminal cerebral influences upon behavior.

Such alerting or arousing influences reach the cerebral cortex via the Reticular Activating System. The R.A.S. is influenced by the great subcortical sensory center, the thalamus; it is supplemented by a thalamic R.A.S., which appears to stimulate more selectively individual cortical areas. The initial source of the impulses in both R.A.S.'s is peripheral, arising from cutaneous, special sense organs and proprioceptors. The brain does not exist for itself alone. It acts as a means of rapid integrated responses to and from environmental changes. Cerebral cortical activity is determined to a large extent by the number of converging sensory impulses that reach the cortex.

The nervous system, therefore, is very sensitive to any alteration in the state of the skeletal musculature. Striated muscle activity has a great deal to do with initiation and content of thought and action. Increased cortical activity can occur as a result of increased muscular tonus. Maintaining a constant postural position will usually produce sufficient sensory stimulation to induce an involuntary shifting of the voluntary muscles.

Frequently the individual may be unable to accommodate his muscles to these sensory messages because of fixation or segmental splinting. As a result, further contracture of the muscles ensues, thereby stimulating increased numbers of proprioceptors in those muscles. Without the induced relaxation, which can be produced by chiropractic manipulation, a vicious cycle of feedback of such impulses occurs along sensory pathways, through the thalamus, to the R.A.S. and thence back to the muscles, perpetuating the muscular hypertonus or the emotional reaction to that tension.

The neurological effects of fixed spinal segmental disrelationship may produce additional effects. When pain is added to the other sensory bombardments, the effects upon the psychic mechanisms and resultant behavioral changes may be even more pronounced. Pain elicits an alarm reaction (General Adaptation Syndrome) with its concomitant autonomic manifestations (Selye, op. cit.). Abnormal behavior, therefore, may be precipitated in this way. Segmental disrelationship with its neurological overtones may explain why certain organs are predisposed to respond to psychic stress in a particular way. Different persons frequently react differently to the same stimuli. Structural differences are well known to the anatomist. A person who reacts to stress with tachycardia may do so because of the way his particular body is constructed or because of the residual muscular tensions which are increased under stress, and not necessarily because of an unconscious symbolic wish fulfillment. In addition, the modifications of posture and locomotion associated with the protection of a painful or mechanically impaired area will readily result in the altered use of adjacent parts. This further changes proprioceptor impulses from the secondarily affected regions and by such alteration increases afferent flow to the brain.

PSYCHOBIOLOGIC REACTIONS OF CERVICAL TRAUMA

We now present further research data substantiating the chiropractic premise that physical trauma can be responsible for mental as well as physical symptoms. Rusk (1969) wrote that it was reported at a conference sponsored by the World Federation of Neurology that "head injuries resulting from automobile, work, home and surfing accidents and from gunshot wounds, are far more prevalent than most people realize." Recent findings by Thompson (1965) indicate that psychoneurosis may be due to post-traumatic injuries. Woods (1960) writes that pre-natal and natal injuries may lay the foundation for psychological disturbances. The research studies of Auerbach *et al.* (1960) signified to them that the sequelae of head injuries may cause psychophysiological syndromes. Ritro (1970) has made an important study entitled, "Neurophysiologic and Biochemical Abnormalities May be the Cause for Infantile Autism and Childhood Schizophrenia." It is mentioned frequently in the literature that traumatic experiences in the cervical region of the spine, such as "whiplash injury alone can result in intracranial lesions, and the development of subdural kematoma." Ommaya (1969A) Experimentations with monkeys have established that, "The clinical results can range all the way from the common minor annoyance of a sprained neck to the rare, but potentially lethal subdural clot on the brain."

The above are only a few examples of the amount of research that is being carried on, not only on the physical symptomatic reactions to cervical trauma, but also on the various emotional and behavioral changes which may occur as a result of these fixations or distortions in this important region of the body.

The neck is the most constricted area in the framework of the body. It is the most mobile and contains the most delicate vertebrae of the spinal column. Within so small an area there are structures that are vital to life itself; the extension of the medulla, the spinal cord within the vertebral canal, large muscles, the trachea, larynx, pharynx, esophagus, carotid arteries, lymphatics, jugular veins, vertebral arteries as well as the thyroid gland. Injuries to that anatomical section of the spine subject the delicate structures of the neck to organismic insult, resulting in a large variety of physical or mental symptoms.

Due to its narrow diameter, the neck is a very crucial area. Any distortion, muscular rigidity, reaction to tension or trauma, which upsets or interferes with this delicate balance, will eventually exert some adverse influence upon the total functioning of the organism. One of the first areas for tension to become manifest is in the posterior cervical and shoulder muscles. Tensions here are quite common and can be determined by cervical palpation and by X-rays. Muscular contraction may also impinge upon the large blood vessels; when the distortion such as a scoliosis is acute, it may interfere with the flow of blood through the vertebral arteries, thereby influencing the arterial supply to the circle of Willis at the base of the brain. Occipito-atlantal or atlanto-axial distortion may initiate many complex vestibular reactions, resulting in abnormal behavior.

Now the mechanics of the subluxation should become clearer, as to how the person can be subject to a variety of complaints, physical or emotional. Just as an emotional insult causes physical response, physical injury may cause emotional response. Some areas of the body, such as the spine, have a more devastating emotional impact when injured than others. An injury that appears to threaten the victim's ability to return to the same level of gainful employment may result in a chain of dysfunctions and symptoms not directly connected to an anatomical basis. Better understanding of the influence of disturbed structure upon the nervous system and the influence of disturbed neural function upon tissues and viscera would decrease the number of mis-diagnoses of hysteric and malingering conditions.

A very common injury is the hyperextension-hyperflexion or "whip lash" trauma to the neck, causing direct physical damage to the muscles, tendons, ligaments and sometimes to the intervertebral discs, especially in the midcervical area. It may also affect the small blood vessels within these structures. In accord with Hilton's Law, the joint injury, through afferent neurones, bombards the spinal cord segment or segments with impulses that cause muscular contractural response, producing the so-called protective "splinting," as well as local referred pain, with alterations in the vascularity of the area. The limitation of movement, local and radiating pain into the shoulder and/or arm are recognized as anticipated neurological symptoms, but a constellation of symptoms may develop which are not so clearly attributable to the area injured. The sudden hyperextension of the neck tends to tear fibres of the thin longus colli muscle against which the cervical portion of the sympathetic chain rests. The resulting hematoma and muscular contraction may bring abnormal pressure upon the chain, resulting in a sympathetic response. There may be irritation of the sympathetic fibres, hence variation in symptoms. Headache is common, due to either referred pain, the pull of contracted muscles on their attachments to the skull, or alterations in blood supply within the cranial vault (Ommaya, 1969). The latter may involve the internal structure of the brain and, therefore, it may be related to personality change as well as many other severe behavioral abnormalities of an unexpected nature. The pupils of the eyes may be constricted if the sympathetic fibres are inhibited, or dilated, if irritation and stimulation result from the injury. Similarly the eyes may sink or protrude slightly if the supporting ocular musculature is inhibited or over-activated. Alterations to the vasomotor fibres of the vascular bed of the arm, forearm and/or hand may also occur with resultant trophic symptoms. In addition, the phrenic nerve, the vagus nerve, the internal carotid artery and the internal jugular vein may also be affected. Disturbance to these structures may produce symptoms such as abnormal function of the heart, lungs, esophagus, stomach, diaphragm, small intestine, proximate half of the colon, the liver, gall bladder, and other organs, depending upon which of its fibers are irritated.

The segmental spinal disrelationships caused by injuries such as the whiplash appear to be most accessible to specific types of chiropractic adjustive therapy. By restoring normal intervertebral joint mobility, it not only affects the vertebral muscles and ligaments, but also the neural bed, i.e., the spinal nerve with its communicating rami to the sympathetic system.

The posterior neck muscles and the muscles of the shoulders insert into the galea apponeuritica, and constriction of these muscles may result in the typical band-like headache (Lowen, ch. 6). The effect of the neuromuscular tension circuit may be compared to electrical modulation. As long as there is continuous input of excessive impulses from striated muscles, the activity of certain portions of the nervous system is modified, and the output from these positions is different from what it would be without the steady barrage of stimuli.

Constantly changing proprioceptive stimuli would allow for normal cortical activity, but a persistent bombardment of excessively strong stimuli from chronic muscle tension results in overactivity of the arousal area. The R.A.S.

parallels sensory pathways, receives collaterals from the sensory pathways, alerts the cortex, and is responsible for emotional reaction to stimuli. In the case of spinal fixations, these stimuli may be subliminal but cumulative.

Due to that constant state of tension, the person simply does not have the flexibility or neurological reserve to cope with the ordinary demands of every day living. Irrational behavior may be the net result because the nervous pathways cannot tolerate any further irritation. They have reached their limit of irritability. Further insult results in a spilling over of these noxious impulses into associated neurohumoral pathways, the response of which is not in tune with the original stimulus. The organism no longer acts or reacts in a harmonious symphonic whole. Responses are spastic, jerky and sometimes bizarre. Reaction may be out of proportion to the stimulus, due to the overactivity of the arousal area.

It is most interesting to note that frequently during the chiropractic adjusting, a therapeutic, relaxing situation is induced in the muscles; it stimulates recollections and memories of either long forgotten emotional or physical traumas that seem to have been stored within those muscle groups. The "muscular armor" described by Reich is released. Lowen (1970) also confirms that when muscle tensions are released painful memories and feelings can emerge into consciousness. This certainly corroborates the hypothesis that feeling and emotion are locked in with muscle rigidity. It is not uncommon for the emotionally distressed patient to cry after experiencing muscular release. This reaction may be the result of momentary relief of painful emotional experiences or the joy of being free of the tension.

CONCLUSION

The aim of chirokinetic therapy is to free the body of neuromuscular-skeletal tensions. Then the person becomes more open and direct, with an increased capacity for appropriate healthy aggression and emotional growth and maturity. In time his voice may become more resonant, and his expressions will soften. He will feel more relaxed, his movement will be free, and the capacity to experience enjoyment in living occurs. Additional positive changes are frequently reported in every aspect of interpersonal relationships. His posture and body-image improve, and the body balance is more near the normal for that individual. The goal level or aspiration index improves. Children in classroom situations achieve more—as reported by parents and teachers. Furthermore, there is a change in the patient's reaction to stressful threatening situations, both emotionally and physically. Cognitive reasoning seems to improve. The cumulative effects upon the patient are positive.

The modern doctor of chiropractic recognizes other causes of emotional illness and the important role of the psychotherapist. He is ready to refer patients to him or work cooperatively with him. Interdisciplinary approach, including chiropractic, is one holding forth great promise for better mental health. Whether cause and effect can be separated at this time is problematical. Research may eventually substantiate the predominant factors. At this time, however, from an empirical standpoint, years of experience have shown that chiropractic manipulation does benefit the emotionally disturbed patient.

REFERENCES

Auerbach, Arthur H. (*et al.*). "The Psychophysiologic Sequelae of Head Injuries," *Am. Psychiatric Assoc.* Atlantic City, May 1960.

Feldenkrais, M. *Body and Mature Behavior.* New York: International University Press, 1949.

Freud, Sigmund. *The Basic Writings of Sigmund Freud.* New York: Modern Library, 1938.

Haugen, G. B., Dixon, H. H., Dickel, H. A. *A Therapy for Anxiety Tension Reactions.* New York: Macmillan Co., Inc., 1958.

Jungmann, M. "Psychopathology Tied to Chronic Gravitational Strain," *Roche Report* (1966), 3:9.

Lowen, Alexander. *Physical Dynamics of Character Structure.* New York: Grune & Stratton, 1958.

Lowen, Alexander. (1970)—*Pleasure.* Coward-McCann, Inc. New York.

Ommaya, A. K. "Whiplash Injuries." A Review of Clinical and Experimental Observations, *Pakistan Medical Review* (October 1969), 4.

Ommaya, A. K. "Whiplash and Brain Damage," *Journal of A.M.A.* (April 22, 1968), 204:285.

Palmer, D. D. *The Science, Art and Philosophy of Chiropractic.* Portland, Oregon: Portland Printing House Co., 1910.

Reich, Wilhelm. *Character Analysis.* New York: Noonday Press, 1949.

Rolf, I. O. "Structural Integration, Systemics," *The Journal of the Inst. for the Comp. Study of Hist., Philo., and Sciences* (1963), 1:1.

Schultz, William C. *Joy.* New York: Grove Press, 1967.

Selye, Hans. *The Stress of Life.* New York: McGraw-Hill Book Co. 1956.

Thompson, George N. "Post-Traumatic Psychoneurosis, a Statistical Study," *American Journal of Psychiatry* (May 1965) p. 1043.

Woods, H. Rachel. "Psychological Disturbances Due to Prenatal & Natal Injuries," *Academy of Applied Osteopathy Year Book,* 1960.

SUPPLEMENTARY READINGS

Bender, Lauretta. "Psychiatric Problems in Children," *Medical Clinics of North America,* May 1958.

Bender, Lauretta. "Psychobiological Problems of Children with Organic Brain Disease," *American Journal of Orthopsychiatry,* July 1949.

Branch, D. H. H. *Aspects of Anxiety.* Phila.: Lippincott, 1965.

Burr, H. S. *The Neural Basis for Human Behavior.* Springfield, Ill.: Chas. C. Thomas, 1960.

Dunn, F. E. "Osteopathic Concepts in Psychiatry," *JAOA* (1950), 50:3.

Fields, A. "The Autonomic Nervous System in Whiplash Injuries," *International Record of Medicine* (1959), 169.

Frank, J. D. *Persuasion and Healing.* Baltimore: Johns Hopkins Press, 1961.

French, J. D. "The Reticular Formation," *Scientific American* (1959), 196:5 and 54.

Goff, W. C. (et al.). *Traumatic Cervical Syndrome and Whiplash.* Philadelphia: Lippincott, 1964.

Kuntz, A. *The Autonomic Nervous System.* Philadelphia: Lea & Febiger, 1947.

Lowen, Alexander. *Betrayal of the Body.* New York: Macmillan Company, Inc., 1967.

Lowen, Alexander. *Depression and the Body.* New York: Coward, McCann & Geoghegan, 1972.

Meares, A. *The Management of the Anxious Patient.* Philadelphia, Pa.: Saunders Co., 1963.

Sappenfield, R. G. *Personality Dynamics.* New York: Knopf, 1954.

CHAPTER 13

THE ROLE OF CHIROPRACTIC IN AN INTEGRATIVE PSYCHOTHERAPY

HENRY GUZE, PH.D.

INTRODUCTION BY THE EDITOR

It was Dr. Guze's intention to write a comprehensive treatise for this anthology. But fate intervened; at the age of 51, the world lost a great human being and an outstanding scholar, and the chiropractic profession lost one of its most devoted friends from the field of behavioral science.

Dr. Guze was an anthropologist, a physiologist, a psychotherapist, and a psychologist. From the vantage point of a mountain top of knowledge, he had a thorough understanding of all the healing disciplines.

From his extensive chapter outline, which Dr. Guze left with the editor, we can surmise what rich and important facts and theories he wanted to embody in this anthology. The outline in part contained the following subject headings:

a. Problems of adaptation and neuromuscular integration;
b. External and internal environmental stress;
c. Concept of Dis-ease;
d. The Visceral Motor System and the Retreat from Reality;
e. The Sensory-Motor Feedback systems;
f. Activation and the Pain System;
g. Foundations for a Theory of Psychophysiological Psychotherapy;
h. The Chiropractic Concept as a Core Theory in Psychosomatic Thinking.

Dr. Guze was aware that around 1895 two profound discoveries were made almost concurrently which, when combined, held out a promise for better and more complete health than the human family had ever dared to hope for. D. D. Palmer found that the cause and effect of disease was always connected with the nervous system. At the same time, in another part of the world, Sigmund Freud discovered that the cause of much mental disorder was within man's subconscious mind or, if one prefers, in neglected or forgotten motives underlying behavior.

Freud taught us that the patient must be understood, that he lives in a world of ideas that are unknown to anyone, not even himself. His thoughts, attitudes, beliefs, and feelings must be uncovered; the patient must gain in-

sight into his characteristic behavior and he can change, if his emotional drive or will to alter his conduct is aroused.

D. D. Palmer, and later, Willard Carver, taught us to look upon the body as a perfectly working machine and that, when illness strikes, the "machine" needs to be adjusted; likewise, that we should look to the nervous system as a significant basis for health.

Both great ideas had their roots deep in history. Chiropractic in one form or another was known and used over two thousand years ago by the ancient Greeks under the name of "Chiropraxy." Similarly, some modern psychological conceptions are traceable to Platonic and Aristotelian discussions of the nature of the human mind and its subtle ways of functioning. Hippocrates was not only acquainted with the cause and cure of many common maladjustments of the physical frame, but is also known to historians as a keen observer and recorder of the accompanying effects upon the "total personality," the peculiar province of psychotherapy.

The distinguished founders of these two schools of thought, D. D. Palmer, a midwestern American, and Sigmund Freud, a central European, had very much in common—more indeed than most of their latter-day disciples realize. They held in common a drugless conception in their respective fields. They regarded health and disease of the body and mind in surprisingly similar fashion. The big ideas with which each was identified captured the imagination of experts and laymen and caused intellectual revolutions of unusual scope and magnitude.

Palmer and Freud were both misunderstood, maligned, and ridiculed. Palmer could very well have joined in this proudly reproachful statement by Freud:

> *"I became familiar early with my destiny—to belong to the opposition and to be proscribed from the 'compact majority.' A certain independence of judgment was in this way developed."*

D. D. Palmer's and Freud's ideas have withstood the test of time. Their concepts have not been changed essentially; they have undergone some modifications—a sure sign of their greatness. Great truths don't alter; time only refines them and modifies them. Truths are flexible enough so that, like sturdy trees, they can bend and sway with the storms of repeated trial, and remain standing as a challenge to man. The very nature of a true principle is that it can be bent and twisted, yet its very essence is so strong that it can stand firmly and accommodate to modifications of time, change and substance. Yet it remains deeply rooted in the soil of virtue and usefulness, because of the unshakeable correctness of its fundamental precepts.

Both disciplines hold one great truth in common which is that we must look to the body and mind for total well-being. Both hold that improvement in a person's physical and mental health depends heavily upon his self-understanding and the freeing of his latent powers. Both chiropractic and modern psychotherapy, while recognizing the influences of an adverse heredity and a distressing environment which are often detrimental to complete health, still hold that health comes from within and look to the patient's "innate" vital forces for a solution to his emotional and somatic dilemma. The greatest aid the doctor can offer any patient is to adjust him physically, advise him nutritionally and help him to understand himself emotionally, so that he can cope with all the organismic and environmental influences, and also learn to take hereditary influences in his stride. The organism then "cures" itself, for to be "normal" is the inevitable goal of all its energies.

It is understandable that the founder of chiropractic had to emphasize that it was a separate and unique new art of healing. In terms of consequences, D. D. Palmer was definitely right in severing chiropractic sharply from all of his former types of therapies such as mesmerism and suggestion (in the same way that Freud divorced himself from hypnotism).

Any inventor or discoverer has to be single-minded in his devotion. He must give all his attention to his discovery and it must not be diverted. To establish chiropractic, Palmer had to circumscribe it into an apparently small one-idea concept. When he said that the cause of disease is subluxated vertebrae he was largely right in basic theory. As the discipline grew and developed that conception broadened, and now all schools of thought in chiropractic accept that there is seldom only one single cause or cure for the ills of man.

If one makes an extended analysis or evaluation of the basic principle of chiropractic as authoritatively expressed by Willard Carver, its promulgator, "Any interference with the receipt, transmission, or application of life force causes all functional abnormality known as disease," one cannot avoid the conclusion that this fundamental tenet is so comprehensive that it plainly includes anatomical distortions, chemical disequilibrium, emotional disturbances, and all sorts of social and environmental stress among the original causative factors in disease.

This broader concept does not negate the initial chiropractic principle in the least. The removal of anatomic distortion, or the elimination of adverse transmissions of nerve impulses or neuromuscular tension, breaks the vicious circle of the interplay between emotional stress and somatic stress, and can be of value in re-establishing proper physiological balance as well as contributing toward normal psychological functioning. It must also be remembered that the removal of anatomical distortion is often hindered because of the emotional involvement which is constantly producing neuromuscular tension and spinal subluxations.

Dr. Guze recognized that it is clearly within the chiropractor's realm to use the apparently more intangible elementary psychological means in the removal or control of adverse nerve interference or irritation. He was cognizant of the fact that the disciples of Freud and Palmer, and the practitioners of movements derived from them have carried on a "cold war" with each other for seventy-five years. Each group has gone its own independent way, sure that it alone was right and the other wrong. Yet in a larger perspective, each had but a part of the full or whole truth. Had the markings of real tolerance been more conspicuous in either school of thought, this insight would have emerged much sooner, to the benefit of all. For in the eyes of later competent and objective critics, both groups have made a definite constructive contribution towards the totality of mental and physical health. In the present decade and beyond, no inherent or artificial conflict need exist in the blending of modern psychotherapy with the broad premise of chiropractic.

It was Dr. Guze's hope that the psychotherapist should gain an understanding of chiropractic and how it can buttress psychotherapy in the mutual goal of advancing better mental health. Therefore, he was instrumental in suggesting to the American Academy of Psychotherapists that they discuss at their 1967 Educational Conference the topic of "Psychopathology and the Healing Systems." What follows are Dr. Guze's conversant remarks regarding chiropractic at the Conference referred to above.

* * *

THE PROBLEM of chiropractic is a very interesting one from a variety of standpoints. If I were going to give an extensive discussion of chiropractic this afternoon, I would discuss some of the sociological and anthropological aspects relating to the field. However, we have with us today a person who is much more competent in this area than I, I refer to Dr. Walter Wardwell of the University of Connecticut.

I am going to chart and to discuss the specific applications and relationships of chiropractic to psychotherapy. I will also touch very briefly on some of the things spoken about by Dr. Kimmel (see ch. 12, Ed.) and introduced into the literature previously by Dr. Herman S. Schwartz who is among our guests today.

I think one of the very important aspects of any healing system is the fact that it offers some kind of a philosophy direct or indirect, to the patient. I am happy that we have in our culture a variety of philosophies and that we have a variety of systems of healing. It is most probable that many of these systems have great underlying similarities.

One of the interesting facts in chiropractic which I have been studying for a number of years is the fact that it offers a kind of psychotherapy to, shall we say, the less sophisticated and less wealthy—those who are not able either for cultural or economic reasons to visit the psychoanalyst two or three times a week; and for those who develop the tensions, irritabilities, the discomforts and "dis-ease."

There is little question that of the 20,000 chiropractors in the U. S. all have served the community in this way, as well as in a variety of other ways. There is certain empirical data which we find chiropractors associated with. These are distinct from the standpoint of objective clinical observations.

We have made it our business to do this objective investigation. By this, I mean we have observed patients in treatment, we have followed their progress, we have examined them electrometrically and we have treated them in psychotherapy concurrently. One of the interesting things which relates not only to chiropractic, but to the general laying on of hands is the fact that the individual in most cases directly responds. There is a closing of the eyes and a general relaxation of musculature. What does this mean? Well, I'm not sure what it means, but the subjective reports of patients very frequently, are that they suddenly feel relaxed, or there is an easing of responsiveness. I have postulated or hypothesized that what happens at this time when hands are laid on, or when the tensed areas are touched or examined is that there is a kind of physical input to an "armoured body" (to borrow a term from

Wilhelm Reich). Thus the inner tension which closes up the organism from the outer world is somewhat dissolved, and we begin to have a possibility for the arousal of the nervous system.

I suppose that one of the points which is important and which Dr. Kimmel has touched upon is that the aspects of tension and armoring is a factor in alienation. As a physiologist I certainly do believe that the body which is ill, whether it's emotional or whether it is due to a bacterium or to any other invading pathogen, armours itself and develops a kind of alienation. Maybe this is what we mean by the development of tension. Muscular tension, where the body closes up, and the individual is then separated from the intruding world, the world which would perhaps stimulate him into a kind of reality of experience. This is certainly open to discussion.

There is considerable evidence that feedback from muscle tension results in a kind of armoring of the individual that resists contact with other individuals. Now it is very possible that the doctor-patient relationship itself in many cases dissolves this armoring. Maybe this is what we mean, to an extent, by the concept of relationship, or maybe it is a kind of transference. One should be indeed interested in the transference relating to someone's touching the individual or someone's maneuvering and dealing with the musculature and the muscular-skeletal system. The effects of movement, and the effects of changes in the vertebral relationships, are very interesting. We have found in examining many of our patients and patients of other practitioners, many pain and tension areas in various parts of the body. These pain and tension areas yield to neuromuscular intervention—by chiropractic. Or perhaps to other interventions.

The patient becomes much more pliable and much more expressive in terms of abreactive material, and I speak indeed as a psychotherapist and a physiologist. Now where there is a consistent blocking of musculature, the organism becomes a closed system. And, as we know the body as a closed system is not adequately functioning. Any healer whether he be a physician or a psychotherapist attempts in some way to make the body a more opened system. Certainly for the psychotherapist this becomes the problem of developing a relationship between the inner body, so to speak, and the outer world. Very often the favorable way of contact, touch or manipulation, and the chiropractic adjustment of areas of tension open the closed system.

I am not saying that this is the only way; it certainly is not. I do not believe there is an *only* way. I'm saying that it is an area which indeed we must investigate objectively. I would say as a psychotherapist who works with psychotics that it is important for the seriously disordered individual to open up to the contact with the outside world. Many of the systems of psychotherapy move towards that goal. In fact, I would say that in one way or another, all of the systems do. The evidence seems to show that during the process of adjusting or of manipulating the patient, he seems to become more susceptible to suggestion and more susceptible to a better relationship with whoever may be dealing with him at the time or whoever is relating to the situation. And perhaps even to whoever comes upon him thereafter. This is not merely a mystical concept; it is a provocative concept and an interesting situation to investigate.

There is a curious story which I would briefly like to call to your attention of the famous manipulative healer of the time of World War II. Felix Gerstein was the private physician to Heinrich Himmler. He was influential in many ways in saving thousands of people from destruction in the detention camps of the Nazi regime. Essentially, it seems that he got most of his favors during the time that he manipulated his Nazi patients.

We can hook up the chiropractic concept to certain concepts of psychotherapy. Perhaps I will have an opportunity to tell you more about this phase later on. Certainly there is a parallel between chiropractic and psychotherapy. It is noteworthy that Morris Fishbein, in a book written in 1930 on "fads, quackery & healing," included chiropractic, osteopathy and psychoanalysis among others. Chiropractic and psychoanalysis started from individual prophets so to speak. On the one hand Freud, and on the other hand Palmer. They developed concurrently, dealing somewhat with different sociocultural aspects, and with different milieus of our society. They spread into a whole variety of upshoots, many of whom contributed greatly to the Mother School. As you know Vienna was the "Fountain Head" for the psychoanalytic movement.

Now I would like to point out that what I am saying is not derogatory either to psychoanalysis or chiropractic. It is a comment on the reality of cults and cultism in the development of human thinking. It is a comment about the reality of the need of human beings for some means of intervention in their difficulties whether physical or emotional.

We certainly have increasing evidence of the relationship between posture and gravity and emotional states. Indeed, no less of a person than William James a long time ago (also about the time that chiropractic and psychoanalysis began) introduced the James-Lange Theory of emotions; the theory said that the posture of fear gives fear, and that when an individual is shocked into action, he first responds reflexly to the action. Then there is a secondary reaction to the organism which is a fear response or an anger response or a sex response as the case might be. In some cases there might sometimes be a vague response. There is no question about the fact that all these are pertinent to the total understanding of the individual. I am going to close our discussion by pointing out that this much maligned system of healing (chiropractic) certainly deserves investigation from thinking and scientific people, on all levels of the interdisciplinary world. I want to thank Dr. Kimmel and to thank you all.

CHAPTER 14

CHIROPRACTIC HEALING AS PSYCHOTHERAPY*

JEFFERSON L. SULZER, PH.D.

SINCE CHIROPRACTIC is the second largest healing profession in America it is surprising how little is known about it by practitioners of the other healing arts. The chiropractor has been stereotyped as a pseudo-professional healer, with a highly reductionistic theory of physical illness and a dubious course of treatment. He is understood to posit "pinched nerves" as a fundamental cause of a variety of ailments, and to treat a multitude of complaints by manual manipulation of the spine. Like most stereotypes this one contains an element of truth, but unfortunately it has led many people concerned with healing to dismiss the chiropractic approach unquestioningly, and without certain fruitful insights.

Chiropractic got its start in 1895 from D. D. Palmer, a grocer from Davenport, Iowa, who had practiced "magnetic healing" for ten years. Chiropractic was born when Palmer apparently cured a case of deafness by "reducing a spinal subluxation." Briefly, having noticed that his deaf janitor had a lump on his back, he massaged and kneaded it; later the janitor regained his hearing. Unhampered by the knowledge that the auditory nerve does not enter the spine, Palmer felt he had made a great discovery. Shortly thereafter he and a lawyer friend, Willard Carver, opened the first chiropractic school in Oklahoma City, offering a short course to all who could pay the tuition fee, regardless of their educational background. From these humble beginnings, chiropractic medicine expanded to become the second largest healing profession (according to the *Congressional Record* of February 8, 1962). The level of training is still below that required of medical students, but many states now require chiropractors and M.D.s to pass the same basic science exams before they are licensed. Courses offered in chiropractic colleges include anatomy, embryology and histology, physiology, biochemistry, pathology and bacteriology, in addition to extensive training in chiropractic diagnosis and treatment.

A popular chiropractic magazine (*Healthways,* May 1962) states that

* The original version of this paper was presented at the Southeastern Psychological Association, Miami Beach, Florida, April, 1963. Printed in *Psychotherapy,* 1965, Vol. 2 Number I. Published by University of Chicago. Eugene T. Gendlin Ph.D. Editor.

Dr. Sulzer is in no way connected with the Chiropractic profession. Dr. Sulzer is head of the Psychology Department of Newcomb College, Tulane University, New Orleans, Louisiana.

600 insurance companies recognize claims for services rendered by D.C.s (Doctors of Chiropractic); all federal agencies accept sick leave certificates signed by chiropractors; the Kerr-Mills Act provides for payment for their services to the aged.

CHIROPRACTIC THEORY

The popular conception of chiropractic is that it involves manipulating the spine. Official definitions of chiropractic (Florida Chiropractic Laws, Section 12, A) confirm this idea. Chiropractic is defined as a "non-combative principle and practice consisting of the science of adjustment, manipulation and treatment of the human body in which vertebral subluxations and other malpositions, articulations and structures that are exerting pressure upon the nerves and thus interfering with the normal transmission of vital energy from the brain to organs, tissues and cells of the body, thereby causing disease, are adjusted, manipulated and treated to their normal position, thereby restoring the normal flow of vital nervous energy which produces normal function and consequent health."

In this clumsy legal definition the naive reductionism of chiropractic's founder may be discerned. Although this is a correct summary of the "official" theory of disease, chiropractors actually apply a wider range of principles derived from dietetics, physiotherapy, neurology, and physiology. This enlargement of chiropractic has become necessary as an increasing variety of somatic complaints are treated. But an undetermined proportion of patients come with emotional problems, and although there is no official theory of mental illness, several recurring emphases may be drawn from articles which have appeared in chiropractic publications.

EMOTIONAL PROBLEMS

In contrast to some psychosomatic theories which stress the "power of mind over body," chiropractic tends to emphasize the importance of body in determining mental and emotional states. Herman S. Schwartz D.C. (1962), writes that chiropractic proceeds ". . . on the concept that the pattern of much emotional illness originates from, and is perpetuated by, nerve irritations caused by structural disrelation. When nerve excitations are perpetuated by hidden nerve irritations the patient may present a constellation of mental syndromes as though stemming only from an emotional or environmental cause" (p. 5). Although this somatic emphasis reflects the fundamental orientation of the chiropractic approach to mental illness it may take on more mentalistic overtones as it is extended. G. T. Crawford (1962), in an article on the effect of posture of personality, takes an interactionist stand. "Posture reflects personality, and the development of posture improves personality." Nevertheless, he places considerable responsibility on the patient as a determining agent. "Health is not the result of succumbing to environment. Health is the controlling of environment." "You either control your environment or your environment controls you" (p. 3). This emphasis on the will, which is far removed from the position of the somatic determinist, provides an important aspect of chiropractic counseling. These three principles, somatic, will power, and body-will interaction, occur in a variety of blends, often under the concept *equilibrium*. F. B. Hamilton (1962) and others suggest various ways in which equilibrium (of body and mind) is related to health, e.g., resistance to stress and disease, lack of anxiety and worrying, and individual autonomy in regard to social forces.

The therapeutic goals of chiropractic medicine have been stated by Paul Mendy (1962, p. 5), who summarizes these aims as follows:

1. Specific adjustive therapy to achieve normal nerve function.
2. Nutrition and dietary guidance to restore normal chemical balance in the body.
3. Rehabilitation procedures to help restore normal physiological functions of the body.
4. Psychosomatic counseling to help the patient achieve a proper balance between the mental, emotional, physiological and mechanical aspects of his person.

In chiropractic treatment symptoms are identified by questioning the patient, encouraging him to mention anything he considers relevant. The practitioner then examines the patient, frequently using x-rays, and makes his diagnosis. If the symptoms and physical examination indicate that physical causes are primarily involved (e.g., spinal subluxations, asymmetry of body or limbs, etc.), treatment will consist mainly of manipulation and realignment. It may also include correction of posture and other deficiency factors, to reduce the probability of recurrence and to improve the patient's general health.

If the patient's complaint is felt to have a psychosomatic or emotional basis, he may be referred to a D.C. who specializes in this area. In such a case the time devoted to identification of symptoms may be extended so that a larger part of each visit is spent "talking it out." As part of the diagnosis the patient is given technical explanations centering around the role of stress, of postural defects and of psychosomatic factors, and he may also be offered psychological encouragement on a non-technical supportive basis, in keeping with his level of sophistication. Treatment and rehabilitation phases may show overlapping. Some manipulation and massage may be used to reduce tension and aid the patient in establishing and maintaining good body tonus, posture, and affective state. This direct treatment may be supplemented with a course of exercises, diet and mental health practices which he is to follow at home. He is advised to avoid excessive worry and stress and to try to maintain an outward orientation, avoiding lengthy periods of introspection. In most emotional cases periodic visits are continued so that the practitioner can reduce any tension or anxiety which may have built up and encourage the patient in the continuation of exercises and other prescribed courses of action. It is likely that the homework assignments tend to maintain the relationship between the patient and the D.C. between office visits, and also give the patient a greater sense of participation in the treatment and a feeling of more responsibility for his own recovery.

THERAPEUTIC CHANGE

Official chiropractic theory has little to say about psychological processes going on within the patient which may account for therapeutic change. Without engaging in too much speculation we may suggest several likely possibilities by drawing from articles by D.C.s and accounts of patient informants. First, the patient achieves an understanding of the nature of chiropractic treatment and of the role of psychological and somatic factors in producing physical and emotional illness. This information provides a frame of reference within which he can interpret future experiences. Second, the patient usually feels that he has established a friendly relationship with the practitioner in which he gains confidence in the practitioner's skill and enjoys a feeling of hope for a cure. Third, the physical manipulation, massage and exercise tend to produce feelings of physical well-being and general optimism. It also seems likely that the physical contact with the practitioner acts to increase the personal element in the relationship. (Some chiropractic patients complain of the lack of warmth in treatment they had received from M.D.s, which may suggest one factor contributing to their choice of chiropractic treatment.) In this connection Braatoy (1954) suggests that in the relaxation therapies physical contact and subsequent relaxation may be unconsciously related to feelings the infant enjoyed when stroked and patted by an affectionate mother. Thus, aside from its possible beneficial effects on the neuro-muscular apparatus and the autonomic system, the physiotherapeutic approach may tend to evoke feelings of infantile comfort and security and, by association, imbue the practitioner-patient relationship with affectionate feelings which were originally directed toward the mother. These feelings, however vague, would tend to weaken the patient's reticence to talk over highly personal problems with the practitioner, and would thus tend to increase openness. Assuming that improved body tonus, release of tension, "talking it out," and openness are all conducive to therapeutic change, the occasions for interaction and increase in these factors afforded by chiropractic treatment may account for much of its apparent effectiveness.

IMPLICATIONS FOR PSYCHOTHERAPY AND RESEARCH

In spite of its somatic orientation, chiropractic, like psychotherapy, has as yet no clear-cut criteria for success and failure. Essentially, treatment is successful if the patient feels he is helped, if his hope in being cured is increased, if he considers his posture and outlook improved, and his resistance to stress and disease increased. Then instead of terminating the relationship he will continue to call upon the D.C. for help with subsequent problems. Failure is admitted only when the patient gives up his expectation of being helped and terminates chiropractic treatment. Generalizing from Frank's (1961) view of psychotherapy, one is tempted to say that therapy is unsuccessful if the patient loses his *belief* in chiropractic. It is also interesting to note that in chiropractic, as in most forms of psychotherapy, responsibility for failure is usually attributed to the patient.

There is virtually no published experimental or observational evidence on the efficacy of chiropractic treatment apart from the few case histories which appear in the *Chiropractic Journal.* Verbal testimonies of cures are readily given by satisfied chiropractic patients, but unfortunately there is no published collection of testimonials to draw from. In this context we might note an article which appeared in *Healthways* (March 1962, p. 23) titled "Don't Be Fooled by Quacks," in which a chiropractor writes: "The whole world of quackery is built on testimonials which are the easiest thing in the world to get or make up." One can only point to the rapid and sustained growth of chiropractic as evidence of the *apparent* success of its approach.

The beneficial effect of somatic therapy on mental and emotional states is taken for granted by a large number of practitioners and writers in the fields of medicine, physiotherapy, and physical education. Jacobson, for instance (1957), and Haugen, Dixon and Dickel (1958) are using *relaxation therapy* in the treatment of apparent neurotic and emotional complaints. Braatoy (1954) has suggested that relaxation technics may be of considerable benefit even in insight or catharsis therapy, particularly during the initial phases, in order to establish rapport more easily and to avoid frightening the patient with a deluge of repressed material bursting forth too early. He also points to the significance of postural attitudes and somatic tension as an indication of "blocked drives."

Therapists who are not catharsis-oriented might use relaxation procedures to reduce the severity of emotional disturbance so that therapy can proceed with a less handicapped, more reality-oriented patient. It may even prove useful to have some patients under the simultaneous care of orthodox "talking" psychotherapists and D.C.s or other somatic therapists. At present no data are available regarding the efficacy or feasibility of such a joint endeavor. There is, however, a growing body of literature which points to a strong relationship between somatic tension and various indices of anxiety and pathology. Plutchik (1954), after reviewing the literature, has suggested that freedom from muscular tension might well be used as a universal criterion of normalcy. It is possible that an index of this sort might be a useful predictor of mental illness or a dependable index of therapeutic improvement. In view of the considerable research effort expended in a search for valid and reliable criteria of health, it is to be hoped that somatic indices will also be subjected to a thorough and systematic investigation.

In addition to the potential applications of its somatic approach to psychotherapy, various features of chiropractic raise interesting questions for sociological and social psychological research. For example, little is known about the socioeconomic backgrounds of D.C.s and their patients, and how such variables as social class, status and general education level may relate to the selection of chiropractors as a source of therapy or the effectiveness of their method.

The foregoing paper is unable to offer more than a brief glance at the chiropractic approach to healing. The extreme paucity of library materials on this topic may also have contributed to inaccuracies or oversimplifications. The writer's purpose will be achieved if the paper awakens investigative interest in the chiropractic approach. The tremendous growth and popularity of chiropractic indicate that it is worthy of serious study by social scientists and members of other healing professions.

REFERENCES

Braatoy, T. *Fundamentals of psychoanalytic technique.* New York: Wiley, 1954.

Crawford, G. T. "How to Improve Your Posture," *Healthways* (1962), 16 (12): 3–6.

"Don't be fooled by quacks." *Healthways* (1962), 16 (10).

Doyle, Kathleen C. *Science vs. Chiropractic.* New York: Public Affairs Committee, 1953.

Flack, M. W. "How to avoid getting ulcers," *Healthways* (1962), 16:10.

Florida Chiropractic Law, Florida Legal Document, 1951.

Frank, J. D. *Persuasion and Healing.* Baltimore: Johns Hopkins Press, 1961.

Hamilton, F. B. "Your road to health may be a quarter of an inch away," *Healthways* (1962), 16 (10).

Haugen, G. B., Dixon, H. W., & Dickel, H. A. *A therapy for Anxiety Tension Reactions.* New York: Macmillan, 1958.

Jacobson, E. *You Must Relax.* New York: McGraw-Hill, 1957.

McClusky, T. *Your Health and Chiropractic.* New York: Pyramid Books, 1962.

Mendy, P. "What is a Chiropractor?" *Healthways* (1962), 16 (9).

Plutchik, R. "The role of muscular tension in maladjustment," *J. Gen. Psychol.* (1954), 50:45.

Schwartz, H. S. "If mental illness strikes," *Healthways* (1962), 17 (1).

Verner, J. R. "The science and logic of chiropractic." Published by Dr. P. J. Cerasoli, 192 31 St., Brooklyn 32, N.Y., 1956, 8 ed.

CHAPTER **15**

THE PSYCHOTHERAPEUTIC EXPERIENCE OF CHIROPRACTIC

HERMAN S. SCHWARTZ, D.C.

INTRODUCTION

HERBERT J. VEAR, D.C.

While chiropractic does not purport to be a form of psychotherapy, nevertheless the psychotherapeutic benefits that have been realized through its application have been notable. The psychology inherent in chiropractic has seldom been explored in our literature. We have often overlooked the fact that, in our unique structural adjustments (aside from its physiological benefits), there are subtle but potent emotional values, which are meaningful and effective to the patient.

An increasing awareness is taking place among mental health specialists that neuromuscular irritations magnify latent mental conflicts which may be the predisposing background of mental and emotional illness.

The doctor of chiropractic diagnoses-analyses the distressed patient and often finds a structural cause for his malaise. While he has in his armamentarium diagnostic tools and therapeutic modalities, he basically depends upon his sense of touch and observation and the fine art of adjusting the human being. The adjustment releases or disperses the neuromuscular irritations and tensions. This indirectly but effectively impresses the patient that here is a doctor who not only can locate some of the causes for his malady, but may give him a measure of immediate relief without any adverse reactions or after-effects.

The chiropractic profession has been accused of claiming too much for its therapy. The fact of the matter is that we have undervalued chiropractic for mental health. The favorable results that we obtain in this field are usually completely unpremeditated and unexpected. Often busy practitioners place all their emphasis upon the correction of the body's distortions, and they do not anticipate positive psychotherapeutic results from their work. This chapter by Schwartz therefore will be enlightening not only to our students and practitioners, but to the concerned public as well.

The emotionally distressed patient reads into the chiropractor's approach of palpation and adjustment a psychological significance. He usually experi-

ences relief from his organismic distress, and at the same time becomes aware of the doctor's empathy and concern for his well-being.

In recent years, the vast proliferation and diffusion of psychological knowledge concerning mental health, complimented by a deeper understanding of the nature of chiropractic itself, has made the doctor of chiropractic cognizant of the role which he can assume in the alleviation of emotional illness, especially when due to spinal subluxations.

* * *

"Every physiotherapist and osteopath receives confessions and more or less intimate information during treatment. Nobody seems to know that this is because *of the treatment, because this aspect is not included in the theory of the manipulations."*

—TRYGVE BRAATOY *

CHIROPRACTIC HISTORY is replete with incidents of recovery from various phases of mental illness. The structural and neurophysiological basis for this phenomenon has already been explored in several of the previous chapters. Before we focus our attention on the distinct psychotherapeutic effect of chiropractic, we must emphatically state that the results chiropractic obtains are primarily due to the neuromuscular structural changes that the adjustment produces, and that the psychology inherent in chiropractic is only a contributory factor.

Let us recall that this basic approach to emotional distress rests upon the awareness that the individual is a complete psychophysiological whole and that unitary reactions govern health as well as illness. Adverse stimuli stemming from the internal or external environment, usually react specifically upon that part of the organism which is already enervated. They manifest themselves as neuromuscular and articular tensions, or frequently in abnormal behavior. The chiropractic muscular and skeletal adjustings definitely tend to release these tensions and noxious nerve cycles of visceral and somatic irritations. This often leads to favorably influencing physical and emotional distress.

Braatoy (P. 157) observed how Paul Roland applied passive movements to the musculature of the neck and face of a chronic catatonic schizophrenic at a Veteran's Hospital in Topeka, Kansas, and obtained remarkable therapeutic results. Braatoy also relates that when a patient in his private psychoanalytic practice was blocked by tension which inhibited his verbal expressions he used ". . . passive movements and concentrates on local muscular tension, I try to help the patient to relax and at the same time release his breathing." (Page 144)

Braatoy's findings substantiate the value of one of the phases of chiropractic care for emotional disturbances, which its practitioners have relied

* Braatoy, Trygve, *Fundamentals of Psychoanalytic Technique,* John Wiley, New York, 1954, p. 144.

upon since the very early days of their practice. Furthermore, Braatoy practically offers an explanation for the effectiveness of musculo-skeletal manipulations. He also substantiates much of the neurophysiological data concerning chiropractic for mental health.

THE DOCTOR-PATIENT RELATIONSHIP

There are inherent in chiropractic care distinct psychological implications which need to be brought into focus. The peculiar events associated with the unique chiropractor-patient relationship have psychological value in their own rights as they help to meet certain basic needs of the emotionally distressed individual.

Let us attempt to understand the patient's frame of mind, when he is coping with persistent organismic symptoms that may have defied previous diagnosis and treatment. Consider the experiences which he may have already undergone: medication, tranquilizers and perhaps shock therapy. He is discouraged and/or depressed, and may think of his continued pain and distress as symptoms of emotional illness. The patient finally decides, after a great deal of hesitation and desperation, to visit the chiropractor.

The first ray of hope that the patient sees may come not only from what the doctor says, but from the effect of what he does. The chiropractor has at his disposal diagnostic procedures and the unique ability to discover, through his specialized art of palpation, the previously unrecognized sensitive areas in the vertebral column, and in the related paraspinal tissues, which may account for his distress. A distinguishing feature of the spinal palpation procedure is that the chiropractor does not usually depend upon the patient telling him where the pain and tenderness is.

The patient is impressed. He may never have undergone a thorough spinal examination of this sort before. He knows that the doctor has found areas of tenderness and irritation in his body that all others have overlooked. The chiropractor continues with his examination and elicits the patient's history; he makes orthopedic and neurological tests, and if necessary, additional radiologic and/or clinical laboratory tests to determine the factors producing the syndromes. He then starts his unique procedure of adjusting the anatomical distortions.

Now let us further consider what the unique approach of chiropractic spinal palpation means to such a patient. From the moment the chiropractor places his calm, relaxed hands upon the patient's neck or shoulders, he senses that he has the attention of a doctor who cares. Every human being has an inborn need for kindness and empathy, especially when ill. From the time of his birth he wants to be cared for, needs protection, needs to feel that he is in a favorable environment. For the infant, affection in various forms is as necessary as food. Ribble (1943), Rule (1967) and Montagu (1957) have shown that an infant can thrive on even a minimum diet, but deprived of loving care, not even the finest conceivable food regimen prevents the infant from becoming ill and he may even die as the result of neglect. The adult, when in mental distress, no less than the infant, needs kind and concerned attention; it is a need that is never outgrown. Wm. McPeak of the Ford Foundation (1960) recognizes this need, in his appeal to the general practitioner to listen to, "The Small Frantic Voice of the Patient."

Due to the patient's low point of toleration to life's stress, he is usually in a disoriented mental state and frequently reacts to stresses in a childlike manner. Chronologically he may be old, physiologically he may be well developed, intellectually he may be a giant, but emotionally his attitude toward life's problems is definitely childish. He feels either weak, anxious, confused, guilty, rejected, frustrated, or is overdemanding. He may be faced with situations which to him seem threatening or which he cannot control. In addition he usually has a very poor image of himself. He may consider himself unworthy of the concerned attention of the doctor. When he finds himself under the care of a humane and competent D.C. who really cares for him, that situation alone may tend to raise his self-esteem and become a force toward his recovery. Possibly for the first time in his adult life the patient perceives that here is a doctor who considers him to be worthwhile; he realizes that the chiropractor is sincere and ready to help him.

When the doctor allows his relaxed hand to rest upon the patient's upper thoracic region for a few moments, it induces relaxation in an important area of the respiratory muscles with the result that the nervous patient's tense, alert, attentive, and restricted breathing is usually eased. Furthermore, this primary contact conveys to the patient much more than words: a friendly, protective, empathic, as well as comforting attitude. Then the palpation and examination can be more accurate, fear of the manipulation is lessened, and the adjustment produces favorable effects.

THE EMOTIONAL EFFECT OF STRUCTURAL DISTORTIONS

It is suggested that the vertebral subluxation itself cannot be considered a pure and simple anatomical distortion—the spine's intimate relationship to the nervous system makes the subluxation a potentially primary source of organismic nerve irritation. We thus postulate that the spinal subluxation, when it persists and especially when the patient superimposes upon it adverse emotions, may become a potential source of psychosomatic distress, or psychopathology.

The following sequence of experiences usually occurs to those who have sustained a whiplash or any other injury which caused a structural maladjustment of a spinal area or to it's adjacent structures.

1. It usually becomes more severe as the nerve irritation increases.
2. It is intensified as a result of fear, worry, and anxiety about the pain or its consequences.

3. As the pain persists, the patient's worry is magnified by the previous doctor's "assurance" that there is nothing to be concerned about.
4. Added inconvenience and pain may persist, and the conventional therapeutic reassurance that there is no pathology to account for it because the X-ray and other tests are negative, may serve as the basis for increased fear and anxiety.
5. Clarity and vigor of mental functions are reduced by palliative narcosis—tranquilizers.
6. The initial nerve irritations, or other soft tissue injury, often started by a physical traumatic experience, when not corrected, may start a "chain-reaction" of total mental and physical stress, which can lead to severe emotional maladjustment.

(For further data on whiplash complications, see Kimmel, Ch. 12.)

THE CHIROPRACTIC ADJUSTMENT

The patient's supine position, the doctor's various gentle maneuvers which he may execute to relax the superficial spinal muscles, all tend to set the stage for a successful and easy adjustment. In this connection, it is interesting to speculate that the chiropractic adjustment, in essence, may evoke what may be considered to be the primary and basic biological reflex of life, the stretch (myotactic) reflex. The patient starts to become more active and alert.

The dynamic chiropractic thrust can be considered as a specifically planned stretch Schwartz (1959), Maigne (1972), of the constricted holding elements of the articulations. It has various homeostatic influences upon the person, depending upon which particular functions are below par. Physiologically the spinal adjustment can alter the mental state by lessening nerve cell fatigue (see Caspersson), raising the pain threshold, increasing circulation, removing neuromuscular tensions, and increasing the oxygen supply to the brain as the result of the release of the muscles of respiration.

The controlled adjustive thrust may perform psychological functions as well. It may lessen noxious neural patterns and help to resolve or diminish troublesome complexes. This in turn frequently tends to release a flood of forgotten memories of drive and earlier hopes of achievement. There can be a new influx into the patient's consciousness of energies long passive which may awaken his sense of well-being and revive his hopes and ambitions. He is now more apt to make meaningful and appropriate decisions about his problems or goals. He senses that his chances of gaining and maintaining better physical and mental health are greatly augmented. The adjustment can pave the way for his more harmonious and better integrated posture and structural behavior. The foregoing accomplishments cannot always be obtained or maintained if there is overbearing mental distress of long standing. But it does hold true for those patients whose adverse emotions are primarily due to neuromusculo-skeletal tensions (spinal subluxations).

Beginning with a subluxated vertebra, or other physical trauma, noxious neural irritations arise, then that person may lose some of his emotional controls. One of these conditions may occur when the person uses a subluxation as an "alibi" or excuse to run away from life's difficulties. He may say "I would if I could, but I can't . . . because of my backache (or headache, etc.)" Here we have a concurrent physical and mental disturbance with the former as cause and the latter unwholesome attitude as effect.

Often the reverse holds, that is, the pain serves to feed the need for overprotection, self-pity, projection, and other unhealthy demands of a weakened ego. This is not to suggest that *all* brooding or depressed moods are ways of capitalizing advantageously upon specific physical hurts since they can also be reactions to unfavorable environmental pressures like domestic, business, social, political troubles, or emotional conflicts.

Every experienced practitioner encounters patients who, just as soon as their nerve irritations are ameliorated by the chiropractic adjusting, may express their attitudinal reorientation to the shocks of existence in the form of casual philosophizing: "You know, doctor, I now realize we all must take the good with the bad in life." One can hardly secure more persuasive evidence of the power of the chiropractic adjustment in its effect of relaxing the patient easily and quickly. The doctor of chiropractic premises his efforts upon the solid principle that there can be a greater easing of disturbed emotions when there is improvement in the ailing body. When a person is free from physical stress, he can rely upon his own thinking and better accommodate to unsatisfactory life situations.

THE EFFECT ON RELAXATION

Mental distress in a cyclical manner reacts adversely upon the body and can initiate, prolong or increase neuromuscular tension and spinal subluxations, and deepen their noxious effect upon the organism. Chiropractic disrupts the vicious cycle of reflex irritation and thus can relieve emotional tensions and induce relaxation.

Jacobson (Ed., 1967), the classic authority in this field, and now many mental health specialists, have reported about patients who recovered from psychosomatic or "psychoneurotic" disorders after learning to relax their bodies thoroughly. His recent anthology, "Tension in Medicine," is a symposium on the subject of relaxation to which 10 behavioral scientists (7 of whom are psychiatrists or psychoanalysts) have contributed. Their researches demonstrate unmistakably the parallelism between psychic events and tension states. One of them, Kendall, a psychoanalyst, cites a number of patients in which psychoanalysis had failed, but which responded exceedingly well (to the point of total recovery) to a supervised program of relaxation training.

This field of investigation has evoked so much interest on the part of psychiatrists that a number of them have abandoned conventional psychiatric methods. Among them, three of the more prominent are Haugen, Dixon, and

Dickel (1960). They prescribe the appropriate exercises that their nurses or attendants supervise. They say:

> "We can handle comfortably in our offices many patients who formerly would immediately have been hospitalized for shock therapy. We can't see now how we ever managed to get along without the relaxation procedure . . . in spite of the decreased demand on our time, we have more dramatic results, and the results last longer."

The success obtained by these psychotherapists in applying the relaxation concept is verification of the basic principles of chiropractic for nervous and mental illnesses. However the chiropractic technique is far different and more efficient. Generally speaking, the dynamic thrust, given by the chiropractor after adequate preparatory measures have been taken, can often effect the transformation from a state of tension to one of relaxation in a matter of a few minutes. The chiropractic approach for mental health is now better understood and appreciated by some psychiatrists and psychologists because of their experience with relaxation, body manipulation, and posture control (see Ch. 13).

Chiropractors specifically promote freedom from neuromuscular tension because they can detect and remove specific spinal subluxations, muscular and fascial constrictions, with their resultant tensions. As long as this premise rests on a reasonable belief founded in both a priori logic and empirical evidence that the tendency to develop persistent emotional stress may be traceable, on the physiological side, to actual musculo-skeletal distortion, chiropractic can be useful as an alleviating as well as a definitively effective therapy.

SEGMENTAL ARCHITECTURAL CORRECTION OF POSTURE

The psychological impact of chiropractic on posture is evident upon close study. The evaluation and extension of structural manipulative efforts in the adjustment of the neuromuscular skeletal frame basically influences posture of the individual. With the correction of his posture, and the lessening of his nerve irritations, there is the possibility that his attitudes towards himself, others, and the vicissitudes of life may become more realistic.

Adverse emotions contribute to poor posture, and adverse posture can and frequently does influence the patient's psychological attitudes (Lowen, 1958, 1967).

Extensive experimentation by Nina Bull (1951) from 1947–1951 at the Psychiatric Institute of New York suggested that the expression of emotions depends upon physical posture. She first conditioned persons to assume physical attitudes of depression, anger, fear, joy, or triumph, they then experienced the emotions and feelings appropriate to that given posture. These scientific findings merely verify everyday experiences that, due to constant low-grade hidden nerve irritations, a usually calm human being may adopt uncalled-for, derogatory, destructive attitudes, panic or anxiety syndromes.

Doctors of chiropractic have been aware of the importance of posture beginning with Willard Carver's exposition of the "typical, complex, opposed rotational scoliosis" (1915). (See Levine, Ch. 8.) This gross prevalent distortion can lay the basis for poor posture. The correction of posture has its influence upon mental health; and a correct mental attitude reveals itself in one's posture. Thus, we apply the word "attitude" with equal emphasis to the position or arrangement of the body, as well as to the mental outlook. The significance of these observations is sometimes overlooked by those who become too deeply immersed in a specific therapy. Rational appraisal of everyday behavior must take in the interchangeable or reciprocating reactions that continually occur in the organism.

THE EFFECT ON FATIGUE

One of the most common and immediate effects of the chiropractic adjustment is the lessening of fatigue. People under stress usually complain that they tire easily or are always weary—which is understandable if their energy reserves are constantly dissipated in wasteful strain or adverse emotions. Indeed, the move from (1) anxiety to (2) fatigue to (3) loss of emotional control may be a standard sequence.

It is common knowledge that certain metabolites and aberrant blood chemicals, are conveyed via blood circulation and affect the nerve cells. The reduced threshold to irritability may arise from such chemical irritants, since it is obvious that the person reacts *more quickly and intensely to petty annoyances when fatigued than when he feels refreshed.* Stimuli that are barely noticed or swiftly absorbed when one is in "top" condition are felt as emotional or physical shocks when one is low. An appeal to universal experience on this point is sound.

Consider, e.g., the disappearance of the chromatin filaments in Nissl bodies of the nerve cells which serves as a sign that an epileptic attack is coming, Boyd (1951, p. 663), Morgan (1950, p. 34). Or note the probably related fact that these same Nissl bodies tend to vanish during extreme fatigue. Positive and inescapable *organic* transformations of such magnitude necessarily affect behavior in at least some respect. The corrective or relieving role of chiropractic then inevitably arises from the powers of the adjustments to (1) remove local or remote nerve irritation, (2) increase bodily elimination, (3) influence blood circulation, (4) release regional or generalized muscular tension. Since chiropractic procedures tend to remove or reduce the effects of fatigue, it gives the central nervous system a chance to recover its tone and freshness. When that occurs, the nervousness evoked by excessive weariness is lessened and the emotional operations are brought more completely under control of the reasoning processes—a result invariably beneficial to all inner awareness and outer behavior.

Caspersson (1948) was able to demonstrate a profound chemical difference between single living cells taken from the nervous system of a person who is tired as compared with those from one who is rested. He noted that "when too much cytoplasmic protein is being produced, or too little, the existence or deficiency multiplied by the number of similar cells also functioning incorrectly results in the symptoms of illness. IT MAY BE A MENTAL OR PHYSICAL AILMENT." Thus there is sufficient evidence that fatigue causes some biological changes in the brain, and it shows up in a change in protein metabolism. The causes of fatigue can come from many sources. But it can be postulated that the chiropractic adjustment quickly lessens its effect. When fatigue is diminished, tension lessens.

WHAT TENSION MEANS

It must not be presumed that "tension" as such is either an inherently undesirable or pathological state of the organism. Actually, it would be impossible for any living creature to respond to any stimulus, i.e., to engage in the most limited experience, without some tension being present. What distinguishes normal from abnormal tension is not solely the difference between *pleasant* and unpleasant strain, but also the contrast between *serviceable* and inappropriate reaction patterns. Some tension occurs in all problem-solving whether that be as minor as computing the sales tax on a purchase or as major as planning a crucial experiment to test an important hypothesis. The kind of tension that is potentially harmful occurs when the autonomic nervous system responds in a total fashion to an emergency—and then fails to subside because the person does not permit the "emergency" to come to an obvious end. (For a full exposition of the relation of tension to maladjustment, see Plutchik, Ch. 7.)

The residual tension discharges eventually into the final effectors—the glands and muscle fibers which may set up psychosomatic reactions. The chiropractic adjustment, by restoring structures to their normal relationships, abolishes habitual motor nerve tensions linked with long-standing mental conflicts. These would eventually produce semi-permanent fascial thickening and shortening in areas where such changes are detrimental to over-all body efficiency. Perseveration from a "winding-base" of stress can be interrupted, thus allowing a fresh start. Critical examination of the concept that disease can stem from anatomical distortions sustains its essential correctness.

The implications of chiropractic for psychological distress, as illustrated here, is historically an evolution along the lines originally envisioned and projected by Willard Carver, D.C. (1915, 1920). It synthesizes the now dominant tradition in the profession with the solid advances of recent physiological psychology to constitute the "link of union" joining the apparent intangible realities of nerve energy, thought, and emotion with a comprehensive conception of the physical frame of man.

Although the present discussion is chiefly centered on the milder cases usually classified as "neurosis," an extension of the logic of this position can apply to more serious disorders. However, the practitioner is strongly cautioned to exercise extraordinary care and prudence when he encounters severely disturbed individuals. In handling these patients, if the problem they present lies outside the doctor's personally tested and socially demonstrated area of competence, he should make referrals freely or enlist the cooperation of qualified and humane psychologists or psychiatrists. (For some interesting examples of how this can be effectively instituted, see Chapter 22.)

The number of simple everyday examples of elementary organic causes or correlates of the standard brand of an emotional upset may be easily understood by personal experiences. Anyone who has had a cinder in the eye, suffered from tight shoes, been made irritable by poorly-fitted clothes or itchy fabrics, or temporarily blocked in emptying a full bladder will recognize that emotional tension of some sort lasts as long as the physical disturbance of the body's equilibrium endures. Anything, therefore, which the organism appraises as a *threat* to its well-being, from a passing minor discomfort to a grim constant peril, is a potential source of an emotional upset. It is sheer folly not to recognize that literally "upsetting" visceral or somatic imbalance, evanescent or persistent, probably may be, and usually is created by every stimulus which the individual recognizes as a menace to his integrity or as an insuperable barrier to some cherished goal. These dangers may either be identified as purely local or segmental, in which case the nervous reaction is roughly proportionate to the importance of the area as judged by the patient; more often, it is total and "organismic" in nature, i.e., imperiling the *entire* psychophysical system in some respect, in which case the *whole* nervous system may be thrown into different degrees of confusion. That intense fear directly harms the nervous system is just as true as that overexposure to a July sun burns a blonde skin; indeed both leave their sufferers feeling "raw." The fact that people "spontaneously recover" after a lapse of time does not do away with the inescapable fact that they have been physically hurt in the first place. Whether the damage is temporary or permanent, the *fact* of tissue injury is clear.

This chapter cannot be ended without a word regarding the phenomenon of suggestion, which is a factor in all kinds of therapy. Chiropractic is not an exception. Every patient under any doctor's care is influenced to some degree by suggestion or autosuggestion.

However, we posit that the improvement the patient experiences under chiropractic adjustments stems chiefly from the removal or alleviation of the neuromusculo-skeletal traumatic distortions (subluxations). This experience does not depend upon what the doctor of chiropractic says, but on what he does, and what effect the spinal adjustments have upon the tissues which had been enervated, irritated, or distorted by the subluxation. Similarly, the feeling that the patient experiences from the extraction of an infected tooth or abdominal obstruction does not depend on the positive suggestion of the dentist or surgeon. Thus, the feeling of well-being from the chiropractic adjustment is the organism's response, rather than the patient's or doctor's wishful or hopeful thinking.

The above observations are not intended to underevaluate the emotional interaction which is often a factor in the patient's recovery; the necessity of the doctor's concerned and empathic listening; his timely well formulated thoughtful words of counsel; nor the essential formuli for healthful living.

REFERENCES

Braatoy, Trygve. *Fundamentals of Psychoanalytic Technique.* New York: John Wiley (1954), p. 144.

Boyd, W. *The Pathology of Internal Diseases.* Philadelphia: Lea & Febiger (1951), p. 663.

Bull, Nina. "The Attitude Theory of Emotion," *Nervous and Mental Disease Monographs* (New York, 1951).

Carver, Willard. *Chiropractic Analysis.* Oklahoma City, Oklahoma: Carver Chiropractic College, 1915.

Carver, Willard. *Psycho-Bio-Physiology.* Oklahoma City, Oklahoma: Carver Chiropractic College, 1920.

Caspersson, T. O. *Cell Growth and Cell Function.* New York: W. W. Norton & Co., Inc. 1950.

Haugen, Gerhard B., Dixon, Henry H., Dickel, Herman A. *A Therapy for Anxiety Reactions.* Macmillan Co., 1960.

Jacobson, Edmund. *Progressive Relaxation.* Chicago: The University of Chicago Press, 1929.

Jacobson, E. *Anxiety and Tension Control.* Phila.: J. B. Lippincott, 1964.

Jacobson, Edmund. *Tension in Medicine.* 1967.

Lowen, Alexander. *Physical Dynamics of Character Structure.* New York: Grune & Stratton, 1958.

Lowen, Alexander. *The Betrayal of the Body.* New York: Macmillan Co., 1963.

Maigne, Robert. *A New Approach to Vertebral Manipulation.* Springfield, Ill.: C. C. Thomas, 1972.

McPeak, William. "The Small Frantic Voice of the Patient," *Postgraduate Medicine* (Jan. 1960).

Mantagu, Ashley M. F. *Anthropology and Human Nature* (chap. 15). "The Mind of the Skin." Boston, Mass.: Porter Sargent Co., 1957.

Morgan, C. T. and Stellar, E. *Physiological Psychology.* New York: McGraw-Hill Book Co., Inc., 1950.

Ribble, Margaret A. *The Rights of Infants.* New York: Columbia University, 1943.

Rule, Colter. "A Theory of Human Behavior Based on Studies on Non-human Primates," *Perspectives in Biology and Medicine.* University of Chicago (1967), 10 (2).

SUPPLEMENTARY READINGS

Agras, W. Stewart (et al.). "Relaxation in Systematic Desensitization," *Archives of General Psychiatry* (vol. 25), December 1971.

Blum, Richard H. (et al.). *Doctor-Patient Relationship.* New York: McGraw-Hill, 1960.

Bull, Nina. *The Body and Its Mind.* New York: Las Americas, 1962.

Dubos, Rene. *Mirage of Health.* New York: Harper Bros., 1954.

Dunbar, Flanders. *Psychosomatic Diagnosis.* New York: Paul B. Hoeber, Inc.

Dunn, Floyd E., "Osteopathic Concepts in Psychiatry," *Journal of A.O.A.* (March 1950).

Ford, Donald H. and Urban, Hugh B. *Systems of Psychotherapy.* New York: John Wiley, 1963.

Gantt, William Andrew Horsley. *Physiological Bases of Psychiatry.* Illinois: Thomas Springfield, 1958.

Gellhorn, E. *Physiological Foundations of Neurology & Psychiatry.* Minneapolis: University of Minnesota, 1953.

Groddeck, W. George. *The Book of It.* New York: Vintage Books, 1949.

Harper, William David. *Anything Can Cause Anything.* W. D. Harper (1966), Box 384, Seabrook, Texas 77586.

Homewood, A. E. (1962)—*The Neurodynamics of the Vertebral Subluxation,* Canadian Memorial Chiropractic College, Toronto.

Kuntz, Albert. *Visceral Innervation and Its Relation to Personality.* Chas. C. Thomas, 1951.

Janov, Arthur. *The Anatomy of Mental Illness.* New York: Putnam & Sons, 1971.

Laing, R. D. and Esterson, A. *Sanity, Madness and the Family.* New York: Basic Books, 1971.

Maslow, A. H. and Mittlemann B. *Principles of Abnormal Psychology.* New York: Harper & Bros., 1941.

Maslow, A. H. *Motivation and Personality.* New York: Harper & Bros., 1954.

Muncie, Wendell. *Psychobiology and Psychiatry.* St. Louis: C. V. Nosby Co., 1948.

Rhodes, W. R. *The Race Between Sanity and Madness.* Fort Worth, Tex.: Privately Printed, 1971.

Roland, Paul. *Recovery from Schizophrenia,* Springfield, Ill.: C. C. Thomas, 1957.

Schwartz, Herman S. "Foundations of Chiropractic Psychosomatics," *Journal of N.C.A.* (June 1949), p. 12.

Schwartz, Herman S. "The Connection Between Nerves and Nervousness," *The Journal of the N.C.A.* (April 1949).

Schwartz, Herman S. "Practical Implications in Psychobiology in Chiropractic," *The Journal of the N.C.A.* (Sept. 1959), p. 71.

Selye, Hans. *The Stress of Life.* New York: McGraw-Hill, 1956.

Stainbrook, Edward. "Behavioral Biology in Medicine," *Psychiatry in Medicine* (1971).

Teitelbaum, H. A. *Psychosomatic Neurology,* New York: Grune & Stratton, 1964.

Thompson, L. Richard. *Foundations of Physiological Psychology:* New York: Harper & Row, 1967.

Verner, Robinson, J. *The Science and Logic of Chiropractic.* Privately Published, 1941.

Weiss, Edward and English, O. Spurgeon. *Psychosomatic Medicine.* Philadelphia, Pa.: W. B. Saunders Co., 1945.

Wenger, M. A. *Physiological Psychology.* New York: Henry Holt, 1956.

CHAPTER 16

AN ANALYSIS OF 350 EMOTIONALLY MALADJUSTED INDIVIDUALS UNDER CHIROPRACTIC CARE

GEORGE W. HARTMANN, PH.D.,*
HERMAN S. SCHWARTZ, D.C.

ALL MENTAL HEALTH DISCIPLINES are still trying to resolve the perplexing question how to positively and scientifically judge the effectiveness of their procedure that aids the emotionally distressed patient. Up to now, we can only rely upon the observations embodied in the final report of the Joint Commission on Mental Illness and Health (1961, p. 55)

> "Good results are discernible in how the patient thinks, feels and behaves—in the subjective conviction of the patient and of his doctor that he is better. These results then remain to be demonstrated to the patient's family and friends, since his continued improvement depends not only on his own behavior but on how others accept him—on his reacceptance as a member of human society."

BASIC ASSUMPTIONS

The National Committee on Psychology of the American Chiropractic Association formerly the N.C.A., developed a pilot study designed to investigate one phase of the problem of mental health. The main assumptions underlying this study may be itemized as follows:

1. It is probable that every chiropractor in the course of an ordinary year's activity deals with a number of patients (a) who either have been at some time in mental hospitals or (b) who would, under a different set of circumstances, seek or receive the attention of a psychiatrist.

2. We take for granted the average chiropractor's competence in applying manipulative therapy, but no one so far knows the degree to which psychotherapeutic techniques, if any, are also employed by him, or how successfully he uses them.

* Originally presented in part by the late Dr. Hartmann in the form of an address to members attending the annual convention of the National Chiropractic Association, Chicago, July 28, 1949. Published in the *NCA Journal of Chiropractic,* November 1949.

3. It is reasonable to believe that the scientific developments of the last generation, plus the recently accelerated educational upgrading of the profession have made most chiropractors aware, in some measure, of the contribution of the psychological factor to the total behavior exhibited by their clientele.

PROCEDURES

This study was designed to be a simple report of the main findings of the survey. The techniques employed in this study involved a community survey, using a mail questionnaire, as a fact-finding device. The mail questionnaire method leaves much to be desired; nonetheless it is often the only feasible procedure in a situation where one must choose between imperfect information or none at all.

A covering letter explaining the general nature of the survey and containing all the motivational appeals that could be packed into such restricted space was sent in successive mailing waves to various selected names of chiropractors in State and Regional directories of association members. The questions posed in the questionnaire are shown in table 1.

RESULTS

The percent return in some geographic areas reached about 20%, but for most "editions" of the questionnaire the rate was much smaller. Gradually, 350 cases were collected and tabulated. These represented chiropractic patients who also exhibited some kinds of mental illness in the judgment of the chiropractor, and in accordance with psychiatric diagnosis before the patient presented himself for chiropractic care.

Table I

CENSUS DATA OF POPULATION

	No.	*Category*	*Percent*
Age	22	Children	6.0
	26	Adolescents	8.0
	211	Military age (18–45)	60.0
	91	45 Years and older	26.0
Sex	194	Females	55.5
	156	Males	44.5
Marital Status	215	Married	61.0
	118	Single	34.0
	6	Divorced	2.0
	11	Widows and widowers	3.0

The experimentally-minded may ask (a) if those who answered constitute a truly random or representative sample or genuine cross-section of all persons actively practicing, and (b) if the cases they chose for transmittal to the research center were highly unusual. The only honest answer to both of these penetrating points is that we just don't know. One may reasonably suppose that the respondents were folks who were both somewhat more interested in, and possibly more informed about, the psychological overtone of their work, with the result that they found it easier to handle these cases. Likewise, it is not unreasonable to believe that in a free choice situation, chiropractors like other members of the human family—tend to recall and relay their "hits" rather than their "misses." Accepting both of these plausible interpretations, our survey data reflects chiropractic at its best rather than at its mid-level or worst. Obviously, even this rigorous self-criticism is not fatal, nor does it weaken the real value of the study, for it still clearly demonstrates what can be done under favorable conditions. It is one of the duties of a profession to try to carry on its functions under optimum circumstances.

With this long-winded background and preliminary caution, let us see what we may learn from first-hand inspections of this valuable group of 350 mentally disturbed patients who visited chiropractors. Some individuals find

Table II

OCCUPATIONS

No.	*Category*	*Percent*
119	Housewives	34.0
35	High school & college students	10.0
28	G. I.'s	8.0
21	Clerks	6.0
17	Mechanics	5.0
18	Farmers	5.0
8	Teachers	2.5
10	Storekeepers	3.5
8	Factory workers	2.5
2	Prizefighters	0.5
84	Miscellaneous	24.0

The occupations represented in our survey group seem on the whole to cover the conventional middle-class range of careers. The most numerous patients were housewives (34%), followed by high school and college students (10%) and G. I.'s (8%). These three classes comprise a majority of the chiropractor's patients suffering some mental disorder.

numbers boring and others fascinating, but any member of an organization with scientific pretensions is under some obligation to consider the strictly quantitative aspects of the realities or phenomena with which he regularly deals and through which he earns his living. Consequently, we offer here no more than the gist of the survey.

The median age of this clinical population is thirty-three. Stress should be laid upon the fact that this composite group includes miscellaneous disorders ranging all the way from mild neuroses to chronic psychoses. As is well known, emotional problems can and do occur at all ages: 6% of these patients were children, 7% adolescents, 60% in what may be called the "military age," range from eighteen to forty-four and 26% forty-five and beyond.

So far as the sex of the sufferer is concerned, a small majority or 55.5% of these cases are female patients, and 44.5% are male. This distribution accords with most physicians' experience and suggests that our sample may be more truly representative of the entire current picture than some of the considerations previously recited might imply. One could speculate on the reasons for this greater percent of female patients with mental symptoms. Is it because women are less happy or emotionally satisfied than men in a masculine-dominated culture and system of values; is it because they have more time, inclination, or money for professional help; or are other forces operating to produce the difference here observed?

Table III

DURATION OF ILLNESS

No.	*Category*	*Percent*
85	1 month to 1 year	24.0
181	1 to 2 years	52.0
31	3 to 7 years	9.0
13	over 7 to 25 years	4.0
40	unknown	11.0

The median length of illness of the patients was slightly more than two years. This suggests that most of the cases fall, as one would naturally suppose, into the chronic rather than the acute category. It is regrettable that the doctor sees the typical patient only after the problem has become well established.

Concerning marital status, the figures show 61% married, 34% single, 2% divorced, and 3% widowed; 130 of the 215 married patients have children.

Table IV
EXTENT AND TYPE OF PREVIOUS MEDICAL THERAPY

No.	*Category*	*Percent*
194	General Medical care	55.5
21	Psychiatry	6.0
60	Unknown	17.0
30	None	8.5
45	Shock therapy	13.0

As one would expect from the socio-historical relationships of the two professions in the ordinary community, an overwhelming majority of the chiropractor's patients with mental symptoms have already seen a medical practitioner. In only one case in twelve was the chiropractor the first specialist consulted. Evidently for many patients, the chiropractor functions as a last resort, possibly on the principle that all else having failed, it will do no harm to give him a try. Fifty-five and one-half percent had previously been under the medical care of a "general practitioner," 13% had already had some form of shock therapy; and 6% were "graduates" of psychiatric or psychoanalytic treatment. Three-fourths of the chiropractor's "emotional" cases, as we may call them, come as a kind of overflow of those in some way inadequately serviced by one or more medical specialties.

Table V
INSTITUTIONALIZED

No.	*Category*	*Percent*
114	Were Institutionalized	33.0
15	About to be committed	4.0
221	Not-institutionalized	63.0

In this population, exactly 33% had been formerly institutionalized and 4% were about to be committed when the intervention of the chiropractor occurred. The remaining 63% were free from any history of formal hospital or sanitarium custodial care. The first two figures suggest that at least one-third of the chiropractor's patients with mental symptoms are desperate cases where the trauma of confinement in a mental institute has occurred or is impending. Since this is about as catastrophic or shattering an experience as the human being ever encounters, it is sobering to consider the responsibilities of consultation in such a crisis.

Table VI
PATIENT RESPONSE TO MEDICAL AND PSYCHIATRIC SERVICE

No.	*Category*	*Percent*
27	Worse	10.0
33	Some improvement	13.0
5	No actual treatment	2.0
195	No change	75.0

Total equals 260 only (since 90—see Table II—had no record of such service).

One important question asked was whether the patient had improved as a result of earlier medical and psychiatric treatment. This is plainly a ticklish item and could probably be most safely, although somewhat cowardly, handled by merely reporting what those who supplied data on this point declared. Taking first the material at face value, we note that 8% said the patient grew worse, 10% mentioned some improvement, 1% said no treatment occurred, and 81% said there had been "no change." Difficult as behavioral criteria in this area undoubtedly are, and hard as it is to get at genuine causal sequences in matters like these, it does not seem objectively likely that four out of five mental patients were left unaltered by the medico-psychiatric attention they received. The patients themselves may have thought so and the chiropractor may well have been susceptible to their strong suggestions, or, not knowing from the beginning the actual course of events, he may have felt on safer ground by proceeding as though the situation had been essentially unaltered since the onset of the disease. This could hold for some of the 81%, but not for all, since that estimate is inconsistent with the magnitude of institutional discharges, which, it is fair to acknowledge, would not have transpired had there not been some change for the better in the prognosis.

To be sure, our respondents may have intended to convey by this unanticipated large figure their opinion that the specific medico-psychiatric stimulation the mental patient received neither aided nor hindered him in coping with the course of his malady. This, however, would get us into a controversy on the nature and frequency of "spontaneous recovery" in such cases, no matter in whose hands the patient happened to be.

We are now ready to introduce one of the high points in the survey. To the key item, "What happened to the patient's mental symptoms following the application of chiropractic?" the following distribution of replies was made: 27.5% reported an immediate change or gain; 23% reported one or more combinations of these patterns: (a) immediate change plus later improve-

Table VII
MENTAL SYMPTOMS FOLLOWING
CHIROPRACTIC ATTENTION

No.	*Category*	*Percent*
96	Immediate change	27.5
14	Immediate change and later improvement	23.0 (Combinations)
26	Immediate change and cumulative betterment	
14	Immediate change, later improvement and cumulative betterment	
26	Later improvement and cumulative betterment	
94	Cumulative betterment alone	27.0
61	Later improvement alone	17.0
13	Nothing noticeable	4.0
4	Somewhat deteriorated	1.0
2	Much worse	0.5

ment; (b) immediate change plus cumulative betterment, (c) immediate change together with later improvement and cumulative betterment, (d) later improvement plus cumulative betterment; 27% mentioned "cumulative betterment" alone; 17% specified "later improvement"; 3% admitted nothing noticeable; 1% confessed their patients became somewhat deteriorated; 5% became "much worse." The much worse in this last category was found on fuller inspection to be a bit of understatement; the two patients involved out of the total of 350 had committed suicide. Such painful failures presumably are traceable to the absence of adequate supervision of disturbed individuals who are risks to themselves or others.

Despite some conspicuous and distressing instances of utter lack of therapeutic success, one cannot avoid being impressed by the fact that the vast majority of patients here described sooner or later showed some reduction in manifest mental pathology following the application of chiropractic, as judged by the chiropractor, the patient and his family.

Assuming that none but easy or lucky situations appear in our laboriously assembled "sample;" assuming that chiropractors are congenital optimists who see some kind of improvement where other observers can detect nothing or remain doubtful; assuming further (what we have no right to assume) that those chiropractors who took the trouble conscientiously to fill out one or more questionnaires for a larger purpose from which they could clearly derive little personal benefit, are bigger liars than politicians or newspaper columnists—assuming all this and more, one would still not be justified in "discounting" all the figures cited. There would remain a hard core of cases indicating that some mentally disordered patients profited in some way from the distinctive chiropractic treatment plus whatever else appeared.

Table VIII

WAS ANY OTHER DRUGLESS THERAPY USED?

No.	*Category*	*Percent*
224	None	64.0
24	Diet	7.0
32	Vitamins	9.0
70	Physiotherapy and Hydrotherapy	20.0

To the query, "Was any other drugless therapy used?" 64% replied in the negative. Of the 36% remaining, 20% used either some kind of physiotherapy or hydrotherapy, 9% used a change of diet. Evidently the D.C.'s concern for the patient's welfare impels him to use other ancillary drugless aids in conjunction with his distinct method.

Table IX

DID YOU USE PSYCHOTHERAPY?

No.	*Category*	*Percent*
147	No	42.0
49	Suggestion	14.0
44	Minor methods	12.5
30	Depth	8.5
23	Not stated	6.5
57	No answers	16.5

To the presumably more basic question, "Did you use psychotherapy?" 42% answered no and 16.5% failed to check this item. However, close to one-half of the chiropractors said they deliberately used some psychotherapeutic technique, i.e., 14% employed suggestion, 12.5% relied on other minor methods, 8.5% applied depth psychology, and 6.5% administered some variety of psychotherapy but did not state what kind. This is a convincing demonstration that about one in every two chiropractors who participated in this preliminary survey recognized concretely the patient's need for counseling and guidance in order to manage more adequately his private reactions to the inner and outer stresses evoked by contemporary living. Some of this usage impresses an outsider as a bit amateurish; and only moderately insightful; nonetheless, it seems like a healthy professional development, particularly if its apparent necessity impels more practitioners to equip themselves more thoroughly in this regard.

Table X

WAS THE PHYSICAL CONDITION PRIMARILY RESPONSIBLE FOR THE MENTAL DISTURBANCE?

No.	*Category*	*Percent*
207	Yes	59.0
115	No	33.0
28	Not stated	8.0

Table XI

WAS THE MENTAL STRESS PRIMARILY RESPONSIBLE FOR THE PHYSICAL DISTURBANCE?

No.	*Category*	*Percent*
115	Yes	33.0
207	No	59.0
28	Not stated	8.0

Because of the fundamental theoretical and practical significance of the nature of the psychophysical relationship in health and disease, it is a matter of deep interest to see how the mind-body interaction appeared to operate within this group. Fifty-nine per cent held the physical condition of the patient to be primarily responsible for his disturbance, while 33% claimed the mental stress to be primarily responsible for the observed physical disturbance. Here we are not concerned with any independent third-party verification of the facts in each clinical picture; what is professionally important is that the "physicalists" outnumber the "mentalists" in a rough two to one ratio. This probably reflects the dominance of a characteristic neurological slant or structural emphasis in the training and thinking of most chiropractors.

A final statement climaxing the entire inquiry appears in the end "results" of the whole process of treatment as administered and appraised by these practitioners. 60.5% of the cases terminated in "apparent cures," 25% were "much improved," 8% were somewhat improved," 5.5% showed "no change," and 1% became worse.

A few additional findings may be casually sketched at this point. It does not appear likely from the data on hand that there is any point-to-point correspondence between the individual's pattern of vertebral distortions and the peculiar mental disorder he exhibits. Beyond noting that the atlas or axis is involved more often than any other spinal region, nothing very enlightening can be said about characteristic anatomical distortions in the emotionally disturbed. Similarly, the total or frequency rate of adjustments has little if any correlation with any measurable variable other than the urgency of acuteness of the patient's condition. The number of adjustments ranged from one to two hundred; thrice weekly was the commonest time pattern for giving them.

Table XII

RESULTS UNDER CHIROPRACTIC CARE

No.	*Category*	*Percent*
212	Apparently cured	60.5
87	Much improved	25.0
28	Somewhat improved	8.0
19	No change	5.5
4	Worse	1.0

Another point brought out by this inquiry is the unsatisfactory nature of the customary classifications of mental diseases. Most of the respondents, perhaps wisely, were unable or reluctant to use formal, academic names for these disorders and contented themselves with vivid descriptions of the most prominent symptoms. It is clearly more valuable to recognize an effective disorder in persistent suicidal thoughts and to take emergency steps to meet this challenge to one's therapeutic powers, than merely to assign the sufferer to such artificial categories as psychasthenia, cyclothymia, or old-fashioned "shell-shock"—all of which may be more useful to the institutional census-taker or to an actuary, than to one trying to restore balance to minds that have temporarily broken under severe stress. While the comparative lack of dependence upon conventional textbook psychopathological groupings may be a mark of deficient scholarship in these areas, it may also be a sign that the practitioner recognizes as primary his obligation to treat an individual who is sick in some novel respect and not to deal with a verbal entity or abstract construct labelled "paranoia." Objectively, too, the fact that many cases of either mild or severe mental distortions involve a diffuse of highly "personalized" emotional response to some literal physical trauma may make them hard to diagnose satisfactorily in rigidly standardized terms. This is especially true when the lessening or elimination of underlying organic "irritations" evoke a corresponding return to normalcy of the "total" organism.

Every single one of the 350 cases described is a fascinating human and potentially valuable scientific document. A brief presentation of a few impressive clinical histories which have been gathered is included in the following pages.

SOME REVEALING CASE HISTORIES OBTAINED IN THIS SURVEY

The following case records are representative of hundreds submitted by doctors of chiropractic throughout the country:

CASE NO. 2

Schizophrenia. Boy, age 13. Subject fell out of his father's car while it was in motion. Soon after the accident he exhibited a decided change in personality. He made animal noises in his throat, bit and scratched. These actions caused him to be placed in a mental hospital where he remained and spent his 21st birthday. His older brother then consulted a doctor of chiropractic. Subject showed heartening improvement from the start and was released from the asylum in 90 days. No further chiropractic care was necessary. Recovery was complete.

CASE NO. 73

Compulsive neurosis. G.I., age 22, single. Ill seven months. Subject complained of terrible pains in head, neck and abdomen. These complaints were labeled "imaginary" by M.D.'s. Subject also suffered anxiety and compulsions. He feared he would harm his brothers and sisters and held his abdomen when walking. Onset of symptoms followed combat explosion, in which subject was blown 40 yards and landed on head, neck and shoulders. He reacted unfavorably to four months of shock treatments and psychiatric service and spent three months in a VA hospital. Subject fully recovered under chiropractic care paid for by the local American Legion post and is now gainfully employed.

CASE NO. 130

Manic depressive-depressive phase. G.I., age 22. Ill since discharge from Navy. Subject was in deep depression most of the time, with prolonged spells of excessive crying, lassitude and despondency. Complained about severe headaches and pains throughout the body. Resented father and brother and feared he would commit suicide or homicide. A dozen electric shock treatments and eight months of psychiatric attention failed to produce any apparent signs of improvement. Subject expressed the wish to be committed to a Veterans Facility, but local VFW service officer recommended chiropractic to subject's father. Patient rapidly improved under chiropractic care and began making own decisions once again. He returned to his draftsman's work, held his job, married and purchased a home.

CASE NO. 103

Schizophrenia. Diagnosis made by a psychiatrist in Bellevue Hospital. Girl, 13½ years old. After a severe fall in 1941, she developed the following mental and physical symptoms:

During the night subject went into a catatonic coma, became completely rigid, fists closed very tightly, eyes wide open, and was obviously impervious to sound, sight, or any outside influence. Remained that way three whole days, was taken to Bellevue Hospital where hypnotism was tried with no success. Institutionalism was then ordered. Against doctors' advice, mother took child home, after signing a document releasing hospital from all responsibility. She consulted a doctor of chiropractic, X-rays were taken, and subluxation in cervical region was adjusted. There was immediate improvement. Had but three adjustings in all and recovered completely. Now married, has two children, and is in perfect health.

CASE NO. 21

Post partum psychosis. Teacher, female, age 28, married, one year-old child. Had been confined to State mental hospital since delivery. She received hydrotherapy and shock treatments. Was gradually becoming worse. Unable to concentrate, would not respond to questions. She was placed under chiropractic care. She received a total of twenty adjustments, given twice weekly. Showed immediate change and cumulative betterment. Was discharged as apparently cured in 1944 and has remained normal in every respect.

CASE NO. 295

Manic depressive. Prizefighter, age 35. On occasions of deep depression, he made a number of attempts to commit suicide. Would often become violent and break furniture. Could not sleep; opiates had no effect. The onset of his difficulty was after one of his bouts with a famous champion (now retired), which resulted in a fractured left jaw that at the same time evidently disturbed the position of the atlas vertebra of the spine. His wife was advised by a medical doctor that it was dangerous to keep him home, that he was "out of his mind," and urged hospitalization. The patient finally was induced to visit a doctor of chiropractic. No more than a slight adjustment was made, and patient immediately fell asleep. Same results occurred on later visits. He made a complete recovery, is now the established owner of a tavern, and in good mental health.

CASE NO. 46

Schizophrenia. Female, 39 years old, married second time. For six months suffered from hallucinations and delusions of nonexisting pregnancy. Had acute anxiety and guilt feelings of living in adultery. Was given to flights of exultation followed by deep depression. Condition became apparent a few months following her re-marriage. Was institutionalized for several months, where electric shock treatments were administered. Their sole effect was that she became progressively worse.

Under chiropractic care, she showed immediate change, and was discharged as apparently cured, after one month of adjustments. Patient has returned to managing a lucrative beauty parlor and exhibits no symptoms whatsoever of any previous mental or physical distress.

CASE NO. 296

Compulsive neurosis. Married woman, age 30. Before coming under chiropractic care, consulted many medical doctors. Complained of severe headaches. Through history-taking, patient also revealed that she suffered from persistent and recurrent compulsions to choke her husband, (due to latent guilt feelings.)

Chiropractic care, plus the suggestion to go back to her church and seek spiritual guidance, resulted in the complete elimination of her physical symptoms and compulsions. Ten years after termination of the spinal manipulations, patient continues to live happily with her husband.

CASE NO. 294

Anxiety hysteria. Female, 35 years old, mother of two children. Ill four years. Was quarrelsome, had a violent temper, uncontrollable compulsions to destroy. Would break mirrors, tear her dress, and also tear at her breasts. Was unjustifiably jealous of her husband. Also complained of headaches. Was in an institution on two previous occasions. Two days before consulting a doctor of chiropractic, she had a very violent spell and preparations were made to have her committed again. After first adjustment, there was immediate change. She improved rapidly under chiropractic care.

Four years later, her father and husband died. Patient showed no signs of emotional unbalance and is in good health. She holds down a job in a broker's office, also takes care of a little insurance business of her own, and manages the house and her two children.

CASE NO. 331

Manic depressive, (depressive phase). Actress, single female, age 40. Ill for many years, with headaches, abdominal pains, insomnia, and loss of appetite. Lost all interest in life and had suicidal tendencies. Underwent hysterectomy. Was under psychoanalysis for six months, with little change in her symptoms. Decided to consult doctor of chiropractic while still undergoing psychoanalysis. The analyst noticed he was able to elicit more psychic information while patient was undergoing chiropractic care. Both doctors cooperated and patient showed steady improvement. A re-check on this case five years later found that the patient had continued to improve.

CASE NO. 151

Manic-depressive (depressive phase). G.I., age 29. The subject had suicidal tendencies. He suffered from headaches, great pain and vomiting. His pain was so intense that the sufferer would beat his head against the wall and pray to die. The onset of the subject's distress was the aftermath to a harrowing overseas experience. He was a tail gunner in a bomber that came down in a forced landing. After the war, the subject was institutionalized for one year in a Veterans Facility. The treatment he received consisted of psychoanalysis three times per week and Murphy drop feeding. When these methods failed to bring about a favorable response, the subject was brought to a chiropractor's attention. Under chiropractic care, the case showed cumulative betterment. Patient was discharged in 1948 as apparently recovered.

CASE NO. 214

General nervousness. G.I., age 26, married. Subject was employed as an assistant hotel manager. Duration of illness: fifteen months. Subject complained of sick headaches, pains in his neck and behind his eyes. He was extremely nervous and given to violent outbursts of temper without provocation. Inability to get along with people spelled a grave defect in his work and lessened his job security. Subject's illness stemmed from a personal fight overseas in which he was knocked down. The medical officer who examined him at point of discharge from service heard the specific complaints. Eye glasses were recommended but brought no relief. Subsequently, under chiropractic care, the subject received ten adjustments and was discharged as apparently recovered. He re-enlisted in the Army and at last report was handling administrative duties capably without a sign of previous distress.

CASE NO. 221

Neurasthenia. Male student, age 23. Illness was of eighteen months duration. Subject complained of severe head and back pains and imagined that he was suffering with a brain tumor. His mental condition was believed to have been precipitated by trying war experiences. Subject served in counter-espionage for several years. This duty was of a consistently dangerous nature and held him in a state of high nervous tension over prolonged periods. Following the war, subject spent two months in a Veterans Facility and showed only partial improvement. A throat specialist referred the case to a chiropractor. Subject responded favorably to the first of a series of adjustments and within six weeks was discharged as apparently recovered.

CASE NO. 248

Schizophrenia. Age 23. Patient believed he was still in a German PW camp where he had been held captive during the war. This camp frequently was under bombing raids by American and Allied planes. Patient would become hysterical and show such strength during attack that several men were required to hold him down. Exhaustion marked the climax of these attacks. Patient was institutionalized for six months. Received rehabilitation and rest treatment. Recovery was not complete. Patient placed himself under chiropractic care. Immediate improvement noted. Doctor of chiropractic handled case for two and a half months. Patient discharged as fully recovered. No subsequent report of breakdown or further treatment.

CASE NO. 280

Acute mania. Male student, age 22. Minister's son. Became violent after an accident to his neck while playing college football. Suffered acute hallucinations. Accused family of trying to throw him into a lion's den. Under care of a number of M.D.'s who diagnosed case as acute mania. Papers signed for subject's commitment. Mother, who had visited asylums in the course of church work, vigorously objected, declaring, in effect, that her son would be better off dead. Patient came under chiropractic care in highly excitable state. M.D. administered anesthetic to facilitate vertebral analysis. M.D. made rectal and urethral examination; strictures broken down. Immediate improvement noted following first adjustment. Subject recovered in four weeks. Returned to Harvard University to complete studies. Became instructor in English literature in another university.

A SUMMARY OF CHIROPRACTIC INSTITUTIONAL CARE

Irrespective of the category into which individuals in distress are placed, chiropractic has been effective when their difficulty stemmed mainly from structural trauma which had a potent effect upon the brain and nervous system. This has been noted in a number of chapters in this anthology.

MENTAL PATIENTS

W. Heath Quigley, D.C., Director of the Clear View Sanatorium in Davenport, Iowa, issued a report in 1954 and in 1958 on case histories of mental illness under chiropractic care (see Chapter 10). His reports state:

> "This selected series of cases represents patients who were mentally ill for the first time and came under Chiropractic care without previous hospitalization, patients who had recurring mental disorders with a history of previous hospitalization and who sought Chiropractic care as an escape from inevitable relapses, and thirdly patients who had been transferred from other hospitals with the hope that Chiropractic could restore mental health. . . . Not only was the psychological aspect of the patient's illness cared for, but an attempt was made to restore the patient to total health, both physical and mental. . . . *The cases presented here have made what we term 'social recovery';* that is, they have been able to return to their home environment or equivalent, possessing the ability to take and hold a job, position, social or professional situation. . . . *They have been able to maintain themselves in society as producing members, rather than dependents in State institutions."* (see Quigley Chap. 10)

JUVENILE DELINQUENTS

There are many hidden causes for delinquency or illness in children, aside from the environmental stresses that they are subject to, either in the home or school, or through the friends they become associated with. Furthermore, there is an ever-increasing body of evidence to support the hypothesis that many children injure themselves and hide it from their parents, and/or they may hide it from their own consciousness. The results of those injuries show up in some physical, mental, or deviant behavior.

In 1932, the Kentucky Houses of Reform in Greendale, Kentucky, instituted chiropractic care for juvenile delinquents, under the supervision of the late Dr. Lillard T. Marshall, one of the founders of the National Chiropractic Association (now the American Chiropractic Association).

The results obtained under chiropractic care were best expressed by the then Superintendent of the Kentucky Houses of Reform, B. W. Hubbard:

> "I have been able to notice a marked improvement in the mental and physical condition of the boys and in school work and conduct; also, there has been a larger number of paroles during that period than any previous period during the past four years." S. E. Duff, Director of Education, said: "I feel that the fine showing in the number of promotions and dismissals from the institution is largely attributable to the very excellent work done by the chiropractors who have almost daily looked after the health and general welfare of these boys. The general tone, the mental alertness and moral and social outlook of these boys have in a large measure been attributable to this very fine cooperation."

Those results were also noticed and attested to by the Chaplain, the Dean of Education, and all the teachers. We can only speculate what it would mean in terms of taxpayers' money, and especially in the rehabilitation of the delinquents, if chiropractic care would be made available to those children who have some hidden physical trauma which may be a cause for their abnormal or deviant behavior. There is a definite basis for chiropractic care for those children whose difficulty may spring from traumatic experiences affecting the nervous system.

In the Public Health Service Publication Number 1152, *Mental Retardation, its biological factors* (1968), it is noted on Page 21 that:

> "Accidents and injuries are putting more children into hospitals than any other cause. A cooperative study of head injuries could lead to prevention of some retardation due to accidents. In one study of children's accidents, the head and brain were found to be injured in 30 per cent of those hospitalized. But much of the retardation apparently arises from a delayed brain reaction a few hours or more after injury."

(For significant additional data on this subject, see Chapter 12, last part, by Kimmel.)

HANDICAPPED CHILDREN

The mentally and physically handicapped children remain a most perplexing problem to all members of the helping professions. The causes are many and often hidden. No one discipline has all the answers. Education, behavioral training, rehabilitation, chiropractic and optimum nutrition have contributed to reversing some previously hopeless conditions, or at least have made it possible for the child to function more comfortably within his limitations.

At the present time, the Kentuckiana Center for Educational, Health and Research, under the direction of Lorraine Golden, D.C., is a most unique center for handicapped children. Here, members of all the helping professions and education join together in the systematic total confrontation for the welfare of these children.

Lorraine Golden, doctor of chiropractic, is aware of the hereditary, genetic, anaphylactic, nutritional, organic, prenatal, natal, or postnatal etiological factors for mental disturbances. She is also aware that falls and injuries may possibly be a cause for some handicapped conditions. This supposition finds verification from some parents, who claim that their child was functioning normally up to the time of a structural injury.

Falls and injuries sustained by young children are quite frequent, according to a study * conducted by Kravitz, Driessen, Gomberg & Korach for the National Safety Council. It revealed that:

> "Unfortunately, babies seem to fall head first. Of the 536 infants involved in the study, 255, or 47.5 per cent, fell from a high place such as an adult bed, a crib, or an infant dressing table during their first year of life. If all infants in the country follow the same pattern as those in our study, we can assume that, during this year, 1.75 million babies will fall at least once during their first year of life."

Chiropractic analysis should be a routine procedure for all handicapped and deviant children, especially when the case history reveals falls or injuries, or the effect of such trauma on the spinal column.

Jerome Smith, assistant professor of social work at the Kent School of Social Work, is exploring at Kentuckiana the all-inclusive contribution of the helping approaches, including chiropractic, in finding solutions for the mentally handicapped. The effectiveness of this total professional teamwork is being evaluated with considerable care and interest.

A significant concept of modern healing is now being tested in Kentuckiana. Is it possible, in planning for the delivery of adequate health services, that only orthodox procedures should or could be depended upon to obtain the maximum health results? Or is it possible that, side by side with the presently accepted methods, other time-tested healing disciplines such as

* ACCIDENTAL FALLS FROM ELEVATED SURFACES IN INFANTS FROM BIRTH TO ONE YEAR OF AGE

chiropractic could also be used? Or must the helpless children not be given the chance to benefit by a healing discipline that has found favor with a large segment of the population for 75 years and is recognized by 48 states?

Dr. Golden has received the support of a large segment of the population of Louisville and its environs. The local press, as well as the University of Louisville newspaper, *The Cardinal,* have given her support through feature stories and editorials. She has inspired volunteer workers to give their free services. Labor organizations are also supporting Kentuckiana from their own funds.

This center has captured the imagination of many students of the Kent School of Social Work. Dean Kenneth Kindelsperger says:

> "Social work has to relate to all phases of life . . . the center provides a unique learning experience for our students. You can't ignore the place (Kentuckiana) . . . We see no conflict in sending students both to the center and to the 'traditional' medical programs."

The Director of Kentuckiana, Dr. Lorraine Golden (based upon her own professional experience), has wisely and humanely incorporated chiropractic in this Center. She is deeply concerned and dedicated to the total health services for these unfortunate children.

Aside from the remarkable results of Kentuckiana's efforts, it can be certain that this center is a vital pilot model proving that:

> It is possible for members of the many healing arts to work harmoniously together with mutual respect for each other and for their respective disciplines.
>
> A staff of divergent people can be inspired to extend their full and free cooperation for the welfare of the unfortunate child.
>
> It is possible to combine a scientific approach with a humanistic approach, thus developing a scientific humanism not only in theory but in practice.
>
> This center is laying the groundwork for the utilization of all disciplines in delivery of total health services.

PART V

BASIC SUPPORTIVE REMEDIAL MEASURES IN PATIENT MANAGEMENT

CHAPTER

CHAPTER **17**

INTEGRATED THERAPEUTIC PROCEDURES WITHIN THE FRAMEWORK OF COMPREHENSIVE CHIROPRACTIC

SCHWARTZ/MOULTON

INTRODUCTION BY EDWIN H. KIMMEL, D.C.

The vast majority of doctors of chiropractic have never adhered to the concept of "one cause and one cure." They have always considered the patient as a person who may be subject to many stresses. While initially relying upon their specialized therapy, they have always used whatever supplementary aids are necessary for the patient's well-being. They have cleaved to D. D. Palmer's credo that "I have never considered it beneath my dignity to do anything to relieve human suffering." Palmer's conception of the causes of disease implies that integrated approaches are sometimes necessary. He also implied that the chief purpose of the doctor should be not to win support for his therapy, but to see that the patient under his care is restored to health. Such a comprehensive view is consistent with the demands of the U.S. Government, the informed and concerned leaders of society, and public-spirited foundations. (F.S.A., 1948) (Blain, 1959) (Ford Foundation, 1960) The general practitioner of all the healing disciplines is being urged and encouraged to gain more orientation and skill to cope with the problems of the patient's emotional stress. (Rennie, 1947) (H.E.W., 1960)

The doctor of chiropractic can be the "first line of defense" against mental illness. He often sees the emotionally disturbed patient before the specialist does. Often he has it within his power to help a patient sufficiently so that specialized psychotherapeutic care or institutionalization may not be necessary. He also sees the half-well, half-sick, tranquilized patients who were formerly hospitalized and do not wish a return engagement or perhaps more electric shock treatments. It can be assumed that those patients are ready and willing to cooperate fully with the doctor.

The procedures that follow, supplement and extend the results that chiropractic obtains for emotionally disturbed patients (see Chapter 16). (They however are not sufficient for the severely disoriented patient.) The doctor lays out a program of activities for him, making certain that the patient understands fully his instructions and advice. This can be accomplished if the doctor asks the patient to interpret or repeat the instructions given him. Following through with this idea has several advantages. The doctor can correct any misunderstandings that the patient may have gathered from his instructions. He also can be assured that the patient fully understands what he should do and when. It can also indicate to the doctor the patient's ability or willingness to cooperate.

The patient's attention should be called to the vital necessity for basic nutrition. This subject is so important that three chapters are devoted to it in this book, headed by Linus Pauling. Next in importance is to instruct the patient in ways of 1) obtaining meaningful periods of relaxation; 2) improving his posture; 3) following through with the tension reduction techniques, as soon as tension develops; 4) emotionally meaningful physical exercises; 5) utilizing psychological aids, and other pertinent physical hygiene factors for his well-being, depending upon the patient's needs. He is reminded and urged to help himself. This lessens the doctor's burden and hastens recovery.

* * *

"There is never one cause for any phenomenon in Nature or in Science. It is always a constellation of causes that brings about the change . . . the mechanisms which the organism utilizes in its continued efforts to cope with stress situations are often strikingly similar, whether the stress situation is of physical (e.g., thermal), biological (e.g., nutritional or allergic), or emotional nature."

GROEN, 1950 *

"The determining causes of disease are traumatism, poison, and (adverse) auto-suggestion."

PALMER, 1910 **

". . . in applied therapeutics, all available means must be used."

HIPPOCRATES

RELAXATION

It is noted in several chapters that the chiropractic adjustment releases specific areas of neuromuscular-skeletal distortions or tensions, and brings about relaxation. This is a most frequent occurrence.

For those patients who are chronically tense, or have basic structural distortions, or are subject to occupational distortions relaxation exercises are a necessary supplementary aid. In order to get the best possible results, it is advisable for the doctor or his assistant to teach the patient how to relax. He is instructed to continue taking frequent relaxation exercises at every opportune time. Gradually, it can become a conditioned reflex which he can use just as soon as fatigue or stress sets in.

The patient can readily recognize that, when neuromuscular tensions set in, the affected part of his body winces or constricts in an attempt to escape the distressing stimuli. These tensions remain, perpetuate themselves and become residual to the point where the patient becomes unaware of them, but they are a constant source of irritation to his nervous system. Teaching the patient to relax places a responsibility upon him to cooperate in his recovery. A persistent and friendly interest can help him to overcome his discouragement, heighten his will to change, and start to face reality.

* LIFE STRESS AND BODILY DISEASE, a Research Publication of the Association for Research in Nervous and Mental Diseases; published by Williams and Wilkins, Baltimore, 1950, pages xvi and xvii, in the foreword by J. Groen.

** SCIENCE, ART, and PHILOSOPHY of CHIROPRACTIC—D. D. Palmer, 1910.

Relaxation procedures are now in use by an increasing number of mental health specialists. Based upon their clinical experience, they have noted that relaxation can often take the place of tranquilizers, shock therapy, or even hospitalization. (Haugen, *et al.,* 1960, p. 34) The chiropractor uses relaxation when indicated not as a main therapy, but as ancillary to his practice, and as homework for the patient. Before starting the relaxation procedure, the patient should be strongly urged to list his various problems and/or the tasks confronting him. The mere listing does not solve anything, but it has an important purpose. It heightens his attention to the task ahead. He can relax with the knowledge that his pressing chores will not be forgotten. The patient has probably been under sustained tension ever since childhood. Hence, it cannot be expected that he will achieve the ultimate in relaxation at the first few attempts. He should not try too hard to make headway; overeagerness will defeat the chief purpose—the achievement of soothing relaxation.

Abbreviated Form of Relaxation

1. Choose a firm bed, a couch, or a blanket on the floor.
2. Loosen all restraining articles of clothing, including collars, bras, belts, garters, compressing hose and shoes.
3. Allot a *minimum* of ten to thirty minutes for this purpose, set the alarm clock or give instructions not to be disturbed.
4. Lie on your back. Perform slow easy stretching exercises of all your muscles at one time, just as one does or should do upon arising from sleep. This would necessarily include easing up all the muscles of the face and forehead, including the eyes, yawning, stretching the muscles of the neck, chest, arms, abdomen, legs and back. Then slowly release all the muscles back into position. The rule is: *always stretch the muscles slowly, against resistance, and then pull them back equally slowly to a comfortable position.*
5. After the exercise, wriggle or shake your body out of the stretch into a position of ease.

   A Basic Rule: Usually the muscles are not relaxed even when one thinks they are. Therefore, keep on slowing easing them up more and more to a state of limpness.
6. Place additional slight support under the nape of the neck or under the knees—if it helps to produce a greater amount of repose.
7. The head and neck must be placed comfortably on the pillow to avert a pull on the scalp muscles. This makes it easier to relax the eyes.
8. Breathing should be slow, regular, and rhythmic.
9. After the patient has become completely relaxed, he commences to think of the word "quiet." With every inhalation and exhalation, he sends down a mental message of "quiet" to further ease up any and every part of the body which failed to relax. He remains in the state of relaxation for as long as his time permits.
10. When finally he is in complete repose, he should become fully aware that within him is a reservoir of intuitive wisdom, power, endurance, and

> strength to cope with his problems. This comforting spiritual awareness brings a full appreciation of his real capabilities, plus a sense that he is playing some useful role in life and in the total scheme of things. The patient can hopefully assume that this newly gained freedom from tension can be carried over in all his endeavors. (Schwartz, 1954, p. 42).

POSTURE

All emotions are reflected in one's posture. The doctor should call to the patient's attention that his posture influences his moods and feelings. When in good posture he not only looks attractive, but he is at ease. Poor posture predisposes him to many ills and makes him subject to depression or increases his depression. Poor posture can set up irritations in the spinal nerve centers or perpetuate the already existing ones. The patient can go a long way in changing his state of emotions by changing his posture.

The correction of posture has its influence upon the patient's attitude, and a correct mental attitude reveals itself in one's posture. Thus we apply the word "attitude" with equal emphasis to the arrangement of our body, as well as to our mental outlook. (Webster's and Oxford Dictionary definitions of "posture" and "attitude" are practically synonymous.)

When the doctor wants the patient to receive the full benefit of the chiropractic adjustment of his spine, he must urge the patient to adopt an evenly balanced, free-wheeling posture. His weight should be equally distributed on both feet. He should wear well-fitted, comfortable shoes. Call to his attention that his abdomen should not sag; his shoulders should not be so far forward as to cause slouchiness, nor so far back as to produce strain on the chest muscles; his shoulders should not be squared or forced upright, giving a rigid, statue-like appearance.

The head is carried evenly balanced on the neck; the chin is not drooping forward and downward on the chest (making the patient appear anxious or depressed). Nor is the head tilted too far backward, giving the impression of looking down upon the world. If the person gets into a habitual way that only part of his muscular and skeletal frame carries the entire weight of his body, then that part of his body undergoes strain and fatigue. Much compensatory shifting and twisting takes place, inevitably resulting in general fatigue. Thinking and feeling in either morbid or healthful phases immediately influences posture and behavior. Conversely and importantly, *it is possible to change feelings by a change in posture*. All that has been stated and much more that could be added may be summed up by saying *the person looks the way he feels,* and *he can feel the way he permits himself to look*.

BREATHING

Shallow breathing is always a concomitant of emotional distress, such as anxiety, depression, frustration, etc. The deeper these emotional states are, the greater the oxygen debt the patient creates. He may think that he is breathing naturally and sufficiently, but he is not. He is usually unaware that he is causing a blocking of his breathing by his tenseness. When breathing is inhibited, the chest becomes sunken and the mood is worsened. When breathing becomes free and easy, the mood can be lightened. Usually the patient's breathing is not full or rhythmical. Inhibited breathing is bound to affect his general health and his emotional outlook on life. The lack of oxygen in the brain can increase depression. Thus, a vicious cycle sets in through continued shallow respiration.

It is important for the doctor to observe the patient's breathing habits. The breathing should be slow, rhythmic and full. At the very beginning of exhalation, the patient should be instructed to start to exhale slowly and fully (Braatoy, p. 176–9). This may serve a double purpose: it will help him to relax, and at the same time, he will exhale more of his residual air, thus creating a vacuum which will be filled automatically by a fuller inhalation. It is also important to suggest to the patient that, in breathing, his teeth should be separated, and the tongue should be slightly receded in the mouth. Yawning is usually an indication that there is an oxygen debt in the body. Braatoy, (1954, p. 62). When the tongue is relaxed-receded, then yawning can be fuller and freer, and is more satisfying.

This test of the importance of correcting breathing can be convincing to the patient. Let him tighten his teeth, press the tongue against the teeth, and inhale several times. Now, suggest that he separate his teeth, even a fraction of an inch, and permit his tongue to recede, and note how much easier his breathing becomes. If he has difficulty in breathing, or feels he has a lump in his throat (barring hyperthyroidism), it is usually due to emotional tension which constricts the respiratory muscles in the throat, as well as in the thoracic region. The release of the respiratory muscles can normalize breathing, and be an aid in the gaining of emotional control.

COPING WITH STRESS

Early in our practice, it was often observed that the emotionally disturbed patient was suffering from muscle tension, and of course would complain about various symptoms. He would talk about his adverse interpersonal relationship with members of his family, or with his co-workers. After a spinal adjustment, the patient's neuromuscular tensions were lessened, and frequently he would spontaneously say, "Well, my wife (or my child, or my boss) isn't so bad, after all." This graphically illustrated that spinal adjustments can often lessen nervous tension to the point where the person can take on a more rational attitude towards people or towards the stress of life.

Such progress was satisfying. In the effort to give the patient some additional procedure for coping with noxious situations, the Tension Reduction Technique evolved. It was taught successfully to patients who had to cope with anger, depression, frustration, fear, or other adverse psychobiological irritations. References to this procedure were made by Schwartz (1954). The requisite for the effectiveness of this procedure must be for the patient to recognize that muscle tension is always present when facing distressing situations or problems.

To prove to the patient that he can either help or worsen his lot, we can ask him to make himself rigid, and notice that, in that state, his problems become magnified; and that, if he becomes completely relaxed, they diminish. The patient will usually notice and be able to relate to the doctor the change in his feeling tone when in a state of tension versus the state of relaxation. This important lesson must be emphasized again and again. Of course, problems cannot be solved that way, but at least they can be coped with in a more rational fashion. When the person becomes proficient in practicing and remembering the Tension Reduction Technique, it can lead to the formation of a conditioned reflex that he can utilize in coping with all sorts of adverse situations, be they from the past, from the present, or in anticipation of a trying situation which he fears may develop in the future.

Tension Reduction Technique

STEP 1

a. Have the patient sit on a chair, holding on tightly to it.
b. His eyes should be closed.
c. His jaw is clenched.
d. His whole body should become rigid—neck, arms, abdomen, back, and legs.
e. Have the patient bring to his mind a stress situation. (He need not reveal the situation to the doctor, unless he wishes to do so.)
f. He stays in that state for five to ten seconds—no longer.

STEP 2

a. He completely loosens his hold on the chair.
b. He continues to keep his eyes closed.
c. He loosens his jaw, separates his teeth; his tongue recedes from the teeth.
d. He relaxes his entire body—neck, arms, abdomen, back, and legs.
e. He breathcs fully and freely.
f. He continues thinking about the same stress situation, in this state of relaxation, for half a minute or longer.

STEP 3

The patient repeats, in every detail, Step #1.

STEP 4

The patient repeats, in every detail, Step #2.

This tension and relaxation technique can be repeated many times, under the guidance of the doctor or his assistant, for five minutes or longer, until the stress situation that he was thinking about has lost much of its impact upon him.

Once the individual has experimented with this procedure, he will find that, after undergoing Step #1 and Step #2 only a few times, the impact of a disturbing experience which he had deliberately brought to mind at the beginning of the procedure had vanished or diminished. This would indicate that, by this technique, a certain amount of mental clarification can ensue almost immediately. The patient must practice this technique under the doctor's direction until he has learned it thoroughly. It is essential to remember that the ratio of time between tension and relaxation should be at least 1:3, i.e., allow not more than ten seconds for him to remain in the state of excess tension, and a half-minute or longer to stay in the state of relaxation. Then repeat until he has noticed its effect upon him.

When the person becomes free from one noxious emotion or experience, then this technique can be used to cope with other stressful situations. It can also be used in preparing oneself for future events, the same as an actor rehearses again and again until he becomes perfect at the role that he has to play. He may use it for situations which he would not otherwise dare to undertake because fear blocks his way to the opportunities that may open up before him. He will notice that, if he visualizes a future situation that he fears while in a state of tension, he becomes overwhelmed by it; but in a state of complete relaxation, he can train himself to more confidently cope with the situation. The technique will be most acceptable to the patient who is eager to free himself from his emotional difficulties. He will readily follow and benefit from this procedure if it is presented to him with patience and clarity.

The tension reduction procedure is not effective for the severely disturbed or disoriented patient, nor is it appropriate to suggest it to him. There is always the possibility that he may create an excessive amount of tension, hold on to it, and become overwhelmed by it; or he may be disoriented to the extent that he simply cannot follow the instructions. Such patients usually cannot or will not grasp the difference between tension and relaxation. This procedure also may not apply to the patient who is full of hostility, or who has come to the doctor under duress, or who is not motivated to overcome his difficulties.

EMOTIONALLY MEANINGFUL PHYSICAL EXERCISES

When the vicissitudes of life have had a strong impact upon the patient, and when he cannot release his emotions either through philosophizing, through spiritual comfort, or through the Stress Reduction Procedure, then it becomes necessary that he release his emotions in a meaningful physical way. A most appropriate way of releasing anger, frustration, or any other noxious emotions, is through joyful constructive activities. The more constructive the physical activity, the more meaning and satisfaction the patients will derive from it.

Another way for the patient to release his tensions is to do some controlled exercises in his home. The exercises could be graduated push-ups, or lying on the floor on the back and simulating active bicycle-riding. This should be controlled and continued in graduated stages, from 2–3 minutes up to 10–15 minutes, depending upon age, condition of the heart, blood pressure, etc. These exercises are to be followed by a period of complete relaxation, so that he may become completely at ease and refreshed. He may also obtain a feeling of accomplishment, because he has learned how to gain control over his noxious emotions, protect his self-esteem, and at the same time avoid being offensive to others.

For the severely disoriented patient, such as the schizophrenic, the procedures in addition to chiropractic, may be grossly insufficient. It is necessary to again remind the reader that while chiropractic has been most effective for some schizophrenics who suffered from a specific vertebral distortion that caused severe interference with the transmission of nerve impulses, it is not effective for others. Most schizophrenics, however, are people whose tension patterns may have developed very early in life, and they cannot relax. The truth is that they dare not relax. They cannot permit themselves to "let go." They are afraid. Should they allow their muscles to relax, their bottled up emotional tensions might come to the fore in hysterical laughter, abusive or obscene language, or violence.

Wilhelm Reich (1949), Francis Regardie (1951), and Alexander Lowen (1958–67), have called attention to the "muscular armor" with which the patient defends himself against the curious who would invade his private world. Lowen (1958) and his associates have been successful with their Bio-Energetic Technique in the recovery of many schizophrenics. Robert E. Palmer (1972) has researched the effectiveness of the use of the Bio-Energetic Technique by Lowen in combination with other techniques on more than 500 hospitalized and non-hospitalized psychotic patients as methods of desensitizing fear of the expression of aggression. But the general practitioner who has not the experience, training or time cannot and should not instruct the patient in this or any other highly technical procedure.

It has also been reported that some schizophrenics recovered through the use of molecular psychiatry, as advocated by Linus Pauling, and by the professional members of the American Schizophrenic Association.

PSYCHOLOGICAL AIDS

Integrated therapeutic procedures of necessity must include some mental health aids. It is not our intent to present here psychotherapeutic techniques that can only be used by the specialist. Those who are in quest of extending their knowledge and interest in elementary psychotherapy for their general practice can find a great variety of techniques in the references given for this chapter. Levine (1947) in "Psychotherapy in Medical Practise", Brussel (1969), and other psychiatrists consider practically anything that the doctor does for the patient to be psychotherapy. The doctor of chiropractic may also choose from some of the seventy-five therapies listed and explained by Small (1970), or Schwartz (1954, 1957).

The psychotherapy that can be used in daily practice is best defined by Strecker (1945A) "willingness to help, affording of security, release of emotional tensions, efforts at clarification, relief of superego tensions, or the giving of inspiration, as the case may be." For a slight elaboration of these basic concepts, and how they are inherent in the chiropractor's work, see Schwartz (1956).

A lack of specialized psychotherapeutic knowledge need not frighten any doctor away from using his good sense, intuitive wisdom, or humane feelings. When he possesses a general knowledge of many practical healing techniques, he may function efficiently in many respects.

The patient may need some mental health guidance and reassurance. He also needs some diversion and entertainment, to suit his wishes or desires. Hobbies are always a great help. If there is too much external strain upon him, due to his occupation or his social life, it should be lessened whenever possible. If he is too engrossed in himself, fostering socialized living by interesting himself in some organization is of value. He may aslo need acceptable outlets for his aggressiveness, such as sports or other physical activities. Ways can be found for him to accept compensations for his inferiority feelings by developing some skills for which he has an aptitude. He must find satisfaction for his frustrated or neurotic needs. (For elaboration of these and other simple procedures, we again refer the reader to Levine, 1947.) The patient must be encouraged to accept his inadequacies, build up his self-esteem, and utilize his potentialities, or learn to live within his limitations.

For the vast number of difficulties or problems that people have, it is not possible to state rules that can be universally meaningful. Every procedure must be modified to meet a given situation. Often the patient is in a dilemma. He suffers in finding solutions to his problems. No matter which course he takes, it may be equally painful. But he, and not the doctor, must make the decision. One way for the doctor to psychologically influence the patient, and yet not take the credit or the blame for it, is to take a lesson from the window dresser. He displays the various objects, and the customer makes the decision. He buys whatever he wants, and he does not praise or blame the merchant for his choice. In presenting alternate courses to the patient, it is best that the practitioner follow a similar pattern.

When the doctor grasps the stressful situation that the patient is laboring under, he attempts to clarify it to the patient. Then, he points out to the patient the various courses he may choose in coping with it, but permits the patient to make his own decision. The patient, with such guidance, may decide to take the course which will be of ultimate or lasting value, rather than a course which will have no benefits. This is probably what Freud meant when he said, "Sometimes all we can do is to remove the agony of neuroticism, and substitute the misery of living."

AUTOSUGGESTION

It is essential that the patient should establish the constructive response mechanisms of autosuggestion. He is living in a world saturated with suggestions of a devastating quantity and quality. Most likely he has been using autosuggestion, consciously or unconsciously, to worsen his lot during a large part of his lifetime. Therefore, the doctor must encourage the patient to apply autosuggestion in a meaningful, constructive way. He should crystalize some powerful suggestive short words such as, "I can, I must, I will;" "I can take it;" "I can do it;" "I will be all right;" "so what;" "I have the strength;" "I can do the job." If he repeats these or similar powerful concepts often enough, it can become a most potent force in his life. But autosuggestion must be based on truth. The patient should not be blind to his unmistakable shortcomings and weaknesses, nor ignore the changes that age or other factors may bring. Merely to suggest to oneself that "I'm well" when he is sick may hinder him from seeking help. To suggest to himself that he has the capacity to do a truly impossible task may only cause him to become further discouraged and depressed. To say to oneself, "I understand myself completely," when he is in need of insight and self-searching, is again doing oneself an injustice. He should strive to uncover the hidden sources of his weaknesses, anxieties, and fears, recognizing that it is usually possible to understand oneself better once one becomes conscious of these weaknesses. Autosuggestions based on unreality or plainly impossible tasks are better not even started; they lead only to disaster.

Holding to a realistic point of view, the patient can do his best under existing conditions by fully appraising and recognizing the powers within him and putting them to use. He makes it his business to emphasize his good points, and to do the things he can do best. He may suggest to himself that it is possible to obtain whatever he needs in the way of motive, skill, or attitude, giving these suggestions to himself at frequent intervals. By relaxing often, he will soon become aware that he has unused resources of wisdom and strength to draw on.

He must guard himself against inertia. It is the greatest stumbling block that constructive autosuggestion has to overcome. The habit of sheer laziness can masquerade as legitimate physical fatigue. It will keep whispering, "What's the use?", "Don't bother," "Leave it alone," "It can't be done." How much easier it is to make no further effort when one meets with reverses than to try again.

He must also remember that he cannot accomplish anything by hoarding his energy. On the contrary, the more active he is,—within his limitations—the stronger he can become. Especially in times of crisis when he is on the verge of an achievement, he can move from "I must," to "I can," and finally to "I will," with no debilitating thoughts dragging at his elbows. This is one reason why *continuous,* repetitious autosuggestion is so vital.

The astounding power of suggestion over the human organism can be easily demonstrated. *The person who finds a new interest is full of enthusiasm.* He doesn't permit weaknesses or weariness to subdue him. He forges ahead effortlessly, powered by fresh vigor. Strength comes to him and flows from him. The doctor focuses the attention of a patient on a worthwhile and possible goal, compliments him for the steps he takes to help himself, and constantly instills in him reasons for optimism. His advice takes the form primarily of *what to do, NOT what not to do.* The doctor finds out what worries the patient most, and then calls his attention to the constructive efforts that are already under way or in the offing through chiropractic and the ancillary health procedures. The doctor may try to convince the patient that one of the surest ways for him to evaluate his own problems is to temporarily become involved with somebody else's problems within limitations.

It is a basic law of nature, which the patient overlooks, that the more active he is, the stronger he can become. The maladjusted usually finds easy and obvious excuses for not following through with some pertinent and helpful suggestions. When it is suggested to him to walk, he will complain, "I feel weak;" to work, he will say, "I cannot do anything," or "I'm not trained;" to smile, he may answer, "When I will be happy, I will smile." But just the opposite behavior can lead to his improvement. When he start walking, he becomes stronger; when he becomes active, he becomes more skillful at work or play; when he starts to smile, even if he is under stress, he gets a pleasant response from others, and it can be a step towards the development of a happier and more hopeful attitude. *Hope* has now become a perfectly respectable concept in the mental health field. (Sipe, 1970, Stotland, 1970, Meissner, 1973.) Frank (1967/8) says that the results of any therapy "can be ascribed in large part to the healing power of hope, which is aroused when the patient finds people doing things he thinks will help him." Such feelings are increased when the patient knows that the doctor of chiropractic is adjusting him and removing his neuromuscular pains and irritations.

The doctor should never forget to inspire the patient with the value of justifiable hope. The patient should be reminded that, throughout the long history of humanity, the person, no matter in what circumstances he found himself, who had hope and a belief in himself, and had sufficient will to survive, was more certain to find a way out of his dilemma than those who simply gave in to their distress and became submerged in the swamp of self-pity, degradation and frustration. Just as soon as a patient learns to enlarge his vision, and becomes interested in other people, or involved in the affairs of an organization, he starts to make progress towards finding more constructive outlets from his distress. Sublimating some of his basic needs into unselfish channels can often be a step towards a more purposeful and meaningful life.

The life and works of Dr. Viktor Frankl (1959, 1969) are an inspiring example of how a person can transfer justifiable hate into love for humanity. Crumbaugh (1971) says Frankl developed *"logotherapy* to indicate treatment through directing the patient in the search for the unique meaning of his personal existence."

Crumbaugh continues:

> "Frankl believes that . . . man's primary need is to find a purpose in his personal existence, a sense of significance in the totality of experience that marks him as a unique individual, different from all others in the entire history of the world. When he finds this, Frankl holds, he can go on against all odds; and when he lacks it, he feels empty and frustrated in spite of whatever else he may have."

When "sure cures" are discovered for mental and emotional stress it will be the general practitioner's obligation to immediately refer the patient for that source of cure. But until that time arrives, it is every doctor's responsibility to seek consultation or cooperation of a mental health specialist; to do everything within his power and knowledge to prevent the patient from being subjected to hospitalization, which is often merely custodial in nature and usually leaves upon the patient a lasting social stigma.

REFERENCES

Blain, Daniel. "Reply to a national survey of 3,500 national leaders regarding medical practise," *Journal of the American Academy of General Practise* (*New York Times,* August 19, 1959).

Braatoy, Trygve. *Foundations of Psychoanalytic Technique.* New York, John Wiley & Sons, 1954.

Brussel, J. A. *The Physician's Concise Handbook of Psychiatry.* New York: Brunner/Mazel, 1969.

Crumbaugh, James C. "Frankl's Logotherapy. A New Orientation in Counseling," *Journal of Religion and Health* (October 1971), 10(4).

Federal Security Administration, Mental Health Series Bulletin (#3), June, 1948.

The Ford Foundation, N.Y. McPeak, William. "The Small Frantic Voice of the Patient", *Postgraduate Medicine* (Jan., 1960).

Frank, Jerome D., *How Do Emotionally Sick People Get Better?* Mental Health Program Reports, U.S. Department of Health, Education & Welfare, National Institute of Mental Health, (February, 1967).

Frank, Jerome D. "The Role of Hope in Psychotherapy." *International Jr. Psychiatry* (1968).

Frankl, Viktor E. *From Death Camp to Existentialism.* Boston: Beacon Press, 1959.

Frankl, V. E. *The Will to Meaning.* New York: The World Publishing Co., 1969.

Groen, J. *Life Stress and Bodily Disease.* Baltimore: Williams and Wilkins, 1950.

Haugen, Gerhard B., Dixon, Henry H., Dickel, Herman A., *A Therapy for*

Anxiety Reactions. New York: Macmillan Co., H.E.W. Report No. 543. July 1960.

Levine, Maurice. *Psychotherapy in Medical Practice.* New York: The Macmillan Co., 1947.

Lowen, A. *Physical Dynamics of Character Structure.* New York: Grune & Stratton, 1958.

Lowen, Alexander. *Betrayal of the Body.* New York: Macmillan Co., 1967.

Meissner, W. W. "Notes on the Psychology of Hope," *Religion and Health.* Institutes of Religion and Health, N.Y. (1973).

Palmer, D. D. *The Science, Art and Philosophy of Chiropractic.* Portland, Oregon: Portland Printing House Co., 1910.

Palmer, Robert E. (in press). "Bioenergetic Assertion for Desensitizing Fear of the Expression of Aggression", *Advances in Behavior Therapy.* New York: Academic Press.

Reich, Wilhelm. *Character Analysis.* Trans. by Farrar, Strauss, Theodore P. Wolfe: Cudahy Press, 1949.

Regardie, Francis. "A Specific Chiropractic Psychiatry" *The Chirogram.* Journal of the Los Angeles College of Chiropractic—Los Angeles, California (1951).

Rennie, Thomas. *New York Times* (April 19, 1947).

Schwartz, Herman S. "What is Chiropractic Psychotherapy?" *The Journal of N.C.A.* (Jan., 1956), p. 31.

Schwartz, Herman S. *Home Care for Emotionally Ill.* New York: Sessions Publishers, 1957.

Schwartz, Herman S. *The Art of Relaxation.* New York: Sessions Publishers, 1954.

Sipe, R. W. A. (ed.). *Hope—Psychiatry's Commitment.* New York: Brunner/Mazel Pub., 1970.

Small, L. *The Briefer Psychotherapies.* New York: Brunner/Mazel, 1971.

Stotland, E. *The Psychology of Hope.* San Francisco: Jossey-Bass Inc., 1969.

Strecker, E. A. & Appel, K. E. *Psychiatry in Modern Warfare.* Macmillan Co. (1945), pp. 46 and 47.

SUPPLEMENTARY READINGS

Barry, Maurice J., Jr. *Non-Neurotic Neurotics.* Postgraduate Medicine, Vol. 43, No. 4, (Mayo Clinic, Rochester, Minnesota, April, 1968).

Burghard, Shirley (ed.). *Constructive Action For Good Health Magazine,* Syracuse, N.Y.

Burton, Arthur. *Modern Humanistic Psychotherapy.* San Francisco, California: Jossey-Bass Inc. (1967).

Eysenck, J. H. (ed.). "The Effects of Psychotherapy." *Handbook of Abnormal Psychology.* New York: Basic Books, 1961.

Ford, Donald H. & Urban, Hugh B. *Systems of Psychotherapy.* New York: John Wiley, 1963.

Fromm, Erich. *Man for Himself.* New York: Holt, Rinehart & Winston, 1947.

Fromm, Erich. *The Forgotten Language.* New York: Holt, Rinehart & Winston, 1951.

Glasser, William. *Reality Therapy*. New York: Harper & Row, 1965.
Goble, Frank G. *The Third Force*. New York: Grossman Publishers, 1970.
Groen, J. "Psychogenesis & Psychotherapy of Ulcerative Colitis" *Psychosomatic Medicine* (1947), 9:151.
Jaco, E. Gartley (ed.). *Patients, Physicians, and Illness*. Glencoe, Ill.: The Free Press, 1958.
Jacobson, Edmund. *Anxiety & Tension Control*. Philadelphia, Pa.: J. B. Lippincott Co., 1964.
Jacobson, Edmund (ed.). *Tension in Medicine*. Springfield, Ill.: Charles C. Thomas, 1967.
Kaelbling, R., Patterson, R. M. *Eclectic Psychiatry*. Springfield, Ill.: Charles C. Thomas, 1966.
Lazarus, Arnold A. (ed.). *Clinical Behavior Therapy*. New York: Brunner/Mazel, 1972.
Lowen, Alexander. *Depression and the Body*. New York: Coward, McCann & Geoghegan, 1972.
Meissner, W. W. "Notes on the Psychology of Hope." *Jn. of Religion and Health*. (1973), vol. 12:1.
Mendel, W. M., & Green, G. A. *The Therapeutic Management of Psychological Illness*. New York: Basic Books Inc., 1967.
Morris, Desmond (ed.). *Primate Ethology*. New York: Doubleday & Co., 1969.
Regardie, F. I. *Be Yourself*. Glouchester, England: Helios Book Service, 1965.
Shulz, J. H. *Autogenic Training*. New York: Grune & Stratton, 1959.
Smallie, Paul. *Chiropractic Management*. (Privately Printed), 1960.
Strecker, Edward A. & Ebaugh, Franklin G. *Practical Clinical Psychiatry*. Philadelphia: Blakiston Co., 1945.
Szasz, Thomas S. *Law, Liberty and Psychiatry*. New York: Macmillan Co., 1963.
Wolberg, L. R. *The Technique of Psychotherapy*. New York: Grune & Stratton, 1954.
Wolpe, J. *Psychotherapy by Reciprocal Inhibition*. Stanford, Calif.: Stanford University Press, 1958.
Zuk, Gerald H. *Family Therapy*. New York: Behavioral Publications, 1972.

CHAPTER **18**

DIETARY MANAGEMENT

RALPH PRESSMAN, PH.D.

THE PURPOSE of nutrition is to furnish every cell in the body and brain with those nutrients which will maintain homeostasis or biochemical equilibrium. This is a basis of good health.

It has been shown that mental illness is often caused by the lack of certain nutrients. The simple expedient of replacing the missing nutrients, i.e., bringing about a biochemical balance, may bring about a remission of symptoms. There are mental disorders that are caused by inborn errors of metabolism. Some of these, too, have responded to supplemental nutrients or vitamins.

At long last, some members of the healing professions are recognizing that poor nutrition can have as ill an effect on the body as viruses and unfriendly bacteria. Indeed one enlightened physician has stated that we all suffer from malnutritional disturbances with resultant physical and mental deterioration.

What is meant by proper nutrition? It certainly does not mean overeating as so many are doing. The people of the United States are the most overfed and undernourished, or malnourished, people in the world. Experiments with animals have conclusively shown that underfed animals live healthier and longer lives than their overfed litter mates. This also applies to humans.

A proper diet should mean balanced meals made up of the three classes of foods—proteins, carbohydrates and fats—in proper proportion at every meal. Each class of food provides something that is nutritionally essential, which the other classes do not provide.

In addition, natural vitamin and mineral supplements should be included since the foods available at the market place today are deficient in some of the nutrients or micronutrients. This is due to the use of pesticides, and to current methods of farming, harvesting, shipping, processing, etc.

In the past, the best sources of protein were considered to be meat, poultry, eggs, fish, milk and milk products. These foods, it was found, had a high biological (USDA 15) value. The biological value of a protein was seen to be related to the composition of the amino acids in it.

It has now been found, however, that meat, poultry and fish can no longer be considered the complete proteins, not because they are less complete (although this may be true), but because of the manner in which present-day animals are raised.

A few words must be said about the raising of the most popular meat, that is, beef. Here are a few paraphrased gems from "The Plain Truth," Ambassador College, Pasadena, California, which happened to come while these pages were being written.

Soon after birth, the calf is given shots of antibiotics and other types of injections, perhaps the most powerful of which is the artificial sex hormone known as Stilbesterol. Then follow feeding programs which force on the calves an unbelievable diet of medicated, often cheap feeds and roughage, including debris and ground newsprint mixed with molasses and sawdust.

The National Observer reports, "Most Americans, if they are to eat much meat at all, must still consume diseased meat and meat from which diseased or unfit portions have been trimmed."

Once meat reaches the packing plant it is subject to a whole new round of additives which preserve, age, cure, tenderize, color, flavor, season and scent the meat—and reduce the processor's costs or increase his profits.

In addition, ninety per cent of our chickens are raised on arsenic treated feeds.

In the Washington Post 8/28/70 we read that the poisons of mercury, lead and arsenic have been found in beef, shellfish and chicken livers. In another issue 10/30/70 we read that mercury from industrial waste and other sources has been found in problem amounts this year in fish, animals or water of 33 States and eight Canadian provinces.

This is a sad picture indeed. We do require protein, but flesh foods need no longer head the list. Those whose lifelong habit has been that of eating meat, and who still insist on eating some meat, should be selective when considering those meats likely to contain the most additives—such as luncheon meats, frankfurters, sausages, etc.

For the more enlightened person there is another class of foods that is relatively high in protein. Included in this class are nuts, such as walnuts, almonds, filberts, brazils, peanuts, cashews, etc., along with nut butters made from any of these. Another high source of protein is seeds, such as sunflower, pumpkin, sesame and sesame butter, and beans such as soy and soy products. Most seed foods are about one-third fat, one-third protein and one-third carbohydrate, making them very well balanced foods. The fat they contain is largely unsaturated in contrast to the saturated fats found in flesh foods.

In view of the poisons that have found their way into flesh foods, a list of the suggested protein foods that should be considered in planning a menu would be, in the order of importance: Milk and milk products, nuts, seeds, nut butters, soy beans and soy bean products, legumes such as peas and beans.

For carbohydrates, we can use fruits and vegetables, many of which can be eaten raw. They become the ideal choice for replacing many of the refined starches and refined sugars.

All fruits and vegetables must be thoroughly washed, so as to remove at least some of the pesticides. Vegetables should not be overcooked, and their juices should be utilized as well as their skins that contain vital mineral salts. The fresh green tops of root vegetables are also rich in minerals; any good cookbook will suggest many attractive combinations. Properly cooked vegetables plus liquefied fruit and vegetable juices are usually palatable. Extra vitamins and minerals as supplementary nutrition are usually necessary to correct possible chemical deficiencies of the body.

An excellent pick-up for the fatigue that often accompanies so many mental disorders can be fruit or fruit juices, or some nuts eaten between meals.

If the patient's digestion is poor, then the foods should be chosen with care, or his nervous system may suffer and his emotional difficulties may be increased. The doctor must remember that every person, to some extent, is a law unto himself as far as the toleration of foods is concerned.

Some of the foods that should be avoided are cakes, white bread, pies, pastries, candies, white sugar, sweetened soft drinks, macaroni, spaghetti, etc.

Fats, which must be a part of every diet, should consist of vegetable oils in the form of salad dressings and in cooking. The oils are rich in Vitamin E and serve as a vehicle or carrier for some vitamins.

FOOD SUPPLEMENTS

As stated above, vitamin and mineral supplements are definitely necessary. The easiest way to take supplements is in the form of a daily capsule or tablet. Some of these products are available in health food stores. They are extracted from natural sources, but in the extracting process some micronutrients may be lost. However, these preparations are definitely more desirable than preparations made from synthetic chemicals found in drug stores.

For those who would have the best form of supplementation the following is suggested:

For Vitamins A and D: Fish liver oil in gelatin capsules. The most common fish liver oil is from the halibut. Each capsule usually contains 5000 units Vitamin A and 400–500 units Vitamin D.

For the entire Vitamin B complex, Brewers' yeast is the best buy. Wheat germ is nearly as good.

For Vitamin C, a natural supplement may be prepared from Rose Hips or Acerola berries or other natural sources, but with the advocacy of massive doses, the use of ascorbic acid, which is produced in the laboratory, might be recommended. It is not, like some synthetic vitamins, a coal tar product.

Vitamin E, like Vitamins A and D, are available in gelatin capsules. While the Shute Brothers, who pioneered work with this necessary vitamin, recommend Alpha Tocopherol, there are many (including the author) who insist on using the mixed tocopherols as they are obtained from the original sources.

Minerals: Three of the most important minerals are calcium, iodine and iron. We recommend that calcium lactate be used as a source of calcium. Kelp may be used for its iodine content. Kelp tablets contain not only iodine but many other organically bound minerals. Another natural source of minerals would be sea salt. Green vegetables should be used as a source of iron.

In a balanced diet of proteins, fats and carbohydrates, milk and milk products would furnish not only protein but the important mineral calcium and some vitamins. Nuts and seeds will furnish, in addition to protein, unsaturated fatty acids, Vitamin E and other desirable nutrients. The oils used in salads would furnish unsaturated fatty acids along with Vitamin E. The fruits and vegetables would furnish carbohydrates, natural sugars as a source of energy along with Vitamin C and a number of important minerals.

Housewives can prepare delicious nutritional drinks in which have been incorporated some of the less easily taken supplements like calcium lactate, yeast, wheat germ, etc. If these are added to milk or fruit juice, a delightful drink can be made that can serve as a between-meal snack or indeed as a meal in itself.

One such blender mixture could contain the following:

½ cup fruit juice—pineapple, berry, etc.
2 T. oil
1 C. milk—start motor
½ C. powdered milk
1 T. yeast or liver
1 t. Bone meal
4 t. Calcium gluconate
½ t. Magnesium oxide
Vitamin—as much as desired.
Slowly increase to 2 T. liver or yeast.
Also see the book by H. E. Kirschner, *Live Food Juices*.

FOOD MAY BE THE PATIENT'S WEAPON

The patient may be emaciated as well as irritable, and may use his abstention from food as a weapon against the family. He knows that, when he eats, they consider him to be better, and may pay little attention to him; if he doesn't eat, they feel that he is worse, and will give him more attention. The most effective countermeasure is a show of indifference.

There is also the possibility that his feelings of guilt, spitefulness, despair, resentment, or physical pain may prevent him from eating. However, a battle of wits should be avoided. Showing either anger or concern may merely serve to encourage his infantile behavior. Therefore, let the aide's first attempt be the use of love and kindness, but no spoiling or yielding to foolish whimsies.

The doctor should instruct the aide to be careful to regulate his own mood, especially at the time of feeding the patient, as anger, disgust or distress can easily communicate itself to him and hamper his digestion.

The ambulatory patient should be advised not to eat when he is exhausted or excessively emotionally upset. A short period of relaxation is then indicated. If he is hungry as well as tired, then a fruit or vegetable drink or broth can reduce his fatigue, as well as subsiding his hunger.

DISPELLING HIS FEARS

If the patient has paranoidal tendencies and imagines that his food is poisoned, the aide may be able to overcome his fear by asking him to open the can of food. If it's juice, the patient may be asked to pour a glass for the aide and one for himself. He should be permitted to help prepare the food, and the two should eat it together, arranging it on both plates in the same order, emphasizing that both *are eating the same food.* When he is confused, instead of urging him to eat, the aide should first eat a mouthful of food from his own plate, then give the patient a mouthful from his. This example will be more persuasive than anything he can say. That and the tempting aroma of the food may persuade him to surrender to his hunger.

Do not be discouraged because the patient is eating little if the *quality* of his nourishment is high. A lack of appetite may be Nature's sign that one shouldn't eat. When the body rebels against food it means that the digestive tract needs a rest. This is Nature's way of declaring that the alimentary canal is either literally too filled with food, or that the energy required to digest it is needed elsewhere. In a long physical or mental disturbance, the organism has a special need for a physiological rest.

FASTING

Having discussed nutrition and mental health, it might be well to consider the absence of nutrition, that is fasting, as a therapeutic approach to health.

Fasting can provide a complete physiological rest if it is combined with a lessening of emotional and mental activities. Fasting is an inner body cleansing procedure. Excess substances of all kinds are eliminated from all the tissues, but none of the vital organs, such as the brain, heart, nerves, kidneys, or glands are affected.

The subject of fasting is replete with human interest. It is no longer open to question that man possesses the ability of enduring a protracted fast without harm to his organism.

Some may never have heard of fasting for other than religious reasons, not realizing that the therapeutic value of fasting was recognized before the days of Hippocrates, the father of medicine. There are authentic records of human beings who endured complete abstention from food over sixty days. Professional fasters have refrained from all nourishment for periods varying from ten to fifty days.

A short fast is definitely indicated for the disturbed and confused patient. However, in spite of his confusion, when food is taken away from him, he may consider it to be punishment for his feelings of sin or guilt, or it may indicate to him that the doctor or loved one is rejecting him. Thus, patience as well as timing should be used in convincing the patient to assume complete responsibility for the fast, of course, under the doctor's direction.

In the last decade or two, a score or more of books and articles has appeared on fasting. To mention a few, there are such names as Carlson (3), Ehret (4), Carrington (5), McCoy (6), Hazzard (7), McEachen (8), Lindlahr (9), and others. DeVries, in his book, *Therapeutic Fasting* (10), lists thirty-three references.

Having written of some of the advantages that might accrue from a fast, it might be well to point out that as one reads books and articles on fasting one soon becomes aware of the lack of uniformity in the recommended methods. Therefore, a method of fasting is proposed with enough built-in flexibility to enable people of varying temperaments and conditions to benefit from a fast.

PROPOSED PLAN FOR FASTING

The plan is of necessity a compromise. It is the result of personal experience, as well as evaluating comments, discussions and clinical experience with doctors who have supervised fasting. On the question of the length of time, ten days are recommended, but this can be reduced to seven days or less, or extended to fourteen days.

For the patient whose elimination ceases during the fast, an enema a day for the first two or three days is indicated. This is preferable to allowing putrescible material to remain in the intestinal tract until "nature" calls.

Regarding exercise, here again no fixed rule need be given. Usually some light exercise should be encouraged. A complete bed rest is seldom indicated. Some people on a fast go to business and follow their usual daily routine.

The suggestions given here are not too difficult for the patient to follow.

A 7-10 or 14 Day Fast

LIQUIDS: 8 to 10 glasses per day, half of which should be vegetable and/or fruit juices, the other half any water except distilled water. In addition to the juices, an herb tea flavored with honey and lemon can be used. If the patient will do everything but give up coffee or tea, submit and let him have it.

VITAMIN SUPPLEMENTS: The easiest, but not the best way, is a prepared daily vitamin-mineral combination. The following products are preferred: Vitamin A–D—5000 & 500 units fish liver oil.

B Complex— Tablets or preferably 1 tablespoon of Brewers' Yeast or 2 to 4 tablets.
Vitamin C— Ascorbic acid—100–200 mgm.
Kelp tablets— 6–8 tablets a day.

If the patient is using additional vitamins to the above, he may continue.

DRUGS: No drugs of any kind during the fast, not even aspirin.

Synthetic vitamins are easy to take. If the patient will not or cannot take the vitamins as suggested, then the synthetic is better than none.

As to juices, here again, it goes without saying that freshly prepared vegetable juice is preferable to canned juice. Where this is a nuisance to prepare, "V8" should make a pleasant substitute.

Breaking the Fast

Having been on juices, breaking the fast need not be a problem. On the day after the fast ends, one can increase the amount of juices. *Eat one of the following suggested foods at a time:* Take yogurt, or vegetable soup; or eat raw fruit and vegetables and some nut butter, crushed nuts or seeds, about 1–2 ounces, and sprouted grains. BE SURE NOT TO OVEREAT. Chew food well.

Each succeeding day the amount of fruits and vegetables can be increased as can also the nut butter, or crushed nuts or seeds. Gradually the patient can phase into a "normal" diet by about the 4th or 5th day after breaking the fast.

When the patient has completed the fast, he will be better able to utilize an optimum diet of wholesome nutrition, which can hasten his recovery.

SUGGESTED READINGS

Abrahamson, E. M. and Pezer, A. W. *Body, Mind and Sugar*. New York: Henry Holt, 1951.

Bragg, P. C. *Toxicless Diet,* Health Science. Burbank, California: 1964.

Bragg, P. C. *Miracle of Fasting,* Health Science. Burbank, California: 1968.

Carpenter, D. L. *Microbiology*. Philadelphia, Pa.: W. B. Saunders Co., 1963.

Davis, Adelle. Several books on Diet and Foods.

DeVries, A. *Therapeutic Fasting*. Los Angeles, Calif.: Chandler Book Company, 1968.

Ehret, A. *Rational Fasting*. Los Angeles, Calif.: Ehret Literature Publishing Company, 1938.

Hoffer, A. and Osmond, H. *Schizophrenia*. New York: University Books, 1969.

Lindlahr, V. H. *Eat and Reduce*. Garden City, New York: Prentice-Hall, Inc., 1946.

Roberts, Sam E. *Exhaustion*. Emmaus, Pa.: Rodale Books, Inc., 1967.

PART VI

A BIOCHEMICAL APPROACH TO MENTAL HEALTH

CHAPTER

CHAPTER 19

NUTRITION AND MENTAL HEALTH

HARRY J. WENDLAND

GOOD MENTAL HEALTH depends upon the proper functioning of the nervous system; which, in addition to its own nutritional requirements, is involved with the nutrition of other organs in the entire body. In fact, no other part of the human body is so intervolved with all the phases of nutrition as the nervous system.[1]

In the complexity of the nervous involvements with nutrition, we have at least two major considerations: First, the effects of nutrition on the brain; and second, the effects of different mental conditions on the use the body makes of food ingested.[2] Like other parts of the body, the brain has its own particular nutrient requirements which are provided through the various systems, organs, cells, etc., which it governs.[1] For its normal functioning the brain is predominantly dependent upon a constant supply of oxygen and glucose. When there is a disruption of supply of these factors the metabolism of the brain is impaired. The specific nature of the alteration determines the symptoms that are produced.[3]

In the secondary consideration, malnutrition of the nervous system may be both a cause and a result of the deranged metabolism of other tissues.[1] The interchangeable relationship between the nervous system and other functioning parts of the human structure, therefore, is important in any consideration of nutrition for mental health.

Heading the nervous system is the brain, which is extraordinarily active metabolically. The normal adult human brain weighs only one-fortieth (about 2 percent) of the body as a whole, but its metabolism accounts for approximately 20 to 25 percent of the total oxygen consumption of the body,[4a] and for about 15 to 25 percent of the resting cardiac output.[3] Although motionless as compared to muscular activity, its oxygen consumption indicates that it is at least ten times as active as that of the average non-nervous tissue.[4a]

In contrast to the extraordinary metabolic activity of brain, it is interesting to note that the rate of entry of many substances from the blood are much slower in nervous than in non-nervous tissue.[5a] The quick and unimpeded passage of oxygen is understandable, since oxygen is necessary for the combustion of glucose to produce energy of which great amounts are consumed in the maintenance of mental life. Deprivation of oxygen for only 15 seconds can result in loss of consciousness, and its interruption for four minutes can cause irreparable brain damage.[6] Highly dependent as the function of the nervous system may be upon an adequate supply of oxygen and glucose, the supply and metabolism of protein and lipids also are vitally important.[1, 8]

Participating in virtually all the metabolic processes that provide energy and structural components for the nervous system are the vitamins, particularly those of the B-complex, which through their coenzymes form a part of the complex enzyme systems, and are particularly essential to carbohydrate metabolism.[1, 8, 13]

Additionally required are the major and minor minerals (trace elements). Vital components of the molecular composite of nerve cells, and necessary for maintenance of electrolyte balance of interstitial fluids, they participate as ionic acclerators of enzyme systems and produce electrical activity through changes of potentials at the cell membrane.[1, 9]

MOLECULES AND MENTAL HEALTH

Since about 1925 when the often referred to "revolution of molecular biology" began there has been a tremendous upsurge in knowledge and understanding of biological systems. New factual, scientific insights resulted in molecular biology exploding on cellular biology. The theory held for more than a century that the cell is the basic structural and fundamental biological unit gave way to the molecular concept, as biology advanced from the cell to its component molecules.[10] With its advance to the molecular concept, the basic principles of biology have not changed; it still is the science of life and a fundamental key to the understanding of disease.

In another chapter in this book Pauling explains that the proper functioning of the mind requires molecules of many different substances. After listing various B vitamins and ascorbic acid (C), he states that mental function and behavior also are affected by changes in the concentration in the brain of any of the other substances that normally are present.

Paul A. Weiss of the Rockefeller Institute in his report to the National Academy of Sciences, Washington, D.C. stated that he believes the ducting of substances through nerve fibers shows how nerves adapt themselves to chemicals, such as a dependency on narcotics or a resistance to drugs.[11]

THE NUTRIENT PROFILE

While certain vitamins in relation to mental health are discussed elsewhere in this volume, a number of vitamins and other nutrients so exemplify the complexities and ramifications of the nutritional processes of the central nervous system that they justify comment here.

Vitamin A, the first vitamin to be discovered, has numerous metabolic roles. Its clinical effects are many and seem to involve all human cells in one way or another.[12] Vitamin A also plays a vital role in the process of the central nervous system in that its deficiency causes pathophysiological changes in the retina, producing xerophthalmia (literally "dry eye") and reducing rhodopsin content.[9]

Each of the vitamins of the B-complex is essential to the proper functioning of the nervous system.[13] This is due to their requirement in a variety of highly complicated enzyme systems which govern and control neural energy. At least five of the B-complex vitamins are components of one or more coenzymes—thiamine, riboflavin, niacin, pyridoxine, and panththenic acid. Coenzymes are catalysts that have important and often related functions in the biochemical processes by means of which nutrients are used for energy and for building up or maintaining the cells and tissues of the body.[14]

Two other B vitamins, folic acid and vitamin B-12 which have antianemic properties, presumably also function as coenzymes.[14]

Thiamine, vitamin B-1, was one of the first vitamins found to be implicated in deficiency states causing neurologic changes of polyneuritis, Wernicke's encephalopathy, Korsakow's syndrome, and beri-beri.[15]

Riboflavin (vitamin B-2) functions as a part of a group of enzymes called flavoproteins, which are involved in the metabolism of carbohydrates, fats and proteins, and is essential for the release of energy within the cell.[18] Riboflavin is necessary before the amino acid trytophan, a source of niacin in the body, can be converted into the active form of the vitamin.[12b] Since a lack of one of the members of the B-complex may upset the vitamin balance and result in manifestations of other deficiencies, the combination of B-complex factors is advocated in treating vitamin deficiency conditions. In pellagra this practice is usually followed.[19a]

Nicotinic acid (vitamin B-3) is also referred to as niacin or niacinamide, although there is a difference of reaction between niacin and niacinamide. Niacin but not niacinamide leads to vasodilating action.[20a] Niacin or a derivative of niacin is required by all living cells. In the body it is an essential component of two important coenzymes, nicotinamide adenine dinucleotide (NAD, coenzyme I) and adenine dinucleotide phosphate (NADP, coenzyme II). More than forty biochemical reactions have been identified as being dependent on them.[20b]

As a chemical substance, niacin has been known since 1867, but its recognition as a vitamin was not fully established until 1937. Its deficiency in human nutrition has long been implicated with various abnormal mental conditions. Some of these, as the psychoses of pellagra and schizophrenia and the favorable effect of niacin, have been described by Pauling in a previous chapter.

The use of niacin in milder mental aberrations, was dramatically brought out in the report of Tom Spies. After showing that the serious mental illness of severe niacin deficiency causing pellagra could be relieved by niacin, Spies turned to the problem of how to relieve the early symptoms of niacin deficiency.[21] In another report, he lists the symptoms in the early stages of the disease, some of which include the following: Periods of depression and apprehension, increased irritability, insomnia, headaches, dizziness, and muscular weakness.[22] Clinically, Spies was able to show that the particular symptoms related to the nervous system could be relieved—and could also be prevented, by giving niacin and vitamin B-1.[21]

The use of niacin has also been suggested as a prophylaxis to prevent or delay the onset of psychoses of senility.[23]

Pyridoxine and vitamin B-6 are similar terms used to denote at least three closely related compounds with analogous physiological actions: Pyridoxamine, peridoxal and pyridoxol. In the form of pyridoxal phosphate vitamin B-6 functions as a coenzyme for many biological reactions, particularly those concerned with the transformation and utilization of amino acids and related compounds.[24] The role of vitamin B-6 in the metabolism of the central nervous system has been the subject of intensive study by numerous investigators. According to their reports there can be no question that an adequate supply of vitamin B-6 is necessary for the normal functioning of the central nervous system in man.[24] Pantothenic acid, another B-complex vitamin, is a key constituent of coenzyme A (A for acetylation) which occupies a central position in metabolism, being vital to all energy-requiring processes within the body. Deficiency in man has been produced experimentally by administration of a pantothenic acid antagonist along with a diet devoid of this vitamin. Resulting deficiency symptoms reported include: Weakness, fatigue, emotional instability, dizziness, impaired motor coordination, nausea, headache, muscle cramps, etc.[25]

Folic acid (also referred to as folacin) participates in many biochemical processes. Its most important activity is the role it plays in the synthesis of purine and pyrimidine compounds which are utilized in the formation of neucleoproteins and transmethylation processes.[26a] Vitamin B-12 appears to be involved with the activity of folic acid coenzymes in many of these metabolic processes.[19b]

Coursin refers to some recent reports that implicate folic acid deficiency with development anomalies in the brain, i.e., hydrocephalus (increased accumulation of cerebrospinal fluid within the ventricles of the brain). Patients in the studies revealed severe mental retardation and dilation of lateral ventricles.[9]

Cyanocobalamin, vitamin B-12, acts in many significant biological roles. Like folic acid, this vitamin in coenzyme form is involved in the metabolism of purines and pyridimines in the synthesis of neucleoproteins, and thereby in the formation of normal red blood cells. Undoubtedly, vitamin B-12 also has an important role in the metabolism of nervous tissue, though its precise mechanism in this respect is unclear.[26b] Ascorbic acid, vitamin C, has a variety of essential roles in the human body. In a previous chapter, Pauling refers to its use in certain mental conditions. In his appraisal of vitamin C in various disorders, Marks mentions that high utilization rates for ascorbic acid have been found in many psychiatric patients and that an improved mental state has been found in controlled trials with high doses of vitamin C.[27]

Vitamin E, also known as tocopheral—alpha tocopheral, beta tocopheral, and gamma tocopheral—is a vitamin of physiological antioxident activity. Studies have shown that it is not only essential for normal muscle metabolism, maintenance of the integrity of the vascular system, but also the central nervous system, as well as some other physiological functions.[5b]

In explaining the use of vitamin E in a variety of diseases, the foremost exponents of this vitamin, Evan and Wilfred Shute, mention the prophylactic role of vitamin E in the arteriosclerotic changes in the brain of the elderly. It helps to prevent clots from forming in blood vessels, and, of course, a clot in a vessel in the brain is what a stroke usually is. The old hypertensive has this danger continually hanging over his head.[28]

PROTEIN IN BRAIN FUNCTION

Protein with its amino acids is vitally important in nutrition for normal brain functioning. This is emphasized, since earlier in this chapter carbohydrate was mentioned as the principle source of glucose, so very necessary in brain metabolism. Protein provides amino acids, which the brain utilizes for the synthesis of protein and phospholipids as do other organs of the body. According to Underfriend, many amino acids which are not deemed necessary to the whole body are required by the brain and are obtainable only in appropriate quantities when the liver and kidney carry out their synthetic processes normally.[29]

MINERALS FOR MENTAL HEALTH

Previous reference in this chapter has indicated that mineral elements are as essential to the functioning of the nervous system as to the rest of the body. Like vitamins, minerals have many physiological functions including important roles in enzyme systems; however, until recently mineral metabolism has been a neglected field of study.[16a]

Minerals, trace elements, etc., have been classified into respective groups. Different authors have designated them by numerous and varying terms, which may be confusing. The official terminological classification by the National Academy of Science in the seventh edition of *Recommended Dietary Allowances* [30] is as follows:

Mineral Elements: Calcium and phosphorus, copper, fluorine, iodine, iron magnesium.
Trace or Microelements: Chromium, cobalt, manganese, molybdenum, selenium and zinc.
Electrolytes and Water: Sodium potassium, and chloride.

CALCIUM is essential for proper control of the excitability of nerve centers,[30a] when blood calcium drops below normal, irritability of the nerves is increased.[32] Thus, it is to be expected that calcium deficiency is generally, but not always [33] associated with irritability and instability of the nervous system.

PHOSPHORUS, which frequently is listed side-by-side with calcium, has more functions in the body than practically any other mineral element.[26c] As a constituent of the phospholipids present in all tissues and which are especially abundant in nerve tissues,[5c] it plays an important part in nervous tissue metabolism. It also has a role in the metabolism of carbohydrates, protein and fat, normal blood chemistry, muscle energy and skeletal growth. Normally, there is an inverse relationship between the serum calcium and serum inorganic phosphate. Little precise information is known concerning phosphorus requirements except for a generalization, based on experience, that phosphorus intake should approximately equal that of calcium, provided the calcium intake is adequate.[26c] Phosphorus equal to that of calcium intake is recommended for all age groups except the young infant.[30]

MAGNESIUM is the fourth most common element in the body, surpassed by only calcium, sodium and potassium. An activator of many enzyme systems, it is closely related to phosphorus, potassium and calcium metabolism.[34] Among its many biochemical reactions, magnesium functions in nerve conduction and muscular activity. The ability to transmit nerve impulse depends on ATP (adenosine triphosphate). The majority of the reactions involving ATP depend on magnesium.[35]

The clinical picture in severe magnesium deficiency is marked by neuromuscular and nervous system hyperirritability. Seen are: tremors (which most often affect the arms) and jerks or twitches which occur irregularly, seeming to wax and wane. Mental changes are striking: patients may be confused and some develop true hallucinations.[36]

One of the provocative facts brought out by Kleiner and Orton is that low levels of either magnesium or calcium in serum lead to the same effect; namely, hyperirritability and convulsions.[17] Interrelationship between the two is also shown by the fact that a high calcium diet worsens the effect of magnesium deficiency; [37] and by the fact that stepping up the magnesium intake, particularly in the presence of adequate calcium intake, improves rather than interferes with calcium utilization.[38]

IRON is present in every cell in the body.[31b] Although the amount of iron present in man is small (about 3.5 grams), it is of vital importance in the living process concerned with the transport of oxygen and with the metabolism of food materials within the cells.[39a] Iron deficiency can result from various causes, and hyperchronic anemia may ensue as a consequence of continued deficiency. Emotional instability may precede or be aggravated by the anemia, as the condition progresses. Apathy, lassitude, unusual anxiety, and irritability have been observed.[40]

IODINE is contained in every cell in the body.[31c] While noticeably present in a number of organs, the thyroid gland is the principal storehouse for iodine;

and iodine and thyroid function are inseparably linked. Iodine is utilized to form thyroid hormone.[39b] The output of thyroid hormone is controlled from the pituitary gland. The thyroid secretions determine the level of metabolism in many cells. If the secretion is deficient, the basal metabolism falls, the circulation is reduced and the whole tempo of the patient's life is slowed down.[41a]

WATER, while it is beyond the scope of this chapter to include data on all minerals, or trace elements that may have some role in mental health, the most important mineral, water, deserves consideration.

The most abundant body constituent, water accounts for approximately 62 per cent of the total body weight. The various tissues within the body differ considerably in water content.[5d] The brain, spinal cord and nerve trunks contain a fraction more than 73 per cent.[42] Deficits or excesses of more than a few per cent of the water in the body are incompatible with normal health.[30]

Next to oxygen water is the most necessary nutrient for survival of man. A person can exist without food for five weeks or more, but without water he can live for only a few days.[43] The German physiologist, Rubner, reported that man can lose all reserve glycogen, almost all fat, and about half of his protein without great danger; however, the loss of 10 percent of the water content of the body results in serious disorders, and that the loss of only 20 to 22 per cent results in death.

NUTRITIONAL NEUROLOGICAL DISORDERS

As intimated in the beginning of this chapter, the integrity and normal function of the nervous system is largely dependent up on the nutritional status of the individual. While that explanation is explicit and seems fairly simple, the relationships between nutrition and mental health are legion and would take a multi-volume treatise to describe adequately.

The group of nervous disorders due to nutritional deficiency is an ever widening one, and is now included in many types of neural degeneration with or without changes in the spinal cord, which formerly were believed to be of another nature. These disorders may appear as obscure features in the background or they may dominate the clinical picture.[45]

Neurological diseases in which malnutrition is of primary etiological importance are listed by Davidson and Passmore as the following: Nutritional encephalopathies and neuropathies associated with pellagra (nicotine acid deficiency), and subacute combined degeneration of the cord (vitamin B-12 deficiency).[41b] Nervous disorders or their symptoms as they relate to vitamin or mineral deficiencies have also been pointed out in previous sections of this chapter.

Nervous disorders in which the state of nutrition plays a secondary role and which sometimes can be influenced by diet are the psychoses and the psychoneuroses.[45] Under each of these two categories there are many classifications, too many to be detailed here. Instead a brief explanation of the terms may be of interest.

The psychoses are a group of conditions dissimilar in their causes, pathology and treatment. Some of them have their origin in manifest diseases of the brain; in others the buffetings of life and the influences of heredity together account for the illness. What the psychoses have in common is an aberration in social behavior and in psychologic attitude.[46] In contrast, the psychoneuroses are considered relatively benign mental disorders, the personality remains socially integrated and the person is able to function. The psychoneurotic person maintains an interest in the outer world and distinguishes between subjective experience and reality. In the psychotic person these abilities are impaired.[47] The psychotic syndrome, schizophrenia, is referred to in another chapter of this book where Pauling points out the noteworthy results secured from the administration of niacin and vitamin C.

DIAGNOSTIC IMPLICATIONS

The account earlier in this chapter of some of the known nutritional processes involved in brain metabolism, and which play a contributing and sometimes prime causal role in nervous and mental changes, would be incomplete without some brief reference to their implications for diagnosis. Campbell points out that recognition of the malnutrition of the human organism or its parts depends not only upon the clinical ability to observe the presenting signs and symptoms of malnutrition, either in specific tissues of the body or in the total behavior; but also upon the nutritional history which, if carefully checked, will reveal the anomaly of normal nutritional health.[1] Determination of past and current dietary intake is a classic method in assessment of the nutritional state,[48] and would seem fairly simple if that was all that is entailed in the diagnosis. There are, however, some complexities and Goldsmith explains that nutritional diagnosis is not easy despite the mass of information published in recent decades. Variation among individuals is great and the line of demarcation between normal and abnormal is not clear-cut.[16b] In his book, BIOCHEMICAL INDIVIDUALITY, Williams gives some insight on the high degree of biochemical individuality that is present in every member of the human family. With respect to many items—specific enzyme levels, endocrine activities, nutritional needs—five to tenfold variations between normal individuals appear to be common.[4b]

The great individual variations have also been emphasized by Sebrell [4a] and other nutritional authorities. However, this should not be discouraging in regard to nutritional diagnosis, since similar difficulties are found in all fields of biologic investigations; and diagnosis of various other types of diseases, including some nonnutritional disorders, are no exception.[16b]

In conclusion, it should be re-emphasized that the whole person, not just a part of him, is affected by his food.[50] Also, diseases of any organ system or portion of the body can adversely affect brain function and cause confusion, delirium, and other signs and symptoms.[51] Despite the inclusion of numerous pathologic entities in this chapter, others of lesser or greater importance have not been included because of space limitations.

The concept of malnutrition is changing, placing it in the category of the metabolic diseases. The doctor must know that he cannot treat any patient in the most effective manner unless he takes into account the patient's metabolic status and he must correct the nutritional and metabolic abnormalities which may have been the result of some other disease.[49] In his closing remarks to the doctor in his report on "Changing Concept of Malnutrition," the noted nutritionalist, W. H. Sebrell, Jr., states the following: "He must learn to use refined methods of diagnosis to pick up the nutritional abnormalities resulting from deranged metabolism. He must have such a knowledge of nutrition that he will do more than merely prescribe a multinutritional preparation without bothering to make a diagnosis in the hope that this will have everything in it and thereby cure whatever nutritional abnormality the patient has. It is more and more evident that specific diagnosis is required and that treatment must be individualized just as in the case with the treatment of other diseases." [49]

REFERENCES

1. Campbell, Douglas G. "Nutrition and Metabolism in Relation to Neurology and Psychiatry," *Am. J. Digest. Disease* (August 1956), 1 (8):333.
2. Bond, Earl D. "Nutrition in the Psychiatric Patient," *Diethotherapy*. Philadelphia: W. B. Saunders Co., 1945.
3. McHenry, Lawrence C., and Valsamis, Marius, P. "Pathophysiology of Cerebro-Vascular Insufficiency," GP: *General Practice* (1966), 33:78.
4. Williams, Roger, J. "Implications for Advance in Psychiatry," *Biochemical Individuality*. New York: John Wiley & Sons, Inc. 1956, a.p. 199, and b.pp. 69–162.
5. Oser, Bernard L. *Hawk's Physiological Chemistry* (14th ed.). New York: McGraw-Hill Book Co. (Blakiston Div.) (1965), a.p. 241, b.p. 735, c.p. 556, and d.p. 543.
6. Wilson, John R. (et. al.). *The Mind.* Life Science Library. New York: Time, Inc. (1967), p. 20.
7. Peterman, Robert A.; Goodheart, Robert S. "Current Status of Vitamin Therapy in Nervous and Mental Diseases," *J. Clin. Nutrition* (Jan.–Feb. 1954), 2:11.
8. Tower, Donald B. "Neurochemical Aspects of Pyridoxine Metabolism and Function," *Am. J. Clin. Nutrition* (July–Aug. 1956), 4:329.
9. Coursin, David B. "Nutrition and Brain Function," *Modern Nutrition in Health and Disease* (4th ed.). Wohl and Goodheart, eds. Philadelphia: Lea & Febiger (1968), pp. 1077–1080.
10. Vallee, Bert L.; Wacker, Warren E. C. "Medical Biology," *Jama* (1963), 184:6:485.
11. Staff report. "Nerve Fiber, A Moving 'River' with Rythmic. Beat," *International Review of Chiropractic* (June 1962).

12. Guthrie, Helen Andres. *Introductory Nutrition* (2nd. ed.). St. Louis: C. V. Mosby Co. (1971), a.p. 190, and b.p. 246.
13. Tower, Donald B. "Pyridoxine and Cerebral Activity," *Nutrition Reviews* (June 1958), 16:151.
14. Goldsmith, Grace A. Vitamins of the B-Complex, *Food—The Yearbook of Agriculture.* U.S. Government Printing Office (1959), pp. 139–149.
15. Spillane, J. D. *Nutritional Disorders of the Nervous System.* Baltimore: E. & S. Livingstone, Ltd., Edinburgh; Williams & Wilkins, 1947.
16. Goldsmith, Grace A. *Nutritional Diagnosis* (pub. no. 356), American Lecture Series. Springfield, Ill.: Charles C. Thomas, Publisher (1959), a.p. 63, and b.p. 7.
17. Kleiner, Israel S.; Orten, James M. *Biochemistry* (6th ed.). St. Louis: C.V. Mosby Co. (1962), p. 594.
18. Mitchell, Helen S. (et al.). *Cooper's Nutrition in Health and Disease* (15th ed.). Philadelphia: J. B. Lippincott Co. (1968), p. 102.
19. Chaney, Margaret S., Ross, Margaret L. *Nutrition* (7th. ed.). Boston: Houghton, Mifflin Co. (1966), a.p. 273, and b.p. 302.
20. Goldsmith, Grace A. "The B Vitamins; Thiamine, Riboflavin, Niacin," *Nutrition, A Comprehensive Treatise,* Beaton and McHenry, eds. (Vol. II). New York: Academic Press (1964), a.p. 173, and b.p. 167.
21. Spies, Tom D. "Some Recent Advances in Nutrition," *Jama* (June 7, 1958), 167:6:675.
22. Spies, Tom D. "Niacinamide Malnutrition and Pellagra," *Clinical Nutrition* (2nd. ed.). New York: Harper & Bros. (1962), p. 628.
23. Gregory, I. "Nicotinic Acid Therapy in Psychosis of Senility," *Am. J. Psychiatry* (June 1952), 108:888.
24. Sebrell, W. H., Jr. "The Importance of Vitamin B-6 in Human Nutrition," *Vitamins and Hormones* (Vol. 22). New York: Academic Press (1964), p. 877.
25. Bean, W. B., Hodges, R. E., and Daum, K. "Human Pantothenic Acid Deficiency Produced by Omega-Methyl Pantothenic Acid," *J. Clin. Investigation* (1959), 38:1421–1425.
26. Burton, Benjamin T. *Heinz Handbook of Nutrition* (2nd. ed.). New York: McGraw Hill Book Co. (Blakiston Div.), 1965, a.p. 106, b.p. 110, and c.pp. 119–120.
27. Marks, John. *The Vitamins in Health and Disease. A Modern Reappraisal.* Boston: Little, Brown and Co. (1968), p. 136.
28. Shute, Evan and Wilfrid. *Your Heart and Vitamin E.* Detroit, Michigan: pub. by The Cardiac Society, p. 65.
29. Underfriend, Sidney. "Factors in Amino Acid Metabolism Which Can Influence the Central Nervous System," *Am. J. Clin. Nutri.* (April 1963), 12:4:278.
30. National Academy of Sciences. National Research Council, *Recommended Daily Allowances* (pub. 1694). Washington, D.C. 1968.
31. Kranz, John C.; Carr, Jelleff C.: *Pharmaceutical Principles of Medical Practice* (7th ed.). Philadelphia: Williams & Wilkins Co. (1969), a.p. 725, and b.p. 535, c.p. 710.
32. Hathway, L. Millicent; Leverton, Ruth M. "Calcium and Phosphorus," *Yearbook of Agriculture.* U.S. Government Printing Office (1959), p. 112.
33. Plank, E. H. "Calcium Deficiency Signs," J. Med. Ass. Alabama (1945), 14:165–167.

34. Hathway, Millicent L. "Magnesium in Human Nutrition," *Home Economics Research Report* (No. 19). Washington, D.C.: U.S. Dept. Agri.
35. Vallee, Bert L. "Clinical Significance of Trace Elements," *Review of Modern Med.* (Jan.–June 1963), p. 102.
36. Grollman, Arthur. *Pharmacology & Therapeutics* (6th ed.). Philadelphia: Lea & Febiger (1965), p. 1003.
37. Shohl, Alfred T. *Mineral Metabolism.* New York: Reinhold Pub. Corp. (1939), p. 164.
38. Seelig, Mildred S. *Am. J. Clin. Nutri.* (June 1964), 14:6:241.
39. Wirtschafter, Zolton T. *Minerals in Nutrition.* New York: Reinhold Pub. Corp. (1942), a.p. 103, and b.p. 117.
40. Farquharson, R. F. "Iron Malnutrition," *Clinical Nutrition* (edited by Jolliffe). New York: Hoeber Med. Book. Div., Harper & Bros. (1950), p. 307.
41. Davidson, Stanley; Passmore, R. *Human Nutrition and Dietetics,* (4th ed.). Baltimore: Williams & Wilkins Co. (1969), a.p. 174, and b.p. 658.
42. Hamilton, T. S. et. al. *J. Biol. Chemistry* (1945), 158:625.
43. Michelsen, Olaf. *Food, The Yearbook of Agriculture.* Washington, D.C.: U.S. Dept. Agri., 1959, p. 168.
44. Rubner, J.: *Lehrbuch der Hygiene* (8th. ed.). Leipzig and Vienna: F. Deuticke, 1907.
45. McLester, James S.; Darby, William J. *Nutrition and Diet in Health and Disease* (6th. ed.). Philadelphia: W. B. Saunders Co. (1952), pp. 545–555.
46. Lewis, Aubrey. "The Psychoses," *Textbook of Medicine* (12 ed.). Philadelphia: W. B. Saunders Co. (1968), p. 1456.
47. Terhume, William B. "The Management of the Psychiatric Patient in General Office Practice," *Med. Clin. N. Amer.* (Nov. 1961), 45:6:1590.
48. Weir, David R.; and Houser, Harold B. "Problems in the Evaluation of Nutritional Status in Chronic Illness," *Am. J. Clin. Nutri.* (April 1963), 12:4:281.
49. Sebrell, Jr.; W. H. "Changing Concept of Malnutrition.", *Am. J. Clin. Nutrition* (June 1967), 20:6:653.
50. Sandstead, Harold H., et al. "How to Diagnose Nutritional Disorders in Daily Practice," *Nutrition Today* (1969), 4:2.
51. Greenhouse, Arnold H.: "Metabolic Encephalopathies," *Current Diagnosis 3* (Conn and Conn, eds.). Philadelphia: W. B. Saunders Co. (1971), p. 825.

CHAPTER 20

ORTHOMOLECULAR PSYCHIATRY*

Varying the concentrations of substances normally present in the human body may control mental disease.

LINUS PAULING, PH.D.

THE METHODS principally used now for treating patients with mental disease are psychotherapy (psychoanalysis and related efforts to provide insight and to decrease environmental stress), chemotherapy (mainly with the use of powerful synthetic drugs, such as chlorpromazine, or powerful natural products from plants, such as reserpine), and convulsive or shock therapy (electroconvulsive therapy, insulin coma therapy, pentylenetetrazol shock therapy). I have reached the conclusion, through arguments summarized in the following paragraphs, that another general method of treatment, which may be found to be of great value, and may turn out to be the best method of treatment for many patients.

Orthomolecular psychiatric therapy is the treatment of mental disease by the provision of the optimum molecular environment for the mind, especially the optimum concentrations of substances normally present in the human body.[1] An example is the treatment of phenylketonuric children by use of a diet containing a smaller than normal amount of the amino acid phenylalanine. Phenylketonuria [2] results from a genetic defect that leads to a decreased amount or effectiveness of the enzyme catalyzing the oxidation of phenylalanine to tyrosine. The patients on a normal diet have in their tissues abnormally high concentrations of phenylalanine and some of its reaction products, which, possibly in conjunction with the decreased concentration of tyrosine, cause the mental and physical manifestations of the disease (mental deficiency, severe eczema and others). A decrease in the amount of phenylalanine ingested results in an approximation to the normal or optimum concentrations and to the alleviation of the manifestations of the disease, both mental and physical.

* Reprinted by permission from the author and the publisher of SCIENCE, 19 April 1968, Volume 160, pp. 265–271. Copyright, 1968, by the American Association for the Advancement of Science.

The functioning of the brain is dependent on its composition and structure; that is, on the molecular environment of the mind. The presence in the brain of molecules of N, N-diethyl-D-lysergamide, mescaline, or some other schizophrenogenic substance is associated with profound psychic effects.[3] Cherkin has recently pointed out [4] that in 1799 Humphry Davy described similar subjective reactions to the inhalation of nitrous oxide. The phenomenon of general anesthesia also illustrates the dependence of the mind (consciousness, ephemeral memory) on its molecular environment.[5]

The proper functioning of the mind is known to require the presence in the brain of molecules of many different substances. For example, mental disease, usually associated with physical disease, results from a low concentration in the brain of any one of the following vitamins: thiamine(B_1), nicotinic acid or nicotinamide (B_3), pyridoxine (B_6), cyanocobalamin (B_{12}), biotin (H), ascorbic acid (C), and folic acid. There is evidence that mental function and behavior are also affected by changes in the concentration in the brain of any of a number of other substances that are normally present, such as L(+)-glutamic acid, uric acid, and y-aminobutyric acid.[6]

OPTIMUM MOLECULAR CONCENTRATIONS

Several arguments may be advanced in support of the thesis that the optimum molecular concentrations of substances normally present in the body may be different from the concentrations provided by the diet and the gene-controlled synthetic mechanisms, and, for essential nutrilites (vitamins, essential amino acids, essential fatty acids) different from the minimum daily amounts required for life or the "recommended" (average) daily amounts suggested for good health. Some of these arguments are presented in the following paragraphs.

EVOLUTION AND NATURAL SELECTION

The process of evolution does not necessarily result in the normal provision of optimum molecular concentrations. Let us use ascorbic acid as an example. Of the mammals that have been studied in this respect, the only species that have lost the power to synthesize ascorbic acid and that accordingly require it in the diet are man, other Primates (rhesus monkey, Formosan long-tail monkey, and ring-tail or brown capuchin monkey), the guinea pig, and an Indian fruit-eating bat (*Pteropus medius*).[7] Presumably the loss of the gene or genes controlling the synthesis of the enzyme or enzymes involved in the conversion of glucose to ascorbic acid occurred some 20 million years ago in the common ancestor of man and other Primates, and occurred independently for the guinea pig and for one species of bat and one bird, in each case in an environment such that ascorbic acid was provided by the food. For a mutation rate of $1/20{,}000$ per gene generation and for even a very small advantage for the mutant (0.01 percent more progeny) the mutant would replace the earlier genotype within about 1 million years. The advantage to the mutant of being rid of the ascorbic-acid-synthesis machinery (decrease in cell size and energy requirement, liberation of machinery for other purposes) might well be large, perhaps as much as 1 percent; a disadvantage nearly as large (less by 0.01 percent) resulting from a less than optimum supply of dietary ascorbic acid would not prevent the replacement of the earlier species by the mutant. Hence, even if the amount of the vitamin provided by the diet available at the time of the mutation were less than the optimum amount, the mutant might still be able to replace its predecessor. Moreover, it is possible that the environment has changed during the last 20 million years in such a way as to provide a decreased amount of the vitamin. Even a serious disadvantage of the changed environment would not lead to a mutation restoring the synthetic mechanism within a period of a few million years, because of the small probability of such mutations far smaller than of those resulting in loss of function.

Moreover, the process of natural selection may be expected later on to lead to the survival of a species or strain that synthesizes somewhat less than the optimum amount of an autotrophic vital substance rather than of the species or strain that synthesizes the optimum amount. To synthesize the optimum amount requires about twice as much biological machinery as to synthesize half the optimum amount. As suggested in Fig. 1, the evolutionary disadvantage of synthesizing a less than optimum amount of the vital substance may be small, and may be outweighed by the advantage of requiring a smaller amount of biological machinery. Evidence from the study of microorganisms is discussed in the following paragraphs.

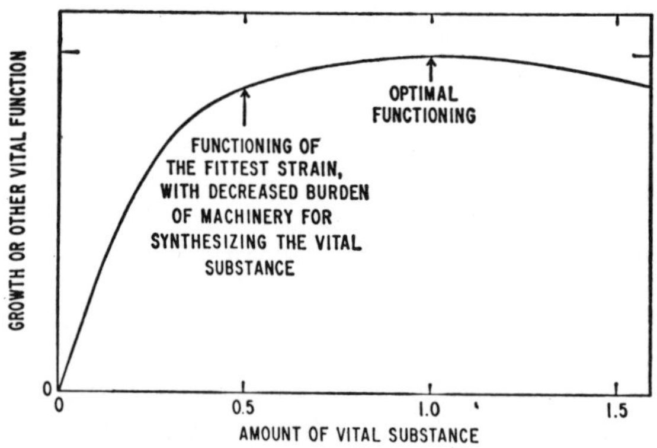

Figure 1. Diagrammatic representation of growth rate on other vital property of an organism as function of the concentration of vital substance in the organism, showing the concentration at which the differential advantage of an increased amount of vital substance is just balanced by the differential disadvantage resulting from an increased amount of machinery for synthesis, and the concentration that gives optimum functioning without consideration of the burden of the machinery for synthesis.

EVIDENCE FROM MICROBIOLOGICAL GENETICS

Many mutant microorganisms are known to require, as a supplement to the medium in which they are grown, a substance that is synthesized by the corresponding wild-type organism (the normal strain). An example is the pyridoxine-requiring mutant of *Neurospora sitophila* reported by G. W. Beadle and E. L. Tatum in their first *Neurospora* paper, published in 1941.[8] Several species of *Neurospora* that have been extensively studied are known to be able to grow satisfactorily on synthetic media containing inorganic salts, an inorganic source of nitrogen, such as ammonium nitrate, a suitable source of carbon, such as sucrose, and the vitamin biotin. All other substances required by the organism are synthesized by it. Beadle and Tatum found that exposure to x-radiation produces mutant strains such that one substance must be added to the minimum medium in order to permit the growth at a rate approximating that of the normal strain. Their pyridoxine-requiring mutant was found to grow on the standard medium at a rate only 9 percent of that of the normal strain. When pyriodoxine (vitamin B_6) is added to the medium, the rate of growth of this strain at first increases nearly linearly with the concentration of the added pyridoxine and then increases less rapidly, as shown in Fig. 2.[9] The growth rate of the normal strain without added pyridoxine is equal to that of the mutant with about 10 micrograms of the growth substance per liter in the medium. At a concentration about four times this value (40 micrograms per liter) the growth rate of the mutant strain reaches a value 7 percent greater than that of the normal strain without added pyridoxine.

The point of maximum curvature of the curve in Fig. 2, at about 3.2 micrograms of pyridoxine per liter (indicated by a cross), may be reasonably considered to mark the division between the region of vitamin deficiency (to the left) and the region of normal vitamin supply (to the right), such as might permit the mutant to compete with the wild type, which has the growth rate

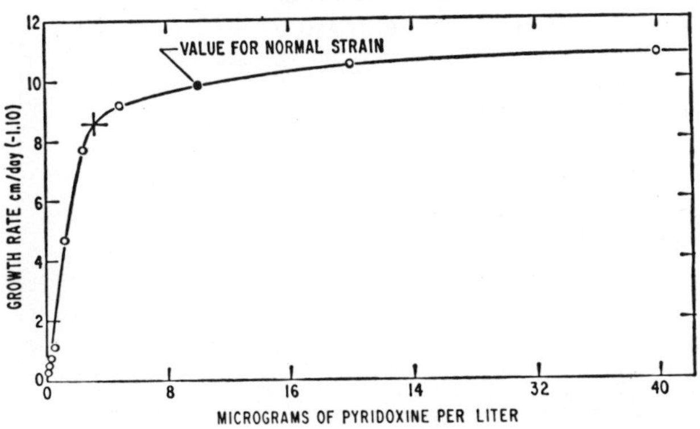

Figure 2. The observed rate of growth of a pyridoxine-requiring Neurospora mutant (Beadle and Tatum, 1941), as function of the concentration of pyridoxine in the medium.

represented by the filled circle in Fig. 2. The point marked by the cross might well correspond to an "adequate" or "recommended" amount of the vitamin, in that the growth rate of the mutant is only 12 percent less than that of the wild strain, and that the amount of the vitamin would have to be increased threefold to make up this 12 percent.[10]

As shown in Fig. 2, quadrupling the concentration of pyridoxine that gives the mutant a growth rate equal to that of the wild type causes a further increase in growth rate by nearly 10 percent. The growth rates of the mutant and the wild type at very large concentrations of the vitamin have not been measured so far as I know, and the optimum concentration is not known. From the work of Beadle and Tatum the optimum concentration may be taken to be greater than 40 micrograms per liter; that is, more than ten times the "adequate" concentration for the mutant and more than four times the concentration equivalent to the synthesizing capability of the wild type. The growth rate of the mutant at the optimum concentration is more than 22 percent greater than that at the "adequate" concentration and more than 9 percent greater than that of the normal strain.

Similar results have been reported for other mutants of *Neurospora*. The values found by Tatum and Beadle [11] for a p-aminobenzoic-acid-requiring mutant of *Neurospora crassa* as a function of the concentration of p-aminobenzoic acid added to the standard medium are shown in Fig. 3. The growth-rate curve is similar in shape to that for the pyridoxine-requiring mutant. The value of the growth rate for the normal strain of *Neurospora crassa* with no added p-aminobenzoic acid is equal to that for the mutant at a concentration of added p-aminobenzoic acid of about 15 micrograms per liter. A value about 4 percent greater is found for the normal strain at 40 micrograms per liter and for the mutant strain at 80 micrograms per liter, as indicated in Fig. 3.

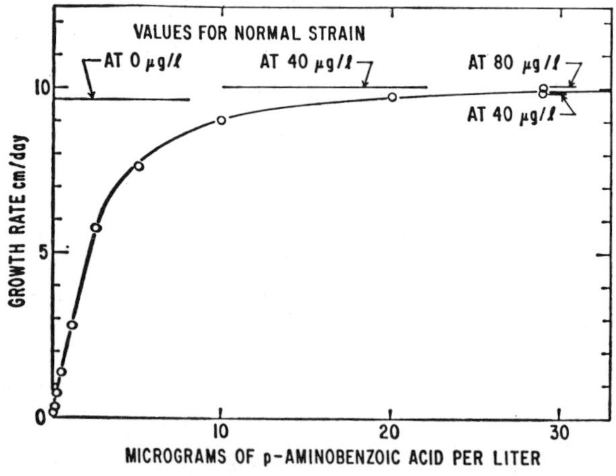

Figure 3. The observed rate of growth of a p-aminobenzoic-acid-requiring *Neurospora* mutant (Tatum and Beadle, 1942), as function of concentration of the growth substance in the medium.

It is customary to plot values of the growth rate against the logarithm of the concentration of the growth substance, as shown in Fig. 4. The amount of increase accompanying a doubling in the concentration of the growth substance is a maximum of 1.25 to 2.5 micrograms per liter, and decreases thereafter to about half the value for each successive doubling.

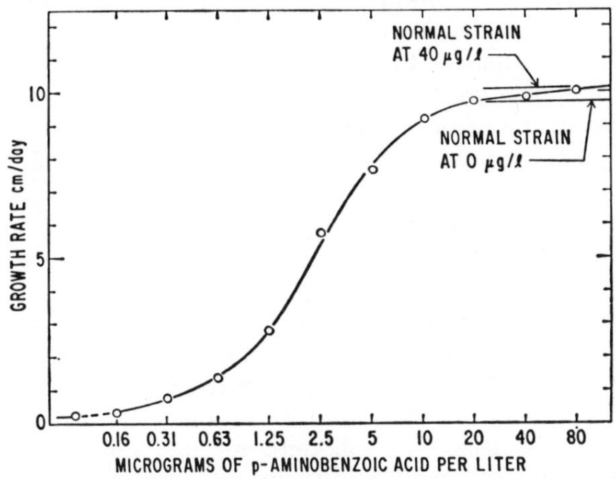

Figure 4. Observed rate of growth of a p-aminobenzoic-acid—requiring *Neurospora* mutant as function of the logarithm of the concentration of p-aminobenzoic acid.

From these two examples we see that there may be a significant increase in rate of growth of the normal strain through addition of some of the growth substance that it synthesizes to the medium in which it is grown; that is, that the amount of the growth substance that is synthesized by the normal strain is not the optimum amount, but is somewhat less—approximately 7 percent less in the case of pyridoxine (with the normal strain of *Neurospora sitophila*) and 4 percent less for p-aminobenzoic acid (with the normal strain of *Neurospora crassa*). Many other examples are known of microorganism that grow more abundantly in a medium containing vitamins, amino acids, or other substances that they are able to synthesize than on a minimum medium.

Evidence supporting the above arguments has been presented recently by Zamenhof and Eichhorn [11a] in a paper entitled "Study of microbial evolution through loss of biosynthetic functions: Establishment of 'defective' mutants." These authors carried out experiments involving competitive growth in a chemostat of an auxotrophic mutant (a mutant requiring a nutrilite) and a prototrophic parent in a medium of constant composition containing the nutrilite. They found that the "defective" mutant has a selective advantage over the prototrophic parental strain under these conditions. For example, an indole-requiring mutant of *Bacillus subtilis* was found to show a strong selective advantage over the prototrophic bacl.—mutant when the two were grown together in a medium containing tryptophan: the relative number of cells of the latter decreased 10^6-fold in 54 generations. They also found that greater advantage to the auxotroph accompanies a greater number of biosynthetic steps that have been dispensed with (earlier block in a series of reactions), with the final metabolite available. They point out that a mutant with a gene deletion would be at a distinct selective advantage over a point mutant, in that not only the synthesis of the metabolite, but also that of the structural gene, the messenger RNA, and perhaps the inactive enzyme itself would be dispensed with, and that accordingly the mutant with a deletion would replace the point mutant in competition. They mention evidence that some of the "defective" strains occurring in nature have lost one or more of their structural genes by deletions, rather than by point mutations.

MOLECULAR CONCENTRATIONS AND RATE OF REACTION

Most of the chemical reactions that take place in living organisms are catalyzed by enzymes. The mechanisms of enzyme-catalyzed reactions in general involve (i) the formation of a complex between the enzyme and a substrate molecule and (ii) the decomposition of this complex to form the enzyme and the products of the reaction. The rate-determining step is usually the decomposition of the complex to form the products, or, more precisely, the transition through an intermediate state of the complex, characterized by activation energy less than for the uncatalyzed reaction, to a complex of the enzyme and the products of reaction, with a rapid dissociation. Under conditions such that the concentration of the complex corresponds to equilibrium with the enzyme and the substrate, the rate of the reaction is given by the following equation [the Michaelis-Menten equation]: [12]

$$R = \frac{d[S]}{dt} = \frac{kE[S]}{[S] + (1/K)} \quad (1)$$

In this equation [S] is the concentration of the substrate, E is the total concentration of enzyme (present both as free enzyme and enzyme complex), K is the equilibrium constant for formation of the enzyme complex ES, and k is the reaction-rate constant for decomposition of the complex to form the enzyme and reaction products. This equation corresponds to the case in which there are no enzyme inhibitors present.

Value of the reaction rate calculated from this equation for different values of K are shown in Fig. 5. The curves are similar in shape to those of Figs. 2 and 3. At concentrations much smaller than K^{-1} the reaction rate is proportional to the concentration of substrate. At larger concentrations, as the amount of enzyme complex becomes comparable to the amount of free enzyme, the reaction rate changes from the linear dependence. At substrate concentration equal to K^{-1} the slope of the curve is one-quarter of the initial slope, and the value is one-half of the value corresponding to saturation of the enzyme by the substrate.

The similarity of the curves of Figs. 2 and 3 to appropriate curves in Fig. 5 suggests that the growth substance may be involved in an enzyme-catalyzed reaction in which it serves as the substrate. The normal strain of the organism manufactures an amount of the substrate such as to permit the reaction to take place at what may be considered a normal rate, 90 or 95 percent of the maximum rate, which corresponds to saturation of the enzyme. As described above, the gain in reaction rate associated with the manufacture of a larger amount of the substrate, with a corresponding advantage to the organism, might be balanced by the disadvantage of the organism associated with the upkeep of the larger amount of machinery required to manufacture the increased amount of substrate. An increase in rate of this reaction could also be achieved by an increase in the amount of the enzyme synthesized by the organism. Here, again, the advantage to the organism resulting from this increase may be overcome by the disadvantage associated with the increase in the amount of machinery required for the increased synthesis. During the process of evolution there has presumably been selection of genes determining the concentrations of the enzymes catalyzing successive reactions such as to achieve an approximation to the optimum reaction rate with the smallest amount of disadvantage to the organism.

The rate of an enzyme-catalyzed reaction is approximately proportional to the concentration of the reactant, until concentrations that largely saturate the enzyme are reached. The saturating concentration is larger for a defective

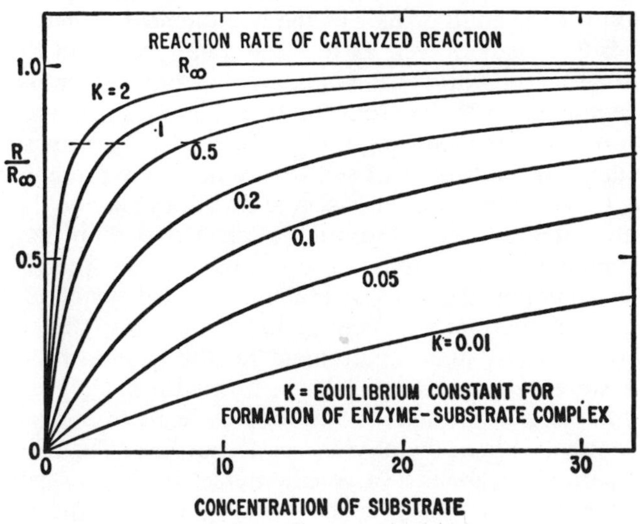

Figure 5. Curves showing calculated reaction rate R/R of catalyzed reaction as function of the concentration of the substrate, for different values of the equilibrium constant K for formation of the enzyme-substrate complex.

enzyme with decreased combining power for the substrate than for the normal enzyme. For such a defective enzyme the catalyzed reaction could be made to take place at or near its normal rate by an increase in the substrate concentration, as indicated in Fig. 5. The short horizontal lines intersecting the curves indicate what may be called the "normal" reaction rate, 80 percent of the maximum. For K = 2 the "normal" rate is achieved at substrate concentration [S] = 2. At this substrate concentration the reaction rate is only 29 percent of the maximum and 35 percent of "normal" for a mutated enzyme with K = 0.2; it could be raised to the "normal" value by a tenfold increase in the substrate concentration, to [S] = 20. Similarly, the still greater disadvantage of low reaction rate for a mutated enzyme with K only 0.01 could be overcome by a 200-fold increase in substrate concentration, to [S] = 400. This mechanism of action of gene mutation is only one of several that lead to disadvantageous manifestations that could be overcome by an increase, perhaps a greater increase, in the concentration of a vital substance in the body. These considerations obviously suggest a rationale for megavitamin therapy.

MOLECULAR CONCENTRATIONS AND MENTAL DISEASE

The functioning of the brain and nervous tissue is more sensitively dependent on the rate of chemical reactions than the functioning of other organs and tissues. I believe that mental disease is for the most part caused by abnormal reaction rates, as determined by genetic constitution and diet, and by abnormal molecular concentrations of essential substances. The operation of chance in the selection for the child of half of the complement of genes of the father and mother leads to bad as well as to good genotypes, and the selection of foods (and drugs) in a world that is undergoing rapid scientific and technological change may often be far from the best. Significant improvement in the mental health of many persons might be achieved by the provision of the optimum molecular concentrations of substances normally present in the human body. Among these substances, the essential nutrilites may be the most worthy of extensive research and more thorough clinical trial than they have yet received. One important example of an essential nutrilite that is required for mental health is vitamin B_{12}, cyanocobalamin. A deficiency of this vitamin, whatever its cause (pernicious anemia; infestation with the fish tapeworm *Diphyllobothrium,* whose high requirement for the vitamin results in deprivation for the host; excessive bacterial flora, also with a high vitamin requirement, as may develop in intestinal blind loops), leads to mental illness, often even more pronounced than the physical consequences. The mental illness associated with pernicious anemia (a genetic defect leading to deficiency of the intrinsic factor (a mucoprotein) in the gastric juice and the consequent decreased transport of cyanocobalamin into the blood) often is observed for several years in patients with this disease before any of the physical manifestations of the disease appear.[13] A pathologically low concentration of cyanocobalamin in the serum of the blood has been reported to occur for a much larger fraction of patients with mental illness than for the general population. Edwin, Holten, Norum, Schrumpf, and Skaug [14] determined the amount of B_{12} in the serum of every patient over 30 years old admitted to a mental hospital in Norway during a period of 1 year. Of the 396 patients, 5.8 percent (23) had a pathologically low concentration, less than 101 picograms per milliliter, and the concentration in 9.6 percent (38) was subnormal (101 to 150 picograms per milliliter). The normal concentration is 150 to 1300 picograms per milliliter. The incidence of pathologically low and subnormal levels of B_{12} in the serums of these patients, 15.4 percent, is far greater than that in the general population, about 0.5 percent (estimated from the reported frequency of pernicious anemia in the area, 9.3 per 100,000 persons per year). Other investigators [15] have also reported a higher incidence of low B_{12} concentrations in the serums of mental patients than in the population as a whole, and have suggested that B_{12} deficiency, whatever its origin may lead to mental illness.

Nicotinic acid (niacin), when its use was introduced, cured hundreds of thousands of pellagra patients of their psychoses, as well as of the physical manifestations of their disease. For this purpose only small doses are required; the recommended daily allowance (National Research Council) is 12 milligrams per day (for a 70-kilogram male). In 1939 Cleckley, Sydenstricker, and Geeslin [16] reported the successful treatment of 19 patients and in 1941 Sydenstricker and Cleckley [17] reported similarly successful treatment of 29 patients with several psychiatric symptoms by use of moderately large doses of nicotinic acid (0.3 to 1.5 grams per day). None of these patients had physical symptoms of pellagra or any other avitaminosis. More recently many other investigators have reported on the use of nicotinic acid and nicotinamide for the treatment of mental disease. Outstanding among them are Hoffer and Osmond, who since 1952 have advocated and used nicotinic acid in large doses, in addition to the conventional therapy, for the treatment of schizophrenia.[18, 19, 20] The dosage recommended by Hoffer is 3 to 18 grams per day, as determined by the response of the patient, of either nicotinic acid or nicotinamide, together with 3 grams per day of ascorbic acid. Nicotinic acid and nicotinamide are nontoxic [the lethal dose, 50 percent effective (LD_{50}), is not known for humans, but probably it is over 200 grams; the LD_{50} for rats is 7.0 grams per kilogram for nicotinic acid, and 1.7 grams per kilogram for nicotinamide], and their side effects, even in continued massive doses, seem not to be commonly serious. Among the advantages of nicotinic acid, summarized by Osmond and Hoffer,[19] are the following: it is safe, cheap, and easy to administer, and it is a well-known substance that can be taken for years on end, if necessary, with only small probability of incidence of unfavorable side effects.

Another vitamin that has been used to some extent in the treatment of mental disease is ascorbic acid, vitamin C. A sometimes-recommended daily intake of ascorbic acid is 75 milligrams for healthy adults. Some investigators have estimated that the optimum intake is much larger: [21] perhaps 3 to 15 grams per day, according to Stone.[22] Williams and Deason [23] have emphasized the variability of individual members of a species of animals; they have reported their observation of a 20-fold range of required intake of ascorbic acid by guinea pigs, and have suggested that human beings, who are less homogeneous, have a larger range.

Mental symptoms (depression) accompany the physical symptoms of vitamin-C deficiency disease (scurvy). In 1957 Akerfeldt [24] reported that the serum of schizophrenics had been found to have greater power of oxidizing N,N-dimethyl-p-phenylenediamine than that of other persons. Several investigators then reported that this difference is due to a smaller concentration of ascorbic acid in the serum of schizophrenics than of other persons. This difference has been attributed to the poor diet and increased tendency to chronic infectious disease of the patients,[25] and has also been interpreted as showing an increased rate of metabolism of ascorbic acid by the patients.[26] It is my opinion, from the study of the literature, that many schizophrenics have an increased metabolism of ascorbic acid, presumably genetic in origin, and that the ingestion of massive amounts of ascorbic acid has some value in treating mental disease.

Other vitamins (thiamine, pyridoxine, folic acid) and other substances [zinc ion, magnesium ion, uric acid, tryptophan, L(+)-glutamic acid, and others] influence the functioning of the brain. I shall review work on L(+)-glutamic acid as a further example. L(+)-glutamic acid is an amino acid that is present at rather high concentration in brain and nerve tissue and plays an essential role in the functioning of these tissues.[27] It is normally ingested (in protein) in amounts of 5 to 10 grams per day. It is not toxic; large doses may cause increased motor activity and nausea. In 1944 Price, Waelsch, and Putnam [28] reported favorable results for glutamic acid therapy for patients with petit mal epilepsy.[29] Zimmerman and Ross then reported an increase in maze-running learning ability of white rats given extra amounts of glutamic acid.[30] Zimmerman and many other investigators then studied the effects of glutamic acid on the intelligence and behavior of persons with different degrees and kinds of mental retardation. L(+)-glutamic is apparently more effective than its sodium or potassium salts. The effective dosage is usually between 10 and 20 grams per day (given in three doses with meals), and is adjusted to the patient as the amount somewhat less than that required to cause hyperactivity; improvement in personality and increase in intelligence (by 5 to 20 I.Q. points) have been reported for many patients with mild or moderate mental deficiency by several investigators.[31]

LOCALIZED CEREBRAL DEFICIENCY DISEASES

The observation that the psychosis associated with pernicious anemia may manifest itself in a patient for several years before the other manifestations of the disease become noticeable has a reasonable explanation: the functioning of the brain and nervous tissue is probably more sensitively dependent on molecular composition than is that of other organs and tissues. The observed high incidence of cyanocobalamin deficiency in patients admitted to a mental hospital, mentioned above, suggests that mental disease may rather often be the result of this deficiency, and further suggests that other deficiencies in vital substances may be wholly or partly responsible for many cases of mental illness.

The foregoing arguments suggest the possibility that under certain circumstances a deficiency disease may be localized in the human body in such a way that only some of the manifestations usually associated with the disease are present. Let us consider, for example, an enzyme or other vital substance that is normally metabolized by the catalytic action of an enzyme normally present in the tissues and organs of the body. In a person of unusual genotype there might be an especially great concentration of this enzyme in one body organ, with essentially the normal amount in other organs. Through the action of this enzyme in especially great concentration the steady-state concentration of the vital substance in that organ might be decreased to a level much lower than that required for normal function. Under these circumstances there would be present a deficiency disease restricted to that organ.

An especially important case is that of the brain. We may, as a rough model of the human body, consider two reservoirs of fluid, the blood and lymph, with volume V_1, and cerebrospinal fluid, the extracellular fluid of the brain and spinal column, with volume V_2. We assume that a vital substance is destroyed in each of these reservoirs at a characteristic rate, corresponding to the rate constants k_1 and k_2, that it diffuses across the blood-brain barrier at a rate determined by the product of the permeability and area of the barrier and the difference c_2—c_1 of the concentrations in the two reservoirs, and that it is introduced from the gastrointestinal tract into the first reservoir at a constant rate. The steady-state concentrations are then in the ratio

$$c_1/c_2 = 1 + (k_2V_2/PA)$$

where PA is the product of permeability and the area of the blood-brain barrier. The steady state corresponds to the following system:

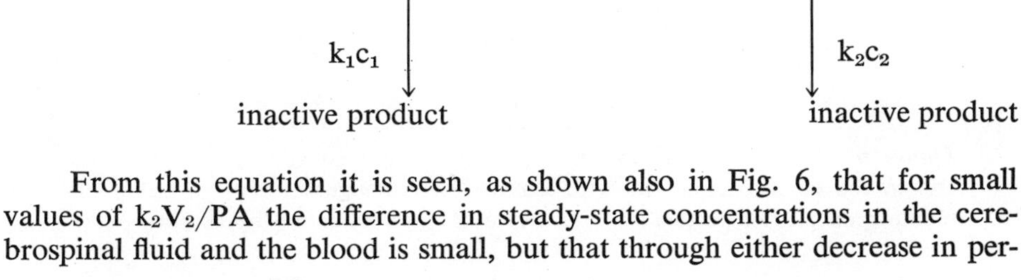

From this equation it is seen, as shown also in Fig. 6, that for small values of k_2V_2/PA the difference in steady-state concentrations in the cerebrospinal fluid and the blood is small, but that through either decrease in permeability of the barrier or increase in the metabolic rate constant k_2 the steady-state concentration in the brain becomes much less than that in the blood.

This simple argument leads us to the possibility of a localized cerebral avitaminosis or other localized cerebral deficiency disease. There is the possibility that some human beings have a sort of cerebral scurvy, without any of the other manifestations, or a sort of cerebral pellagra, or cerebral pernicious anemia. It was pointed out by Zuckerkandl and Pauling [32] that every vitamin, every essential amino acid, every other essential nutrilite represents a molecular disease [33] which our distant ancestors learned to control, when it began to afflict them, by selecting a therapeutic diet, and which has continued to be kept under control in this way. The localized deficiency diseases described above are also molecular diseases, compound molecular diseases, involving not only the original lesion, the loss of the ability to synthesize the vital substance, but also another lesion, one that causes a decreased rate of transfer across a membrane, such as the blood-brain barrier,[34] to the affected organ, or an increased rate of destruction of the vital substance in the organ, or some other perturbing reaction.

It has been suggested by Huxley, Mayr, Osmond, and Hoffer,[35] partially on the basis of the observations of Book [36] and Slater [37] on the incidence of schizophrenia in relatives of schizophrenics, that schizophrenia is caused by a dominant gene with incomplete penetrance. They suggested that the penetrance, about 25 percent, may in some cases be determined by other genes and in some cases by the environment. I suggest that the other genes may in most cases be those that regulate the metabolism of vital substances, such as ascorbic acid, nicotinic acid or nicotinamide, pyridoxine, cyanocobalamin, and other substances mentioned above. The reported success in treating schizophrenia and other mental illnesses by use of massive doses of some of these vitamins may be the result of successful treatment of a localized cerebral deficiency disease involving the vital substances, leading to a decreased penetrance of the gene for schizophrenia. There is a possibility that the so-called

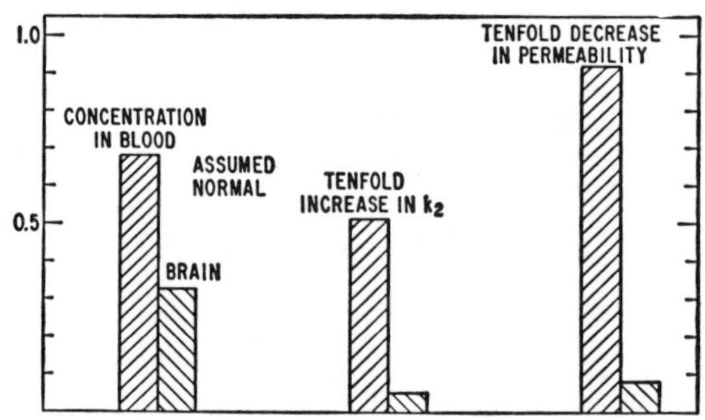

Figure 6. Values of the concentration of a vital substance in the blood and in the cerebrospinal fluid for three different assumed sets of value of blood-brain barrier permeability and rate of destruction in the cerebrospinal fluid.

gene for schizophrenia is itself a gene affecting the metabolism of one or another of these vital substances, or even of several vital substances, causing a multiple cerebral deficiency.

I suggest that the orthomolecular treatment of mental disease, to be successful, should involve the thorough study of and attention to the individual, such as is customary in psychotherapy but less customary in conventional chemotherapy. In the course of time it should be possible to develop a method of diagnosis (measurement of concentrations of vital substances) that could be used as the basis for determining the optimum molecular concentrations of vital substances for the individual patient and for indicating the appropriate therapeutic measures to be taken. My co-workers and I are carrying on some experimental studies suggested by the foregoing considerations, and hope to be able before long to communicate some of our results.

SUMMARY

The functioning of the brain is affected by the molecular concentrations of many substances that are normally present in the brain. The optimum concentrations of these substances for a person may differ greatly from the concentrations provided by his normal diet and genetic machinery. Biochemical and genetic arguments support the idea that orthomolecular therapy, the provision for the individual person of the optimum concentrations of important normal constituents of the brain, may be the preferred treatment for many mentally ill patients. Mental symptoms of avitaminosis sometimes are observed long before any physical symptoms appear. It is likely that the brain is more sensitive to changes in concentration of vital substances than are other organs and tissues. Moreover, there is the possibility that for some persons the cerebrospinal concentration of a vital substance may be grossly low at the same time that the concentration in the blood and lymph is essentially normal. A physiological abnormality such as decreased permeability of the blood-brain barrier for the vital substance or increased rate of metabolism of the substance in the brain may lead to a cerebral deficiency and to a mental disease. Diseases of this sort may be called localized cerebral deficiency diseases. It is suggested that the genes responsible for abnormalities (deficiencies) in the concentration of vital substances in the brain may be responsible for increased penetrance of the postulated gene for schizophrenia, and that the so-called gene for schizophrenia may itself be a gene that leads to a localized cerebral deficiency in one or more vital substances.

REFERENCES AND NOTES

1. I might have described this therapy as the provision of the optimum molecular composition of the brain. The brain provides the molecular environ-

ment of the mind. I use the word mind as a convenient synonym for the functioning of the brain. The word orthomolecular may be criticized as a Greek-Latin hybrid. I have not, however, found any other word that expresses as well the idea of the right molecules in the right amounts.

2. A. Felling. *Nord. Med. Tidskr.* (1934), 8:1054. *Z. Physiol. Chem.* (1934), 277:169.

3. See, for example, D. W. Woolley. *The Biochemical Bases of Psychoses.* New York: Wiley, 1962.

4. A. Cherkin. *Science* (1967), 155:266.

5. L. Pauling, *ibid.* (1961), 134:15. S. Miller. *Proc. Nat. Acad. Sci. U.S.* (1961), 47:1515.

6. The literature is so extensive that I refrain from giving references here.

7. For references see I. Stone. *Amer. J. Phys. Anthropol.* (1965), 28:83. The only other vertebrate known to require exogenous ascorbic acid is the red-vented bulbul *Pycnonotus cafer.*

8. G. W. Beadle and E. L. Tatum. *Proc. Nat. Acad. Sci. U.S.* (1941), 27:499.

9. The points in Fig. 2 represent my measurement of the slopes of the growth curves shown in Fig. 1 of reference (8). They agree closely with the points of fig. 2 of reference (8) except for one point, that for 1.2 ug/liter, which may have been misplotted.

10. The reported growth rate for the normal strain in a medium with 40 ug of added pyridoxine per liter is 3 percent greater than that for the basic medium, as shown by the slopes of the lines in reference (8), fig. 1.

11. E. L. Tatum and G W. Beadle. *Proc. Nat. Acad. Sci. U.S.* (1942), 28:234.

11a. S. Zamenhof and H. H. Eichhorn. *Nature* (1967), 216:465.

12. L. Michaelis and M. Menten. *Biochem. Z.* (1913), 49:333.

13. A. D. M. Smith. *Brit. Med. J.* (1950), 11:1840.

14. E. Edwin, K. Holten, K. R. Norum, A. Schrumpf, O. E. Skaug, *Acta Med. Scand.* (1965), 177:689.

15. T. Hansen, O. J. Rafaelson, P. Rødbro. *Lancet* (1966), II:965. Report serum B_{12} concentration below 150 pg/ml in 13 of 1000 consecutive patients admitted to a Copenhagen psychiatric clinic; J. G. Henderson, R. W. Strachan, J. S. Beck, A. A. Dawson, M. Daniel, *ibid.,* p. 809, report that nine of 1012 unselected psychiatric patients in a region in Scotland were found to have B_{12} deficiency, in addition to five pernicious anemia patients in the group.

16. H. M. Cleckley, V. P. Sydenstricker, L. E. Geeslin, *J. Amer. Med. Ass.* (1939), 112:2107.

17. V. P. Sydenstricker and H. M. Cleckley. *Amer. J. Psychiat.* (1941), 99:83. References are given in this paper to some earlier work on nicotinic acid therapy.

18. A. Hoffer, H. Osmond, M. J. Callbeck, I. Kahan. *J. Clin. Exp. Psychopathol.* (1957), 18:131. A. Hoffer. *Niacin Therapy in Psychiatry.* Springfield, Ill.: Thomas, 1962.

19. H. Osmond and A. Hoffer. *Lancet* (1962), I:316. Review of a 9-year study.

20. A. Hoffer and H. Osmond. *Acta Psychiat. Scand.* (1964), 40:171. A. Hoffer. *Int. J. Neuropsychiat.* (1966), 2:234.

21. For example, E. D. Kyhos, E. L. Sevringhaus, D. R. Hagendorn. *Arch. Int. Med.* (1945), 75:407. Found that for some subjects 1.5 to 2.8 grams per day were needed for saturation.

22. I. Stone, *Perspect. Biol. Med.* (1967), 10:135. *Acta Genet. Med. Gemell.* (1966), 15:345.

23. R. J. Williams and G. Deason. *Proc. Nat. Acad. Sci. U.S.* (1967), 57:1638.

24. S. A. Akerfeldt. *Science* (1957), 125:117.

25. J. D. Benjamin. *Psychosom. Med.* (1958), 20:427. S. S. Kety. *Science* (1959), 129:1528, and 1590.

26. A. Hoffer and H. Osmond. *The Chemical Basic of Clinical Psychiatry.* Springfield, Ill.: Thomas (1960), p. 232. M. H. Briggs. *New Zealand Med. J.* (1962), 61:229.

27. H. Weil-Malherbe. *Biochem. J.* (1936), 30:665.

28. J. G. Price, H. Waelsch, T. J. Putnam. *J. Amer. Med. Assn.* (1944), 122.

29. H. Waelsch. *Amer. J. Ment. Defic.* (1948), 52:305.

30. F. T. Zimmerman and S. Ross. *Arch. Neurol. Psychiat.* (1944), 51:446.

31. A recent survey of the role of glutamic acid in cognitive behaviors has been published by W. Vogel, D. M. Broverman, J. G. Draguns, E. L. Klaiber. *Psychol. Bull.* (1966), 65:367. Many references to earlier work are given in this paper.

32. E. Zuckerkandl and L. Pauling. In *Horizons in Biochemistry* (M. Kasha and B. Pullman, eds.). New York: Academic Press (1962), p. 189.

33. L. Pauling, H. A. Itano, S. J. Singer, I. C. Wells. *Science* (1949), 110: 543.

34. It has been suggested by B. Melander and S. Martens. *Dis. Nerv. Syst.* (1958), 19:478. *Acta Psychiat. Neurol. Scand.* (1959), 34:344. A. Hoffer and H. Osmond. *Int. J. Neuropsychiat.* (1966), 2:1. The effects of taraxein [R. G. Heath, S. Martens, B. E. Leach, M. Cohen, C. A. Feigley; *Amer. J. Psychiat.* (1958), 114:917], may result from changing the permeability of the blood-brain barrier.

35. J. Huxley, E. Mayr, H. Osmond, A. Hoffer. *Nature* (1964), 204:220.

36. J. A. Book. *Acta Genet. Statist. Med.* (1953), 4(1). *Proc. Int. Congr. Genet. 10th* (1958), 1:81.

37. I. E. Slater. *Acta Genet. Statist. Med.* (1958), 8:50.

PART VII

HOME CARE FOR THE EMOTIONALLY ILL

CHAPTER

CHAPTER 21

PROPOSALS FOR REFORM IN THE MENTAL HEALTH FIELD*

THOMAS S. SZASZ, M.D.

> *The only purpose for which power can be rightfully exercised over any member of a civilized community, against his will, is to prevent harm to others. His own good, either physical or moral, is not sufficient warranty.*
>
> —JOHN STUART MILL (1859, p. 13)

IN MANY PARTS of this book, I criticize our present legal and psychiatric practices with respect to mental patients. Although the suggestions for improvement are implicit in the criticisms, the reader is entitled to a systematic exposition of my views on reforms in the mental health field.

My objections to many current practices, as well as my suggestions for reforms, rest on a fundamental proposition: We should value liberty more highly than mental health, no matter how defined.

THE PRESUMPTION OF CRIME AND OF MENTAL ILLNESS

If a society wishes to combat some type of evil, it must have proper techniques for detecting it. Such things as crime, witchcraft, bodily illness, and mental illness have been regarded as socially undesirable, and hence worthy of a community's remedial efforts against them. Each of these categories denotes a departure from socially approved norms of law, religion, medicine or psychiatry. However, they differ, first, in the specific norms violated; second, in the methods used to establish the violation; and third, in the techniques employed to combat the deviation.

Comparing our practices with legal deviation will prove instructive. In Anglo-American law, a person is considered innocent until proved guilty. We tend to take this rule for granted. It is, however, an arbitrary rule. In past ages, the accused rarely enjoyed such protection. Some contemporary

* Reprinted by permission of author and publisher—The Macmillan Co., *Law, Liberty and Psychiatry,* 1967.

legal codes also do not adhere to this principle. Finally, let us not forget that even in England and the United States, this formula was reversed in witch trials; the accused was considered guilty unless he could prove his innocence. In witch trials, individual liberty mattered not at all. The rule was: better to burn a thousand innocent men at the stake than let a single guilty one escape. With such immoderate emphasis on never missing a diagnosis of witchcraft, it was inevitable that brutal diagnostic methods would not only be used but accepted as legitimate.

Physicians face a similar problem of uncertainty. As judges and juries must decide whether a person is guilty or innocent, so physicians must decide whether a person is sick or well. Unfortunately, the rules governing the medical game are less explicitly formulated than those determining criminality. Physicians are taught always to suspect illness. Thus, they usually follow the rule that once a person is suspected of being ill, he should be considered sick until proved healthy (Szasz, 1961, page 100).

Before the special problems posed by so-called psychiatric diagnoses can be considered, two other issues deserve comment. First, the object of medical investigation is usually a consenting patient. In other words, the patient hires the physician to search for and detect illness, and pays him to use all "reasonable" methods necessary to accomplish this. If a person prefers the risk of undetected sickness to the dangers of certain diagnostic procedures, he is free to so decide. Thus, a person may avoid physicians altogether, or having consulted one, may consent to some procedures but not to others. He can therefore control, to some extent, the dangers of pursuing too aggressively the possibility of his sickness. In contrast, the involuntary patient lacks the authority to refuse diagnostic procedures and is therefore unprotected from its hazards.

The second issue is the social and legal consequences of a medical diagnosis. Sometimes, medical diagnoses remain confidential. Frequently, however, the nature of a person's illness is communicated to other people. When President Eisenhower suffered a coronary occlusion, his illness was public knowledge. However, medical diagnoses of this type, unlike legal judgments of criminality, do not damage the person's reputation and status in life. Hence, from a social point of view, there is no harm in falsely suspecting such illnesses. The mental anguish which a false medical diagnosis might cause may be regarded as a risk the patient assumes for wishing to take advantage of the opportunities that modern medicine offers.

The logical difficulties and social dangers of making so-called psychiatric diagnoses were discussed in detail in Chapters 2 and 3 (Szasz, 1967). It should suffice here to summarize the main problems.

1. Inasmuch as there are no clear or generally accepted criteria of mental illness, looking for evidence of such illness is like searching for evidence of heresy; once the investigator gets into the proper frame of mind, anything may seem to him to be a symptom of mental illness.
2. Frequently, the person suspected of mental illness does not consult the

psychiatrist voluntarily. In this respect he differs from the ordinary medical patient, and resembles instead the person suspected of witchcraft or crime.

3. A diagnosis of mental illness may not serve the patient's interests, as he sees them.
4. The social and legal consequences of psychiatric diagnoses are unlike those of ordinary medical diagnoses.

What are we to conclude from these characteristics of the psychiatric diagnostic process? The consequences of labeling a person mentally ill may be indistinguishable from the consequences of bringing criminal charges against him and securing his conviction: in both cases the person will be incarcerated against his will. Accordingly, we shall be bound to inflict grave injustices on people if we apply the rules of the medical-diagnostic game to psychiatry: that is, if we readily suspect (mental) illness, and, once having suspected it, assume that it is present unless it is proved absent. If we are to respect human dignity and rights, the model for the rules of the psychiatric-diagnostic game must be our traditional legal maxim: Every person should be considered mentally healthy (innocent) until he is proved mentally sick (guilty).

My proposals for reform are animated by the wish to extend to the so-called mentally ill the traditional safeguards for personal dignity and liberty embodied in the Constitution.

I have divided my suggestions into two groups—long-range and short-range objectives. Practical necessities require this division. It is inadvisable to depart suddenly and radically from habitual methods of handling social problems. For example, one of my suggestions is to eliminate involuntary mental hospitalization. As a short-range goal, this is impractical. However, as a long-range goal it is not. If, then, some of my short-range proposals fall short of the ethical ideal which libertarian thinkers have set for us, and which I support, it is because I agree with Popper [1945], that "piecemeal social engineering" is the most desirable method for effecting social change.

LONG-RANGE GOALS

The underlying purpose of these reforms is to restore to the hospitalized mental patient the full range of his constitutional rights.

1. *Involuntary Mental Hospitalization Should Be Abolished.* All provisions for involuntary mental hospitalization should be abolished. Like the institution of slavery, the institution of hospital psychiatry, as we know it, must go.

This is a radical idea. But it is a goal worth attaining. The full import of my recommendations cannot be appreciated unless it is contrasted with other approaches to this problem.

Most important among these is the American Bar Foundation's proposal. This group urged that "The degree of mental illness which justifies involuntary mental hospitalization should be clearly expressed in the statutes"

(Lindman and McIntyre, Jr., 1961, page 40). This seems reasonable, but it is not. It disregards the fact that thus far jurists and psychiatrists have been unable to agree on even a qualitative definition of mental illness. It is therefore unreasonable to ask for a quantitative definition of the severity of mental illness precise enough for the purposes of law enforcement.

Despite the good intentions, such a proposal, if enacted into law, would only invite more verbal gymnastics from psychiatrists. The result would be greater psychiatric discretion and less justice.

Legal provisions for so-called psychiatric emergencies are, of course, necessary. I believe that the existing provisions for dealing with medical emergencies and with crimes are adequate. Psychiatric emergencies fall into one of two categories. The passive, stuperous, uncommunicative patient is one type. Legally, he should be treated like the unconscious medical patient. The other is the aggressive, paranoid person, who threatens violence. Legally, he should be treated like a person charged with an offense; psychiatrically, it would be desirable, of course, if he were not incarcerated in an ordinary jail, but in a prison-hospital, where he could receive both medical and psychiatric attention.

True psychiatric emergencies are rare. They constitute only a small proportion of cases of involuntary hospitalization. Moreover, in this group, the patient often suffers from bodily illness or intoxication; for example, brain tumor or diabetic hypoglycemia. Such patients should therefore be hospitalized in medical, not mental, hospitals. Like hospitalization for medical emergencies, this type of confinement should last only until the patient regains his powers.

In the scheme I am proposing, two classes of people could no longer be forced to submit to psychiatric hospitalization. The first is composed of persons threatening to commit suicide; the second, of those considered mentally ill by others, who refuse to submit to psychiatric treatment. Later, I shall discuss the individual who is said to be "dangerous to himself and others."

2. *The Hospitalized Mental Patient Should Not Lose His Human Rights.* Mental hospitals, both private and public, should be restricted to the care of consenting, voluntary, adult patients. Both the hospital and the patient should be treated as independent, contracting parties. Patients should be free to enter or leave the hospital at will. Similarly, psychiatrists and psychiatric hospitals should be free to refuse to accept patients they do not want. In brief, the power of both patients and psychiatrists should be curtailed. Thus, patients should be deprived of the power to coerce psychiatrists, for example, by a threat of suicide; psychiatrists should be deprived of the authority to coerce patients, for example, by a threat of commitment. The power of both parties should be limited by law to persuasion. If persuasion fails, each should be allowed to act autonomously, in its own best interests.*

* So long as hospitalized mental patients are regarded as children, and psychiatrists their parents, who are largely responsible not only for their welfare but for their conduct toward society as well, the psychiatrists shall be compelled to exercise autocratic controls over their

The therapeutic tasks of such voluntary psychiatric institutions might range from social rehabilitation to intensive individual psychotherapy. However, protection of the public from harm by so-called mental patients would not be one of them. There would be no need, indeed, it would be absurd to copy the penal model. Psychiatric hospitals, like school dormitories, medical hospitals, museums, or personal homes, would be at once "open" and "closed." Like the inhabitants of these places, those in mental hospitals would be fully responsible for their acts. Mental hospital personnel should have no more concern about the antisocial conduct of their patients than should, say, a medical school faculty have of its students.

The mental hospital should be a new kind of institution, resembling neither prison nor medical hospital. Its purpose would be to provide the kind of help rendered today by many psychiatrists, psychologists, and social workers. These services are more comparable to those obtainable in certain schools, hotels, vacation resorts, and aboard ocean liners, than to those furnished by ordinary hospitals. Accordingly, in mental institutions (the term "hospital" would only be distracting) few physicians would be needed, and they would care only for bodily diseases. Until new standards are developed, personnel for this sort of organization should be recruited from those who demonstrate interest and skill in this type of work, not from those who meet the existing, but irrelevant, institutional qualifications.

This type of institution would be unsuitable for many persons who are now confined in mental hospitals. Those who break the law, but are now classified as mental patients, should be held in what I call "prison hospitals." Children regarded as mentally ill would also require another kind of facility. Minors do not have the legal rights of adults. Hence, a "therapeutic" program designed especially to safeguard the legal rights of adults would be inappropriate for them. Finally, the mentally retarded, whether child or adult, would also need a different type of institution.

3. *The Insanity Plea Should Be Abolished.* The reasons for not considering mental illness an excusing condition for crime were set forth in Chapter 10 (of *Law, Liberty and Psychiatry* Ed.'s note). Not only do I believe that mental illness should never be accepted as a release from criminal responsibility, but also that it should never be the ground for a refusal to try a person charged with an offense. Everyone accused of breaking the law should be tried. This sweeping statement requires clarification.

I believe we should continue to adhere to the principle that a person should not be tried unless he can understand the charges against him and can assist in his own defense. It might be argued that if a person is in a catatonic state, i.e., mute, immobile, and perhaps unable even to feed himself, he should not be put on trial. The point of my argument is this: the reason for not trying such a person is that he is unable to assist in his own defense, not that he is schizophrenic.

charges. The basic structure of the bargaining situation (Schelling, 1960) between these two parties is faulty and requires change.

My thesis is that psychiatric considerations as such are irrelevant to the conduct of a trial. The psychiatric expert may be allowed to testify on certain facts or observations, but not on psychiatric disease or criminal responsibility. Because such a modification would, in effect, abolish the special psychiatric plea (the insanity plea), and the special psychiatric disposition (not guilty by reason of insanity), there would be little need for psychiatric testimony. Extreme psychiatric conditions, such as a catatonic stupor, make it obvious that a person is unfit to stand trial; hence no psychiatrist is needed to make that determination. On the other hand, such conditions are usually temporary, and lead either to death or a remission of symptoms. Trial would thus be postponed only until gross behavioral incapacity disappeared. A person with "mental illness" of less than extreme proportions should not be declared unfit to stand trial. No two people are equally capable of defending themselves against criminal charges. Hence, even if some so-called mental illnesses should impair a person's capacity to defend himself—others, however, might improve it—it would be no more logical not to try a person for this reason than for relative lack of education. Surely, a cleaning woman, accused of political subversion, cannot defend herself as well as a professor of political science. This, however, does not prevent us from trying her. Thus, even if so-called mental illnesses were to impair a person's ability to defend himself, we could not, on this basis alone, declare him unfit to be tried, unless we were to limit the privilege of standing trial to the most highly educated members of society.

In sum, then, all persons charged with offenses, except those grossly disabled, should be tried. The emphasis here is on gross disability: it should be readily apparent or easily explicable to a group of lay persons, like a jury. The claim that trial may endanger a defendant's physical or mental health seems to be preposterous. Such a claim can always be made, and therefore, except for gross disability, should never be allowed. If found innocent, the defendant should be set free, even though considered mentally ill. If he is found guilty, he should be sentenced, according to the law. Finally, if the accused is declared both guilty and "mentally ill" he could be cared for in institutions suitably equipped and staffed.

Comments. The scheme I have outlined would eliminate the confusion between mental sickness, defined as an illness-like phenomenon—and criminality, defined as lawbreaking. Obviously, these concepts and phenomena are not mutually exclusive. However, we must distinguish between mental illness and crime, not because our theories of human conduct demand it, but because the ethic of a free society requires it. The hybridization of mental hospitals with jails undermines the security of every person's constitutional rights. The undoing of this hybridization, with the consequent separation of institutions for voluntary care from prisons, will guarantee that if a man keeps within the law, he cannot be deprived of his liberty. And it will guarantee, also, that if he does break the law, he will lose his liberty for a limited period only.

Such reforms will be difficult to implement if we maintain our hypocritical attitudes toward the problem of mental illness, and especially toward suicide. The standard contemporary justification for involuntary mental hospitalization is that the person is "dangerous to himself and others." This phrase combines two quite unrelated issues. In a free society, a person must have the right to injure or kill himself. I think Mill was right when he asserted that there is no moral justification for depriving a person of his liberty in order to treat him. If a man wants to kill himself, he can always do so. Thus it is actually impossible to deprive men of their "right" to kill themselves. Some efforts to prohibit suicide, like those of the Roman Catholics, are at least honest. In the United States, however, the attitude toward suicide is hypocritical. If a person kills himself, his suicide tends to be viewed as evidence of mental illness, and as an event that might have been prevented. In the mental hospital, however, the occurrence of suicide is accepted with equanimity, as a risk inherent in "mental illness." To see the problem of suicide only from the medical point of view is to be blind to its moral and psychosocial aspects.

While being "dangerous to oneself" should never be considered a legitimate reason for depriving a person of his liberty, being "dangerous to others", if it involves breaking the law, is the best reason for doing so. One of the main functions of society is to prevent violence among its members. Thus, if so-called mental patients commit violence, or threaten to do so, they should be treated for what they are: lawbreakers.

Judicial sentencing of lawbreakers does not deprive us of the opportunity of also trying to help them. Even if we accept the argument that many criminals are mentally sick, it does not follow that they should be in mental hospitals rather than in prisons. Mental hospitalization of offenders should not be, and cannot be, a substitute for prison reform.

If we sincerely desire that prisoners be rehabilitated, so that they become useful members of society, instead of hardened criminals, what is to prevent us from doing so? As Bixby [1961] pointed out, this can be achieved by decent and humane treatment of criminals. It need not be done under the guise of quasi-medical psychiatric therapy.

While we go to great lengths to cut off a prisoner's contact with free society, the European nations do everything possible to minimize isolation from the outside world. Visiting and mail regulations are liberal; furloughs to go home are not unusual; and many prisoners are on a status of *semiliberté* which allows them to go out daily to private employment and return at night without escort. These practices, together with shorter sentences, extensive use of open institutions, and a genuine effort to give prisoners as much freedom of choice as possible, serve to reduce the danger of turning men into convicts (Szasz, 1967 p. 7).

The desire to treat decently those who break our laws does not require or justify turning prisons into mental hospitals. Mental hospitalization of offenders, however sincerely advocated, can only aggravate an already bad situation in both our penal and psychiatric institutions.

SHORT-RANGE GOALS

The basic aim of the short-range goals which I suggest is to improve the bargaining power of the mental patient in his dealings with psychiatrists and others.

1. *The Antagonistic Character of the Relationship Between the Involuntary Mental Patient and the Psychiatrist Should be Frankly Recognized and Publicly Acknowledged.* We must begin by candidly acknowledging the role of the hospital psychiatrist vis-à-vis his patient. Such a psychiatrist, especially if he works in a state hospital, is not the patient's agent. The law, the mental patient, and the public must cease to look on hospital psychiatrists—and perhaps even on current psychiatry as a profession—as the patient's helpers and friends. To be sure, sometimes they try to be. But more often they are the patient's adversaries. Perhaps this is a shocking statement. I shall try to explain it.

The relationship between hospital psychiatrist and mental patient is one of oppression disguised as benefaction. The institutional psychiatrist, though not necessarily the patient's enemy, is neither his friend nor his therapist. I believe that there is a conflict between them.

Let us compare this with the struggle between industry and labor at the turn of the century. To solve that problem, American legislation embraced the principle that workers have a right to organize and strike. I believe that mental patients should have a similar opportunity to protect themselves against the psychiatrists who coerce them.

One reason why this has not happened is that mental patients despised their own identities. (Until recently, the American Negro had the same problem.) This has led them to dissociate themselves from their fellows, and to identify with their aggressors. Clifford Beers's (1908) life story, including his founding of the National Committee for Mental Hygiene, is a good example of this. Though ostensibly wishing to help mental patients, Beers actually despised them. When Beers was first hospitalized, only an attendant treated him with decency and kindness. Nevertheless, he despised attendants. He showed interest only in psychiatrists, especially prominent psychiatrists.

Wrote Beers (1908): "Of course, an insane man is an insane man, and while insane *should be* placed in an institution for treatment, but *when that man comes out,* he should be as free from all taint as the man who recovers from a contagious disease and again takes his place in society" (italics added; page 218). Facts are said to be stubborn, and indeed they are. Launched under what seem to me false pretenses, the Mental Hygiene Movement has had no ameliorative effect on the plight of the mentally ill in America. I suspect it may even have retarded worthwhile efforts in this field. It is significant, perhaps, that this movement should have been started by a man who admired authority and force, and was contemptuous of human rights.

Like Beers, few mental patients care to think of themselves as mental patients. They prefer to believe that there never was anything wrong with them, or that they have recovered. Beers spoke of having "found his mind."

This implies that mental patients *qua* mental patients do indeed deserve the bad treatment that has traditionally been their lot: they deserve something better only if unjustly committed or if recovered. This posture robs the mental patient, and those wishing to help him, of arguing effectively that he is deserving of human rights, even in his role as mental patient.

The mental patient's disdainful attitude toward the mentally ill also robs him of the incentive to unite with his fellows. Benjamin Franklin warned the Founding Fathers that if they fail to hang together, they shall hang separately. Mental hospital patients have consistently failed to hang together. As a result, they have indeed hanged separately. Nevertheless, psychotherapeutic efforts with mental patients—directed at educating them to revolt for independence—might yet instill in them the understanding and the hope, that their rights may be secured, not only by assimilation into the more privileged majority, but also by effective protest.

The problem of "liberating" the hospitalized mental patient from his psychosocial, religious, and legal shackles is exceedingly complex and difficult. It calls to mind the socioeconomic problems of so-called underdeveloped nations. Because of a low level of education and industrialization, it is extremely difficult for such nations to get going in a cycle of increasing education, increasing industrialization, and increasing democratization. Similarly, it is often a lack of social feeling or interest that causes a person to become a mental patient. This deficiency prevents him from engaging in organized social activity with his peer group. Hence, he remains isolated, and the benign circle of organizing, learning, acquiring new skills, approaching equality with his superiors, never begins. Like underdeveloped nations, mental patients need "foreign aid." But such "aid" can easily be destructive. The mental hospital patient needs help, but not in the form of housing, food, and tranquilizers. Such aid only perpetuates the infantile, disabled role for the patient.

In my opinion, what the mental hospital patient needs is to acquire the spirit of liberty and, indeed, of revolt. To foster this, I propose that we supply him with an agency.

2. *A Watchdog Agency Should Be Created to Protect the Rights of the Mental Patient.* The mental patient needs an agency to counteract the power of the hospital psychiatrists. It should consist of a corps of lawyers, psychiatrists, social workers, and perhaps others, and be independent of the department which operates the state mental hospitals.

This agency would assist persons threatened with commitment and those already hospitalized. For instance, when a wife files a petition to commit her husband, it would be the duty of this agency to provide capable persons to investigate the possible alternatives to commitment. They could help the husband obtain a separation or divorce from his wife, or help him rebut her accusations of mental illness.

This agency would thus be entrusted with the task of promoting the "mental patient's" interests as he defines them. The hospitalized mental patient could call on the resources of this facility if he should wish to leave the hospital, obtain a driver's license, or secure any other lost rights or privileges which he is ill-equipped to regain.*

Lack of commitment to this enterprise, or inadequate financial support for it, could lead only to failure. However, if properly implemented, I am confident that such an agency could foster a significant improvement in the conditions of the mentally ill in America.

3. *Mental Hospitals Should Cease to Be "What Else" Institutions.* When people do not know "what else" to do with, say, a lethargic, withdrawn adolescent, a petty criminal, an exhibitionist, or a difficult grandparent, our society tells them, in effect, to put the "offender" in a mental hospital (Becker, 1962).

To overcome this, we shall have to create an increasing number of humane and rational alternatives to involuntary mental hospitalization. Old-age homes, workshops, temporary homes for indigent persons whose family ties have disintegrated, progressive prison communities—these and many other facilities will be needed to assume the tasks now entrusted to mental hospitals. Some of the money and effort spent on mental hospitals should be devoted to such enterprises. As matters now stand, mental hospitals only waste our valuable human resources and funds. They also endanger our trusted political institutions and our personal liberties.

4. *The Hospitalized Mental Patient Should Retain as Many of His Rights as Possible.* At present, the involuntarily hospitalized mental patient is virtually without any rights. In theory, the committed mental patient is not incompetent. In fact, however, he may be treated as if he were. If the hospital psychiatrists decide to deprive the patient of a right, there is little he can do about it.

As an alternative, we could experiment with partial deprivation of liberty for the mental patient. In this connection, involuntary military service may serve as a model. A person conscripted for military service loses some of his freedom—for example, the freedom to pursue his occupation, to select his home or clothes, to move about freely, and so forth. He retains, however, the right to marry and divorce, to enter into valid contracts, to vote, and many others. The point is that the conscripted soldier surrenders only those rights which are required by the duties of soldiering. The deprivation of rights that cannot be justified on this ground—for example, censoring the serviceman's mail or reading materials—offends our sensibilities. It would also be unconstitutional.

The same principles should apply to the loss of freedom incurred by the involuntarily hospitalized mental patient. Let us suspend only those freedoms which are necessary for settling the dispute that caused him to be defined as mentally ill. For example, instead of committing the alcoholic husband who abuses his wife, the court could order him to cease annoying her. Subsequent

* There is a similarity between the agency I am proposing and the practice of supplying defense counsel to indigent persons accused of crimes, by federal courts, by local bar associations, and by legal-aid societies. [See in this connection Gellhorn (1961, p. 38)].

violations of such orders could be treated by judicial, not psychiatric, penalties. The court would thus regulate only the patient's relationship with his wife. His liberty would remain otherwise unimpaired. Accordingly, the husband would not be forced to submit to psychiatric treatments he does not want; nor would he be prevented from working, making telephone calls, writing letters, and so forth. Current commitment laws deprive such a person of all these freedoms. In sum, the committed patient's loss of rights should be partial rather than almost total.

5. *Involuntary Mental Hospitalization Should be Discouraged.* Frequently, when people do not know what to do about a human problem, they may try to resolve it by committing one of the parties to the conflict to a mental hospital. Thus, husbands may prefer committing their wives to legally separating from them or divorcing them. Physicians may prefer committing a difficult patient to withdrawing from the case. Policemen and district attorneys may prefer committing certain offenders to prosecuting them. And so forth.

In each of these instances, commitment offers—at least temporarily—an easy solution to a difficult situation. If, however, we consider involuntary mental hospitalization a serious evil, we should search for more effective means of coping with these problems. Moreover, if we do not discourage easy commitment, there will never develop the social tension which may be necessary for creating adequate facilities for, say, indigent old people.

The present practice of admitting to the state mental hospitals people of all sorts, whether "mentally ill" or not, represents the persistence of an old habit: this was the function of the insane asylum in the eighteenth century. This practice cannot be justified any longer. Under the same roof, how can psychiatrists provide for the needs of such diverse persons as juvenile schizophrenics and indigent old people dying of cancer, drug addicts and depressed housewives, petty criminals and religious paranoiacs? They cannot—but often justify what they do by humanitarian motives and the pressure of social needs. In the long run, however, inadequate or misdirected stopgap measures of this kind serve only the self-seeking interests of psychiatrists for whose services such tactics generate an ever increasing demand. At the same time, the welfare of the sufferers is sacrificed.

6. *People Should Be Educated About the Dangers of Mental Hospitalization.* My final proposal, if adopted, would reverse many current practices in mental health education. Instead of comparing mental health to physical health, and exhorting people to use psychiatric services as much as possible, I suggest clarifying and emphasizing the differences between them. These I consider the more significant. Likewise, I suggest stressing the similarities between the roles of prisoner and mental hospital patient. If we expect people to conduct themselves responsibly, we must tell them not what is "good" for them, but what is true.

I believe further, that so long as our mental health facilities are inadequate, we should not urge people to use psychiatric help as much as possible.

Instead, we should emphasize the risks. Curiously, psychiatrists seem to be quite immune to the hazards that threaten nonpsychiatric physicians and various medical facilities (such as hospitals and pharmaceutical companies). Radiologists and surgeons, for example, who do not inform a patient of the dangers of a procedure, fail to secure "informed consent" (Hirsch, 1961). This renders them liable for damages if the patient is harmed as a result of their actions. In other words, the physician will be liable for damages even if his performance was faultless, and the patient suffered merely as a result of risks inherent in the procedure.*

This principle was the basis for awarding compensation to the persons who contracted poliomyelitis from injections of Salk vaccine manufactured by the Cutter Laboratories. "In the Cutter suit, no judge or jury has found the laboratory negligent in its manufacture of the vaccine, but damages were awarded on the grounds that *Cutter had breached an implied warranty since the vaccine caused the disease it was intended to prevent.*" (Italics added. *Modern Medicine,* December 11, 1961, p. 2.) Because the public was not warned of the risk of contracting polio from the vaccine, the court held the manufacturer responsible for an "implied warranty."

The Cutter affair, tragic though it was, is a relatively minor instance of injuries incurred by patients as a result of their having been misinformed. The faulty polio vaccine affected less than fifty persons, some only slightly. Compared to the thousands, perhaps hundreds of thousands, who have been injured by mental hospitalization without having been fully apprised of the risks inherent in this form of "treatment", the Cutter affair will seem like a raindrop in the ocean. Approximately a quarter-million people are hospitalized in mental institutions every year. A significant proportion is injured as a result. Nevertheless, contemporary mental health propaganda (it cannot very well be called "education") is silent about the hazards to which a person exposes himself when he enters a mental hospital, or to which he exposes those whom he causes to be hospitalized. It may be argued that there are certain unavoidable risks inherent in mental hospitalization. Indeed there are. But this only emphasizes that all those responsible for recommending or providing this type of care ought to be duty-bound to inform the patients, and the public, of the exact dimensions of this risk. If, instead of providing accurate information, they indulge in spreading propaganda—then, I submit, they should be held legally responsible for the damages that may result from mental hospitalization.

Indeed, this may be the best way to improve the social position of the mental patient. For attorneys specializing in cases of personal injury resulting from medical procedures, there is a large, unexploited field for suits for dam-

* I think this is entirely reasonable. A person cannot intelligently decide whether to avail himself of medical help if he is apprised only of the potential benefits, but not of the dangers of the treatment to which he contemplates submitting himself. The physician who exaggerates the beneficial effects of a particular form of therapy, and minimizes or withholds information about its dangers, misleads his patient. If, as a consequence, the patient is injured, it is only fair to hold the physician responsible.

ages caused by psychiatric action. To be sure, suits for false commitment are almost always ineffective. In such cases, compliance with the form of law protects the psychiatrist. However, there is no such protection for the psychiatrist whose patient enters the hospital voluntarily, and then discovers he cannot leave, or is otherwise injured. It is against the rules of the psychiatric hospital game, as it is currently played, to give prospective patients, or their relatives, accurate information about the social dangers (for example, from loss of civil rights, injury to chances for future employment, and so on) inherent in mental hospitalization. Hence, patients incurring such injuries would, I think, have valid cause for civil action against the psychiatrists responsible for not informing them.

CONCLUSIONS

Pinel may have struck the chains of iron from the hospitalized mental patient, but the chains of the law are still fastened on him. Who shall sever these legal restraints? Perhaps it will be attorneys. They have already helped the medical patient in his struggle against coercive practices by (nonpsychiatric) physicians. Although unpleasant for doctors, malpractice suits fulfill two important functions. First, they secure money damages for patients injured as a result of certain medical procedures. Second, they underscore the fact that a person's body belongs to himself, not to his physician. The latter assumes paternalistic control over it at his own peril.

In psychiatry, and especially in the hospital practice of it, physicians frequently exert paternalistic control over their patients. Perhaps through litigation, attorneys could dislodge this oppressive relationship. An individual's personality, no less than his body, should belong to him, not to his self-appointed psychiatric guardians. Anything that would move us toward this goal would contribute immensely to the furtherance of human liberties, and hence, in my view, to better "mental health" as well.

SUPPLEMENTARY READINGS

Becker, E. *The Birth and Death of Meaning: A Perspective in Psychiatry and Anthropology*. New York: The Free Press of Glencoe, 1962.

Beers, C. W. *A Mind That Found Itself: An Autobiography,* 1908 (7th ed.). Garden City, N.Y.: Doubleday, 1956.

Bixby, F. L. "Treating the prisoner: A lesson from Europe." *Federal Probation* (1961), 25:7.

Gellhorn, W. *American Rights: The Constitution in Action.* New York: Macmillan, 1961.

Hirsch, B. D. "Informed Consent to Treatment," *Tort and Medical Year Book* (vol. I). Indianapolis: Bobbs-Merrill, 1961.

Lindman, F. T., and McIntyre, D. M., Jr. (Ed.). *The Mentally Disabled and the*

Law: The Report of the American Bar Foundation on the Rights of the Mentally Ill. Chicago: University of Chicago Press, 1961.

Mill, J. S. *On Liberty* (1859). Chicago: Henry Regnery, 1955.

Popper, K. R. *The Open Society and Its Enemies.* Princeton, N.J.: Princeton University Press, 1945.

Schelling, T. C. *The Strategy of Conflict.* Cambridge, Mass.: Harvard University Press, 1960.

Szasz, T. S. *The Myth of Mental Illness: Foundations of a Theory of Personal Conduct.* New York: Hoeber-Harper, 1961.

CHAPTER 22

PHYSICAL, PSYCHOLOGICAL AND ENVIRONMENTAL AIDS*

HERMAN S. SCHWARTZ, D.C.

"The physician must not only be prepared to do what is right himself, but also to make the patient, the attendants, and the externals cooperate."

—HIPPOCRATES

"There is also a need to extend the domiciliary care of patients in their own homes. With the extension of education on psychiatric topics, more and more relatives have developed sufficient insight to be able to tolerate the patient in home surroundings, provided they are given (professional) help. . . . It is not always advisable to admit the patient to a hospital if his family is prepared to maintain him in the close emotional relationships of the home."

—World Health Organization Technical Report, Series No. 73, Expert Committee on Mental Health; Third Report, Geneva, September 1953

EMOTIONALLY DISTRESSED patients are problems to every doctor of the healing arts. He may question himself, "How can I find the time and energy to give the patient the attention that he needs to prevent possible mental hospitalization?" The answer may be found in applying the ancient wisdom of Hippocrates.

The cooperation of the family may be the determining factor in adequately caring for the patient as well as possibly preventing mental hospitalization. The information contained here can be useful for the mildly distressed emotional patient as well as for those who are severely disturbed and who require more than the application of any specialized discipline.

* Condensed and reprinted from *Home Care for the Emotionally Ill,* 1957, by the permission of author and Session Publishers.

If the doctor accepts a severe problem patient, he must assure himself of the full cooperation of the family and to use his prerogative of obtaining consultation and/or cooperation of a mental health specialist. Schwartz (1957) says that many authorities, including Dr. Harry Solomon, Professor of Psychiatry at the Harvard Medical School, emphasize the value of home care. Solomon points out that the patient responds best when he is the center of attention and that "in no hospital, as hospitals exist today, are they likely to be." It is mentioned in the same reference that Dr. Stevenson of the National Association for Mental Health, believes that "service to masses of people is never as satisfactory as the individualized care that is provided at home."

This is understandable. The nurse or the attendant who is often responsible for hundreds of patients has little time to talk with or even listen to the patient and find out whether or not his requests are reasonable. So it is much easier to assume that his mind is not clear and that he does not know what he wants. While it is true that his mind is frequently confused, at other times it is very clear. Often only by individual attention and by giving the patient the benefit of patience, kindness, and understanding, may his recovery be hastened.

ADVANTAGES OF HOME CARE

Experts now agree that it is not only possible but often advantageous to keep the mentally ill at home. They are beginning to realize that the patient's environment is often a more important factor in his recovery than the possible treatments that he obtains in most institutions (usually he receives only custodial care). They realize that he can regain his emotional control more quickly when he is not uprooted suddenly from his familiar background, providing his home life is at all bearable. In any case, *if the patient is going to continue living at home after he has returned from an institution,* he and his family need to learn to adjust to each other. When they give themselves the opportunity to do so when under stress, their familial relationship has a better chance to be strengthened.

The strong emphasis on the prophylactic value of home care for the emotionally ill is finally being more fully explored. Pasamanick (1967) conducted an extensive study that was designed to determine whether home care for the schizophrenic patient was feasible. He found that:

> "Despite the inherent risks and the difficulties encountered in the execution of this experimental Home Care study, the unequivocal findings and their enormous potential for more effective and practical care of the mentally ill requires a categorical verdict of dramatic success for the enterprise."

Yalles (1967), referring to that study in the introduction to the above book, says:

> "This study of an experimental Home Care program for the treatment of schizophrenics provides specific evidence that many schizophrenics—the

> feared, the shunned, the isolated—need not be hospitalized if they are adequately treated in their home communities."

(Two brief case histories, the first dating back to 1922, are noted in this chapter illustrating the effectiveness of this approach.)

WHEN HE MAY BE KEPT AT HOME

An important advantage of giving the patient an opportunity to recover in his own surroundings is that he does not need to make the readjustment to everyday life that is inevitable for one who has been in a mental institution. Another advantage is that the patient and his family are saved from the stigma of "insanity". The late C. C. Burlingame, former Chairman of the Committee of Public Education of the American Psychiatric Association expressed himself publicly that the emotionally disturbed patient can only fulfill his destiny as a useful member of society if he is trained to develop and use his powers in the work-a-day world outside of the mental hospital. He questions whether a patient is re-educated for a useful life in the institution where all he learns is making baskets, weaving rugs, and polishing its long corridors. Will such a patient be making baskets, weaving rugs or polishing floors when he is returned to the community? (Schwartz, 1957, p. 5.)

The doctor may be willing to aid the family in keeping the patient at home, for a time at least, under conditions such as these: if the patient is not destructive; if the family honestly wants to do everything possible to take care of this patient; if there is room and necessary facilities; if the doctor can obtain the cooperation of a mental health specialist. Though each emotionally ill person is a unique case, and his difficulties are legion, the probable course of the more common mental illnesses can often be predicted. Before the doctor or specialist can venture to make a fairly definite diagnosis, however, he needs a period of time in which to observe the patient. Certainly during these weeks, the patient can be observed better at home. Moreover, it is a matter of record that many "spontaneous" cures often take place during the initial few weeks.

Many emotional illnesses, it is now agreed, respond well to home nursing. One of them is the most common illness of all, the "nervous breakdown." In this condition, the patient has given way under the strain of a situation from which he sees no possible escape. So what does he do? He may retire into himself, refusing to face the reality that is too painful for him to bear. He divorces himself from everyday life, he turns his face to the wall, he becomes confused and miserable, afflicted not only by depressions but by pseudo-heart attacks and many other physical symptoms that often have no organic basis. Unless the situation that has driven him to this state is in the home itself, he will recover much more quickly surrounded by loving personal attention than he will in an institution which impresses on him every waking moment that he is mentally ill.

Another condition that responds well to home care is the disturbance brought on by sudden emotional shock. Although the attack may appear violent, the chances are that the patient may recover as quickly as he became ill, when kept at home—under surveillance if necessary. If he is rushed to an institution, the additional shock of seeing what is going on around him and realizing that he is identified with disoriented patients may further disturb him. In his confusion his fears are exaggerated. He is distressed by the strange surroundings and strange, very strange people. Fear dominates his thinking, and exaggerates his lonesomeness and helplessness. The dread of being crazy is increased by being treated as crazy. He may become worse before he slowly begins to recover.

Doctors know that the woman who becomes emotionally upset after childbirth often makes a quick recovery (as indeed do some women who have received other emotional shocks). The terror that disturbs them is often dissipated after the birth of the child. The extreme exhaustion that some women suffer during or following a difficult pregnancy or delivery brings on a condition much like that of sudden emotional shock, and the mental distress is comparable. Edward A. Strecker (1945) reports a typical case of post-puerperal psychosis, and a case of toxic psychosis due to lobar pneumonia. Both patients made complete recoveries after being in the institution for only a few weeks. They received no psychiatric care except hospital rest and some medication. Could not such cases have been kept in the favorable home environment?

Akin to these conditions are mental disturbances (delirious or toxic psychoses) caused by infectious diseases such as pneumonia. Temporary psychoses may also be due to some drugs. In such cases, when patients receive a rational therapy, are kept quiet, fed well, and not antagonized, they usually recover quickly.

Patients who suddenly become deranged from a fall or an injury can make a startling recovery when the proper anatomical corrections have been made at the doctor's office or in the patient's home. Many of the D.C.'s dramatic results occurred with such patients.

Many patients suffering from paranoia are not dangerous, and although they may be a greater or lesser annoyance to the family, they can safely be kept at home. As Hugh Cabot, the renowned Boston physician, observed as long ago as 1916, most of the paranoids "need not be put in asylums." When the general practitioner in the chiropractic or medical profession cannot make those decisions, consultations are necessary.

WHEN HOSPITALIZATION IS NECESSARY

The doctor may be influenced in favor of hospitalization if he finds the head of the house is panicky or in poor health; if the patient was *always* queer, irrational, and irresponsible, or has a history of recurrent mental disturbances (for then his mental disturbance may be of a long duration).

There are certain other conditions under which it would be difficult to keep the patient at home. If he is so sunk in depression that he may be a suicidal risk, he will need constant watchfulness and could probably receive better 24-hour protection in an institution (unless the proper custodial care can be arranged in the home). If he is so excitable that his behavior is a constant embarrassment or threat to the family; if he is openly hostile to the family or community, because he suffers from delusions or hallucinations; if it becomes obvious that keeping him at home will be a great burden, financially and otherwise; if the rest of the family is a constant source of irritations to the patient and especially if it is his will to go away—under any one of the above conditions, the mental institution may be the better place for him.

However, if the family pleads with the doctor to stand by, and is willing to follow through with his recommendations, which may include active cooperation with a mental health specialist, and also institute custodial care in the home, it is still possible that the patient may make a recovery under the comprehensive care of the many integrated therapeutic approaches suggested in this volume. As bad as a family life may be, when mental illness strikes, it is still often possible and feasible for the family and the patient to live together under the wise and informative guidance of the doctor. The family that has a measure of wisdom, courage, and a willingness to free itself from the outworn notion of the disgrace of mental illness, will seek help, and the doctor who wants his efforts to be most effective must become involved with the family. He will give them emotional support and guidance as part of his professional care.

The doctor may have to reckon with the family's over-protection as well as its feelings of guilt, shame or blame. They may introject those adverse feelings into themselves or project them upon the patient. The doctor will need to establish a fine balance of involvement between the patient and the family. In his attempt to obtain the cooperation of the family, he should gain information as to the relationship existing in the home atmosphere. An inadequate environmental situation and an antagonistic family attitude toward the patient may negate the best care the doctor can give.

Best results may be expected when a triad is established between the doctor, the patient, and his family or the aide.* Responsibility for recovery rests not only on the doctor, but on the family and the patient. This triad of responsibility makes it easier on all and binds them together, all working toward the goal of bringing about recovery. There must be mutual respect for each other.

The use of paraprofessionals in helping the "mental patient" has undergone extensive research and demonstration in 185 projects involving 10,000 people. Their effectiveness has been definitely established. "Generally, project directors reported that their nonprofessionals were ready and willing to learn, to act, and to undertake more than was expected of them." (Sobey, 1971.)

The aide can be a significant help in the recovery process. The responsibility of caring for the patient however, must never fall upon one helper. The

* Aide refers to a para- or nonprofessional, a member of the family, practical nurse, neighbor, attendant or anyone who is able to carry through the doctor's instructions. This task must not fall upon one person.

patient's difficulty may last for a long time. Several people should share the tasks so that no one will become exhausted or discouraged. The ideal aide, the paraprofessional, must function under the doctor's direction. This one additional step may negate mental hospitalization of many. Consultation with a specialist should also be available to the general practitioner. With all these supports, the doctor's burden is greatly lessened, his responsibility is shared and the possibility for the patient's recovery is increased.

The social workers are of important help. They interest themselves in the patient. Many not only know the techniques of occupational therapy, but are also aware of many other resources in the community that may be helpful to the patient. It is indeed regrettable that there is a shortage of these highly skilled and humane specialists.

WHERE TO GET HELP

When such expert help is not obtainable, there may be someone in the neighborhood who will be glad to work with the patient for a while, on a part-time basis. A clergyman may be the most appropriate personage to contact when help cannot be obtained from any other source.

The Reverend Harry C. Meserve (1971) says, "We underestimate the capacities of people to help others. While there is and will ever be a need for professionals of all kinds in the fields related to religion and mental health, help often comes most readily from the thoughtful human being who has no special professional skills, but who cares and is intelligent and discreet."

Now is the time to mobilize the idle but humane army of women who no longer have the burden of caring for their children, and of the even greater army of retired workers who still want to be useful. They can be taught the rudiments of mental hygiene and psychiatric nursing so that, when a mental emergency occurs, they can aid the doctor in giving the patient satisfactory care. Let us capitalize on their inherent kindness, wisdom and humaneness in helping the family to nurse their loved ones back to health. (Schwartz, 1957.)

When a doctor evaluates how distressed personalities were successfully cared for under chiropractic with only the addition of ancillary aids, he may come to the conclusion that he could do likewise. Caring for a person in distress and seeing him improve can be a great satisfaction, but results do not always come about merely by the best of individual professional care.

The very nature of emotional distress and all the possible complications and traumatic experiences that the patient may have been subjected to, make it impossible to state specifically what procedure may be helpful in a given situation. Thus, a number of procedures are presented here. There are no absolutes to instructions. What is best or desirable for one situation may not apply to another.

TWO CASE HISTORIES

It is fitting at this time to relate how home care procedures can most adequately buttress chiropractic in bringing about good results. The first mental patient that came to the author's attention was at the beginning of his clinical practice in 1922.

A male student age 21, sustained an injury to the cervical spine while playing football at Harvard University. He became highly excitable, hallucinations set in and he became paranoid. He was diagnosed by a psychiatrist as suffering from acute mania (schizophrenia) and was brought back to his home in New York under guard. Commitment papers for hospitalization were signed, however, the mother refused to send him to the hospital.

Because of the mother's insistent pleadings, the patient was accepted for chiropractic care. It was found necessary to obtain the help of an M.D. to anesthetize him in order to facilitate vertebral analysis.

Chiropractic examination revealed a severe subluxation of the upper cervical vertebrae. The first adjustment was performed under an anesthetic because of the patient's violent condition.

Next, the home was organized for proper surveillance. It was obvious that the patient should never be left alone. The mother willingly slept in her son's room at night, and for a daytime attendant she engaged a retired fireman who lived in the neighborhood. The fireman had sympathy for the boy, and regarded him as his own son. He was both humane and intelligent. He quickly understood the meaning of the doctor's list of instructions and abided by them. They were simple but they defined well what the attendant's attitude should be to his patient.

They were:

1. Never argue with the patient.
2. Satisfy all his reasonable demands. Remember that he is not confused all the time.
3. Don't force him to do anything against his will. Use gentle but firm persuasion in making him dress, wash, eat, and walk.
4. Remember that the patient is often unreasonable and uncooperative, and will tax your patience.
5. Keep yourself busy by reading, writing, or doing jigsaw puzzles.

The ex-fireman mastered these instructions and soon was able to control his patient fairly well without allowing friction to develop between them.

The mother pleaded with the M.D. and the D.C. to cooperate fully in helping the boy. They complied, and then they waited hopefully for results. They were rewarded, for his recovery occurred as suddenly and dramatically as had his derangement. Within ten days he became completely rational. His appetite returned; he gained weight rapidly. In the autumn of the same year he returned to Harvard and graduated with honors. Later he became an instructor in literature at another leading university.

Now we skip practically 47 years of practice to present another limited sketch of a recovery that occurred in 1969. A 76 year old woman was in the throes of a severe attack of agitated depression. The onset was the aftermath of influenza. Suddenly her early memories of shame and guilt plagued her to the extent that she could find no rest during day or night. Twice before in her adult life she had been confined to a mental institution. The patient developed a mortal fear of being again confined, this time for what she thought would be permanent. Then the patient came under chiropractic care. She was anxious to cooperate fully with every suggestion and procedure. The chiropractor obtained consultation of a mental health specialist. He also consulted with a local M.D. and arranged for constant surveillance by a practical nurse, who also acted as her companion.

Full agreement as to procedure and care was established by these members of the healing arts. The patient was adjusted daily. A nutritious diet was arranged. The necessary medication was prescribed (in two weeks it was greatly diminished, and then entirely eliminated).

The nurse was briefed as to her behavior toward the patient. The patient was given the necessary encouragement and reassurance. A daily schedule for all physical care, diversions, other mild activities and rest periods was established and adhered to. By degrees the patient was induced to become more active, to do whatever she could do for herself. Improvement set in slowly. She learned to take in her stride her slight recurrent periods of depression. Considering the patient's age, the results were gratifying to all concerned. When severely disturbed patients can recover at home under comprehensive care, surely less disturbed patients can also recover.

THE DAILY SCHEDULE

The doctor will emphasize that the chief role of the family in the recovery process should be to help the patient to help himself. If he is physically unable, then the primary concern of the patient's family is to make him as comfortable as possible. For the emotionally ill, his body-mind interrelationship is exaggerated and distorted. No matter what the cause of his difficulty, his entire organism is soon disturbed, and so is his outlook on the world. By taking good care of his physical needs, the family can play a vital role in improving his mental attitude. Good physical care is one of the best ways of impressing upon the patient that he is not "rejected" by his family. This is especially effective if he feels that he is a burden to them. It may have less effect on those patients who have strong guilt feelings, who are gravely depressed, too deeply engrossed in self-pity, or too far out of touch with external realities.

The aide (family, etc.) could try various ways to influence the patient. One way to overcome sluggishness and resistance is to start an act and entice the patient to complete it. The aide might begin the process, whether it is cleaning, working, or playing and then ask the patient to help, or urge him by saying, "Let's both do it." Or, the aide may ask the patient how to do something he knows the patient is efficient at doing. Often, by participating in an activity that appeals to him, the patient can be lifted out of an ugly mood. The attendant should be kind, but firm, giving the patient enough help so that he can assume responsibility. He should never permit himself to show fear, anger, disgust, or discouragement; such reactions only increase the patient's inner turmoil.

If the patient is indifferent or exceedingly despondent, it may often be effective for the aide to schedule certain routine procedures to follow, especially if the patient is unwilling or temporarily incapable of helping himself. Such loss of ordinary initiative is common with persons suffering emotional distress, melancholia, or psychosomatic illness. With the dull or disturbed patient, talking, requesting or "ordering" isn't always sufficient.

Even though it is kept flexible, a daily schedule is advisable. It helps to keep the patient occupied, it answers in advance the question of what to do next, and it is also a time-saving device for the aide. The schedule must be arranged in accordance with the person's former normal activities. It will fit the needs of the individual and will vary according to his sex, age, former habits, attitudes, and present inclinations. Whenever possible the daily or weekly schedule of activities should be worked up with the full and free cooperation of the patient. Thus the patient feels important and will have something to look forward to—a factor in restoring his hopeful attitude.

A normal daily schedule should list the many minor activities that we take for granted: bathing, dressing, drinking water or fruit juice, taking a walk, writing a letter, making a telephone call, making social visits, attending church, participating in recreation and periods of relaxation, watching particular TV programs, reading, and eating meals.

Even though a precise time may be listed on the schedule as a guide, it is not necessary to follow it strictly. It is just as important for the patient to feel free and at ease as it is for him to know how to spend his time.

Appearance. Another primary consideration will be the patient's appearance. Moods can often be sharply altered through a change in dress. When the patient is not too confused or depressed, he will usually get some pleasure out of presenting a pleasing appearance. This is especially true if he has been nursing a feeling of unworthiness, rejection, or has the idea that the family is indifferent to him. A new hair-do for a woman, a shoeshine for a man, neat, clean, pressed clothes, especially with a bright new touch of some kind, are splendid morale builders.

Physical Positioning. If the patient has been bedridden or physically inactive for a considerable time, the muscles of his feet (like the muscles of the entire body) have been weakened through comparative disuse, and may have caused his arches to flatten. The encroachment of the bony foot structures upon delicate nerves will heighten his irritability; it is often noticeable in his anxious and strained facial expression when he starts to walk. If the patient evidences difficulty in walking or complains about his feet, the doctor may deem it advisable to suggest to the aide that he gently massage his feet and encourage him to take some foot exercises.

When the patient is bedridden, the aide should be alert as to the position of the patient's head and neck when he is lying down. He will be most comfortable with only one or two pillows under his head. If he has hypertension, it is advisable that his head be raised. Additional pillows can be put under the mattress or blocks of wood under the legs of the head of the bed. Thus, the head is kept higher yet the incline is gradual and there is no sharp break in the curve between the head and body to cause muscular strains. If the head is elevated too high, his chin will drop toward his chest, and cause strain. When the patient rests or sleeps without pillows, his head goes too far backward and his chin upward. The curve of the neck is increased. This position will both interfere with brain circulation and cause diffuse muscle and nerve strain.

The best average temperature for the sick room is approximately 70–74 degrees F., depending upon the patient's level of resistance and feeling of comfort. The room should be well ventilated and the lighting should be soft and diffused. A night light usually is sufficient after dark.

Exercise. The importance of controlled and graduated exercises for the emotionally disturbed patient cannot be overlooked. It tunes up the muscles and quiets the nerves. It is particularly beneficial for the mentally disturbed because it helps to work off some of the glandular energies generated by excessive emotion.

When the patient is able to walk, the aide should emphasize the advantage of good posture. He should be encouraged to "walk tall", with an evenly balanced movement. The head should be evenly poised on the neck and the patient should be encouraged to breathe freely and fully. As a rule, the patient's ability to exercise moderately should be taken for granted and should be increased gradually. No matter how emotionally ill he may be, he should not be permitted to get into a long-continued helpless, inactive or bedridden state. He should be persuaded to be as active as his physical condition permits. Confinement may lead to more serious behavior difficulties. While it is true that fatigue is a part of most illnesses, he must not be allowed to use it as an excuse to be totally inactive.

If he is forced or chooses to remain in bed, he becomes weak and mentally dull, and will not recover as quickly as he should. Therefore, it may be imperative for the doctor to suggest to the aide that he begin to help the patient with some form of exercise as soon as possible. Between the exercises, while he is resting, the patient should be taught to take slow, deep, rhythmic breaths. Deep breathing is a help to stabilize his nerves, activate his abdominal organs, and keep his temper even; in addition, it gives his brain a steady and abundant supply of oxygen. This most important exercise can help the patient to start his mental motors functioning better.

Music. Another valuable, yet simple, therapy is music. Through it, the person who is emotionally disturbed may redirect his resentment, frustration, eroticism, or whatever upsetting emotion is dominating him. It stills the turmoil within him, and it also obscures the noises from the home or outside the home. The thoughts that were going around in his mind in the same old groove, now have a chance to be subdued, as his mind keeps in tune with the music.

Instruct the aide to let the patient choose the music, as long as it is not too exciting or depressing. Should he choose selections which perpetuate his mood, then either a more soothing melody or a more exciting one could be suggested. If he wants something light and humorous, by all means it should be permitted. Even if the patient's emotions are at the bursting point and he expresses himself through loud singing or violent dancing, these are clearly better outlets than uncontrolled destructiveness. And if he selects sad music, a mingling of his own particular sadness with that of the music gives it a wider, infinite meaning and becomes a catharsis. He may no longer feel isolated in his loneliness. *Laughter* is one of the best "medicines" in any nurse's kit. It removes the cobwebs from the brain and raises our spirits. Storytelling or jokes, or listening to the patient's jokes will make him feel that he is accepted and liked.

Then too, laughter has a definite physical value. We all know how it exercises the diaphragm, floods the lungs with fresh air, increases the circulation and gives all the underused bodily organs exercise they don't get in any other way. A good laugh not only relieves tension, but it is recreation and exercise as well. The actual muscular motion of laughter brightens one's mood. When the patient is despondent, the aide should wait for the chance to encourage him to try a self-produced laugh. No one can laugh without experiencing some relief of neuromuscular tensions.

THE HEALING VALUE OF WORK AND PLAY

The doctor should suggest to the aide enough activities for the patient. It need not be a difficult problem. The aide should explore the patient's strongest interests. As long as the patient retains even the smallest reserves of energy, he may be able to find in some kind of activity an outlet for his emotional stress. Everything constructive that he can learn to do with his hands diverts his attention from himself, takes him out of his shell and helps him to identify himself with others. Likewise, when he plays a game with either children or adults, he momentarily forgets himself and acts in a social way. Putting his vital forces to work is bound to be helpful. The most tragic thing that can happen to him is that he be kept in a state of uselessness.

So, no matter how confused the patient may be or how sick he is, the aide should induce him to do something. Even though he is depressed, egocentric or deeply frustrated, he may still have vague yearnings to be useful and creative. He will be capable of making the effort if someone has the patience to help him.

The work he should be encouraged to undertake should be useful but not strenuous, and at the beginning should be relatively easy, increasing in complexity as his ability increases. Both work and play should be adapted to his particular needs and personality. They should be designed to calm him when he is agitated, and to stimulate him when he is apathetic. In either case, they will prolong his rational periods.

Simple weaving and elementary needlework are good for the excitable person, as is any repetitious work that is not too boring—provided the patient does not rebel against such tasks. Even if he is severely depressed, he should be encouraged to do something, almost anything active, such as carpentry, playing an instrument, playing ball—to arouse him from his lethargy. Any kind of activity can help him increase his zest for recovery.

FRIENDS CAN HELP

Often, friends can be helpful in persuading the patient to participate in activities. He may be in the depths of despondency, but let some good friend come and smilingly urge him on to do something and one may note the change almost immediately. With tact, an almost reluctant, embarrassed, duty visit to the patient can be turned into a pleasant social event.

Friendly suggestions can include almost anything, for instance, "Come on, let's take a ride," or "Come and have dinner with us." For the patient who feels unworthy and forsaken, such a stimulus can have a dramatic effect upon him. It is surely more potent than trying to arouse his will power or appeal to his logic.

The aide could suggest that visitors play a game of cards or Ping-Pong with the patient, or have them ask him how to do a thing that he liked, or in which he was proficient before his illness. Understanding friends may be trusted to take him for a walk in the park or go window shopping, or perhaps they will plan a quiet picnic or a call on a mutual friend. The companionship of others strengthens the patient's self-esteem. He often accepts suggestions from friends that he may not take from anyone else. Friends probably will be anxious to help if they are made to realize that they are doing something that really counts. The doctor must urge the family not to "suffer in silence" with their disturbed patient. Mental illness is no disgrace. If the family will arouse its courage to tell friends about the difficulty, the friends may help.

If the patient is in no danger of harming himself or others, then even a child may help. Every period, no matter how short, in which the patient is taken away from his morbid thoughts, pain or troubles, is a definite gain. When a youngster approaches the patient and says: "Dad (or uncle or aunt), please help me," "Please fix this," "Do you think this is all right?", "How shall I do this?", the appeal is all but irresistible. The patient is taken out of his doldrums momentarily. The simple request convinces him that he is not as weak or ill as he thought. The fact that he is accepted and can be of use, and especially the thought that the child trusts him and is not afraid of him, gives him a tremendous lift of spirits.

The child could eat with the patient, visit with him, tell an interesting happening at school, or read to him. The teen-ager also can be remarkably helpful by making the patient a partner in his activities, showing interest in him and demonstrating that the patient has earned his respect.

PSYCHOLOGICAL AIDS

The doctor may instruct the aide that when making a suggestion to the patient he should first formulate the suggestion in as few and as simple words as possible. Then, when the suggestion is given, he should not demand an immediate answer. It may be more effective to end the suggestion by saying, "You think it over," and quickly, pleasantly but unobtrusively leave the patient's presence. The aide should understand that often the patient is in a dilemma. He may have difficulty in following a procedure as well as in not following it. It resolves in the question "damned if he does and damned if he doesn't". As an example, a friend may invite the patient to come for dinner. He feels that he doesn't want to accept the invitation because he may be clumsy, uncomfortable, poor company or be embarrassed. However, if he does not accept and stays at home alone, he will feel sad, suffer loneliness and may regret his decision. So, the aide can point out which is the best alternative for him—to share a meal with friends, even though they will realize his incapacities, or stay at home and feel left out.

He may point out to the patient that he understands his dilemma, but that in the long run, he will gain more by accepting the invitation. If it is possible for the host to make the invitation, either by phone or in person, then it is more effective. The aide or host must show a great deal of patience and perseverance in getting the patient out of his lethargy. By not accepting the patient's negative response, but by waiting calmly and silently, a positive response can be expected. It is worth waiting for.

When the patient is cooperative he will be eager to do what is suggested, but if he is lethargic or suspicious, the aide will have to proceed indirectly and by easy stages. Remember that the confused person is frightened by anything new and different. Suggestion is an effective way of re-orienting a distraught patient. It is a powerful help in gradually changing his mental attitude. The doctor's advice should be given to the aide as to when and how he should attempt to influence the patient. No one should attempt to give a suggestion to the patient when he is angry, moody, heavily depressed or agitated, as it will fall on deaf ears. At a moment when the patient is rational, that is, able to control his responses, one can discuss the immediate situation with him and encourage him to arrive at fairly reasonable conclusions. Whatever the aide wants him to do should be suggested in the form of an indirect question such as: "Shall we go for a walk now or later?" "Should we do this before or after lunch?" "Do you want to start writing now or later?"

Constructive hints are most helpful when the patient is permitted to take his own good time in following them. The "let's-put-it-up-to-you" technique is one of the clinical psychologist's most effective methods. It is better to plan with the patient rather than force ideas upon him. In trying to influence him, one should be realistic and avoid impossible objectives that will lead to disappointment. Suggestions should be grounded on the truth and on the chance of a reasonable early fulfillment.

Among the most powerful tools of suggestion are words. Choosing words that imply health, strength, power, ability and tranquillity serve to counteract the adverse suggestions that are continually bombarding the patient. It should always be kept in mind that he usually is strongly suggesting to himself sickness and despair, discouragement and guilt, such as "I'll never get well," "I'm no good anymore," "I'm not wanted." So, not only by your words, but also by your manner, posture and behavior, he can be convinced that he is wanted. He needs the assurance that he is distinctly worthwhile and that he has sufficient strength within himself to overcome his difficulties.

The patient's feeling of self-importance should not be injured. If he does not respond right away to suggestions, it may be that he is repelled by a hint of dominance on the aide's part. His self-respect may prevent him from complying even when he knows that what is suggested is for his own good. His sense of pride is usually as strong when he is ill as when he is well, and perhaps more sensitive because of his increased dependency upon others. No matter how confused and weak he may be, he will usually attempt to protect his self-respect. Except in an emergency the aide should never resort to a direct command, for to do so may defeat the purpose—which is to activate the patient's power of self-mastery.

THE POWER OF SILENCE

The doctor may advise the aide that, when prompting or urging the patient to change his abnormal behavior has no effect, he can sometimes control or influence him by silence. This approach varies in its effectiveness: some patients respond to it slowly, some quickly, and others, especially those severely disturbed, may not be affected by it at all. The method of applying silence is very simple, but one has to use it with perseverance. It is certainly worth trying before other drastic steps are taken or before despair overtakes the aide. The procedure of silence must not be undertaken lightly. It should never be attempted when one is exuberant, tired, discouraged, or angry. At the beginning silence can be an ordeal. It should be used for only about fifteen to thirty minutes at a time and repeated after an interval. The aide must emotionally prepare himself by auto-suggestion such as, "I can take it," or "He is not going to upset me." Keep from showing gaiety, scorn, ridicule, anger, fear, or even compassion or love.

The aide shows no frigid attitude, but a serene calm. It should not prevent one from being responsive to the patient's reasonable wishes even though one must be firm when the patient is unreasonable and forces a showdown. Should he become agitated and yell, "Get out of my room!", do not take issue. Leave him alone. But exit with a calm gesture. Your attitude and posture are more important than words. Before entering the sick room, make a very short written list of the things the patient is expected to do, such as: get out of bed; get dressed; eat; go for a walk. Upon entering the room tell the patient calmly what to do, or sit quietly for a while and wait for a favorable opening.

Sit with the light at your back so that your expression can be relaxed while at the same time you will be better able to observe the patient. Look in his direction but not directly at him. Never stare in his eyes. He should be only a small part of your total field of vision. This exhibition of serene but firm restraint may subdue the excited patient, or arouse the lethargic one. Keep your arms limp at your sides or folded across your chest or your hands quietly clasped in your lap. Make yourself impenetrable to all possible rebuffs from the patient as well as irritations from your own body. Suggest to yourself that nothing can upset your equilibrium. Your expression neither condemns nor approves. While your patient refuses to budge, talks incoherently, or does childish things, you remain motionless and emotionless. Hold this position as long as you can do so comfortably.

When the aide is in this relaxed and controlled mood, he will be likely to know what to do or the way to do it at the proper time. This type of treatment is in part a battle of wits. You are not attempting to frighten or browbeat the patient. Rather, your calmness is designed to distract your patient and arouse him to talk or act. By focusing his attention on an external problem you may decrease his exaggerated concentration on himself. Surprise is perhaps the most important element of this method. Sometimes the patient may be so puzzled by his inability to shock or upset you with his negative behavior that he may abandon it, either because it doesn't work or because his attention has been withdrawn from it.

Should he express hostile feelings toward you, you soon learn to accept them without reacting to him in kind. You can also learn to accept your hostile feelings toward him and yet not be disturbed by them or show them in your expression or behavior. When your patient is confused he may mistake you for someone else, or may misjudge your motives and actions. You will learn to overlook much and to forgive much. Guard yourself against anticipating that your patient will become distraught. Anger or fear is bound to show itself on your face. It is thus most important that you should develop a tranquil mood. No matter what feelings he expresses, accept them without reacting to them.

Impressed by your steadiness and firmness, he may be drawn to you as a tower of strength about which he can regroup his shattered forces. If he realizes that he cannot get the better of you while at the same time he need not fear you, he may switch to relying on you and thus take one step toward appropriate behavior. When the patient starts to comply with your reasonable and necessary requests to which he has persistently failed to respond—when he says, "I'm sorry," "What do you want me to do?" or "All right, I'll eat (or go to bed, or get dressed),"—you will know that you have gained your objective. By your silence and reflection you may be able to obtain some insight as to the patient's moods or needs. You may detect some clues as to his regression or progress. Such information is valuable to you as the aide and to his doctor. With his faith buttressed by silence, you will be able to rise to each situation and to use your knowledge, compassion, and patience to affect his mood. Every time you have lessened his negativity, you may be sure that you are gently but firmly propelling the patient a little further along the road to recovery.

A STARTLING RECOVERY

An illustration of the home care principles at work was reported in a significant paper by A. Querido (1954) of Amsterdam, President of Social Medicine and President of the Dutch Federation for Mental Illness. He reported on how the application of good psychiatric common sense led to the prevention of hospitalization: A police report was received in the Mental Health Center about an excited patient. The social psychiatrist quickly responded. He found neighbors around the door of the house. In the living room the furniture had been thrown about. Two massive policemen guarded a boy 26 years old, tied with rope, lying on the floor; female relatives were crying. The psychiatrist suggested that the police go outside and disperse the crowd. The patient was asked if he would behave if the ropes were loosened. He nodded and sat up; the story unfolded. He was a minimal mental defective. He was working. He came home with his pay considerably docked and was reprimanded by his father. A quarrel started; he hit his father, then a neighbor. They subdued him and tied him up.

The talk continued between patient and doctor. Gradually, the father turned from being sullen to being ashamed. The mother came in and placed a timid hand on her son's shoulder. The boy felt the support from the doctor, who assured the boy that an easier job would be found for him. He was asked what his plans were for the night. He replied, "Go to the Mandolin Club." The doctor told him that if he hurried, washed, and dressed, he would take him to the club.

> "And so half an hour later our dangerous lunatic, hair slicked, face washed, and clad in neat blue, walks quietly out of the house, the mandolin under his arm. Next week he was tested, a job was found for him at one of the factories which cooperates with the department, (Dept. of Mental Hygiene) and during the follow-up, no serious trouble was reported."

CONCLUSION

The emotionally disturbed patient is perhaps the hardest of all to understand. He suffers pain that has no apparent physical cause and is full of seemingly unjustified suspicions and complaints. This may make us feel that he is just being stubborn or unreasonable. It is hard for the healthy person to realize that the mental patient suffers as much as someone with a broken leg. Although the original cause of his trouble may have been a particular event such as a structural distortion, it would not have affected him severely if to begin with he had not been emotionally weak. The cause may also have been a slowly cumulative desire to escape from some responsibility that he could not bear; biochemical irritations, glandular imbalance, or nutritional deficiency may have been the trigger. Fatigue also could be either a cause or symptom, the "last straw" that finally produces the "mental breakdown." The practitioner of the healing arts should be fully aware that the patient may not be a neurotic after all. M. J. Barry, Jr., of the Mayo Clinic (1968), in his thought provoking article entitled "Non-neurotic Neurotics," cautions doctors of all the healing disciplines to rule out every possible organic disorder of the brain or body before making the final diagnosis that the patient is a neurotic.

When the patient is suffering, he cannot be expected to try to grapple with the situation that frustrates him. The more pronounced his symptoms, the more sympathy he demands, and the more preoccupied he becomes with himself. So, his illness becomes a way of thinking, a habit, the strongest one of his life pattern. The neurotic thinks of himself as extra special. He persistently and constantly cries, "Why should it happen to me?" When he cries, "Why am I so ill? What can I do to get well?", he may mean, "What can others do for me?" Unconsciously, he may not want to help himself, or perhaps he cannot.

No one, not even the most experienced expert, can give exact instructions as to how the patient can be shown the ineffectiveness of his way of thinking and make normal living attractive to him. Every person is a unique problem. But the patient's chances for improvement can be influenced by scattered encouragement and helpful guidance. The aide may never know what casual remark may help to break the log jam in the patient's mind and arouse him to an understanding of his condition. If in a moment of clarity the patient is fortunate enough to hear a potent word or phrase, he may be brought out of his ego-centered world.

Although each patient is different, there are certain attitudes, in any number of combinations, that are more or less common to the emotionally distressed. He most likely will be hypersensitive, inconsistent and lacking in self-confidence. The roots of many a serious emotional difficulty lie in a deep-seated feeling of inadequacy. One of the most irritating characteristics of the neurotic is his concentration upon his symptoms. He is thoroughly convinced that they are unusual, exceptionally interesting, and that no one understands them. Magnifying his complaints to prove that he is unique not only salves the patient's ego, but justifies his demand for sympathy. The best that anyone can do for the patient is to be both firm and sympathetic and to assure the patient that his troubles are not uncommon.

Whenever possible, the patient should be encouraged to make his own decisions. The sooner he copes with even his minor problems, the quicker his recovery. When he is physically able, he should be allowed to do as many things as possible for himself. This will help to build up his confidence. There will be times when the patient doesn't want to be annoyed by having people ask him questions, or do things for him, or even to have anyone around. His moods should be respected and his wishes should be granted when they are not harmful. The emotional difficulties of the chronic patient are in many ways similar to those of the neurotic. Physical illness may awaken the patient's dormant psychological maladjustments. Often he has an unconscious tendency to use his symptoms as an excuse for demanding excessive attention and affection, or for escaping responsibilities. Before the patient's condition became chronic, he may have been acutely ill. When that happens a person is given a great deal of attention and his childhood selfishness is reawakened; if he then becomes chronically ill, it continues to assert itself.

The patient's former normal attitudes and ethical and social values by which he functioned when he was well, are the ones that can help him now. He must be induced in every way possible to become responsible for his behavior. Alertness, confidence, and infinite patience are the attributes for which the doctor and the aides will have the greatest need. It is surprising how many emotionally disturbed personalities make a complete recovery when they are handled wisely by the doctor, the nurse, the family, and friends. Above all we should not forget the query raised by John Rosen (1953): "Who would suspect that man's humanity to man could be a medicine?"

Over 2,000 years ago, Hillel addressed three questions to mankind:

> "If I am not for myself, who is for me?"
> "And if I am only for myself, what am I?
> "And if not now, when?"

His words can remind every member of the helping professions that if we are to improve our personal human conditions, we must act for ourselves; that if we are to achieve full humanity as healers, we must regard the patient no less worthy than ourselves; and that when extra measures, time or help become urgent, we must act now, for there may be no tomorrow. This is a heavy charge, indeed, but one that we cannot escape.

REFERENCES

Barry, M. J., Mayo Clinic, "Non-Neurotics", (1968).

Meserve, Rev. Harry C. (ed.). *Journal of Religion and Health.* New York: Jan. 1971.

Pasenanick, B., Scarpetti, R. F., Dumtz, S. *Schizophrenics in the Community.* New York, N.Y.: Appleton-Century-Crofts, 1967.

Rosen, John N. *Direct Analysis.* New York: Grune & Stratton, 1953.

Sobey, Francine. *The Nonprofessional Revolution in Mental Health.* New York: Columbia Univ. Press, 1971.

Strecker, Edward A. and Ebaugh, Franklin G. *Practical Clinical Psychiatry* (5th ed.). Philadelphia, Pa.: Blakiston Company (1945), pp. 288–290.

World Health Organization Technical Report, Series No. 73, Expert Committee on Mental Health; Third Report, Geneva, September 1953.

SUPPLEMENTARY READINGS

Ackerman, N. W. *The Psychodynamics of Family Life.* New York, N.Y.: Basic Books, 1958.

Blain, Daniel. *The Use of People in Mental Health Activities.* Calif. Dept. of Mental Hygiene (M. Klutch, 2 vols.). Calif.: June 1967.

Burton, Arthur. *Modern Humanistic Psychotherapy.* San Francisco, Calif.: Jossey-Bass, Inc., 1967.

Field, Ninna. *Patients Are People.* New York, N.Y.: Columbia University Press, 1953.

Greenblatt, Milton, M.D. (et al.). *The Prevention of Hospitalization.* New York: Grune & Stratton, 1963.

Guerney, B. G., Jr. *Psychotherapeutic Agents.* New York, N.Y.: Holt, Rinehart & Winston, 1969.

Grosser, Charles; Henry, William E.; Kelly, James G. (eds.). *Nonprofessionals in the Human Services.* San Francisco: Jossey-Bass, 1969.

Hawxhurst, Donna. "Patients Helping Patients," *Mental Hygiene* (July 1970), 54(3).

Mayerhoff, Milton. *On Caring.* New York: Harper & Row, 1971.

Morrissey, James R. *The Case for Family Care of Mentally Ill.* New York: Behavioral Publications, 1967.

Nagy, Boszourmenyi Evan. *Intensive Family Therapy.* New York, N.Y.: Hober Publishing, 1958.

Parad, H. J. *Crisis Intervention.* New York: Family Services Assn. of America, 1965.

Querido, A. *Experiment in Mental Health.* World Mental Health Bulletin, W.F.M.H. (London: Dec. 1954), 6(4):206.

Rapoport, L. *Working With Families in Crisis: An Exploration in Preventive Intervention.* Social Work V7 (1962), 3:48–56.

Render, Helena Willis. *Nurse-Patient Relationships in Psychiatry.* New York, N.Y.: McGraw-Hill Book Co., Inc., 1947.

Richardson, Henry B. *Patients Have Families.* New York, N.Y.: The Commonwealth Fund, 1948.

Rosen, John. *Direct Analysis.* New York: Grune & Stratton, 1953.

Schachnow, J. & Matorin, Sue. "Community Psychiatry Welcomes the Nonprofessional," *The Psychiatry Quarterly* (1969), 43:492.

Schwartz, Morris S. and Shockley, Emmy Lanning. *The Nurse and the Mental Patient.* New York, N.Y.: Russell Sage Foundation, 1956.

Silverstein, M. *Psychiatric Aftercare.* Philadelphia, Pa.: University of Pennsylvania Press, 1968.

Southard, Samuel. *The Family and Mental Illness*. New York, N.Y.: Westminster Press, 1946.

Tulipan, A. B. and Dietrich, W. H. *Outpatient Psychiatry in the 1970's*. New York, N.Y.: Brunner/Mazel, 1970.

Zuk, Gerald. *A Triadic-Basic Approach*. New York: Behavioral Publications, 1972.

CREDO OF A BIOLOGIST*

RENÉ DUBOS, PH.D.

THE LEGEND of the Golden Age is so universal and ancient that it must have a base of truth. From the beginning of recorded time, men have believed in some form of Arcadia, a happy land where their ancestors led an Orphic life devoted to the enjoyment of natural pleasures and of external nature. In *Works and Days,* written almost 3,000 years ago, Hesiod evokes the Golden Age when "men feasted gaily, undarkened by sufferings . . . and all good things were theirs."

The name Arcadia might symbolize the pastoral scenery and semi-tropical climate of the East African plateaux, where the human species probably emerged under environmental conditions that most people still find enjoyable. Arcadia could have been located also in one of many other regions that were occupied by man during prehistory and where abundance of game, nuts, and fruit assured him a life of plenty without much effort.

As recently reported in the symposium devoted to *Man the Hunter,** there still exist a few archaic populations that derive adequate sustenance by hunting small game and collecting wild plants. The bush-men of the Kalahari desert, certainly one of the least favored regions of the world, do quite well on a few hours of work a week. Ignorant of agriculture and free from the curse of organized labor, they spent most of their time in social intercourse and other enjoyable pursuits. Since most Stone Age men lived in areas where game and vegetation were varied and abundant, their lives may not have been as nasty, brutish, and short as they are commonly imagined. Indeed, photographs of life among contemporary, archaic people suggest that gaiety, comradeship, and love for children are quite compatible with extremely primitive conditions.

René Dubos, Ph.D., Professor of Pathology and Microbiology at Rockefeller University, New York, was assistant, associate and member of the Rockefeller Institute for Medical Research from 1928 to 1956. Recipient of many honorary degrees and awards for scientific achievement, he is widely known as an author and a seminal thinker about man's relation to the natural world.

Reprinted by permission of the author and publisher, The Academy of Religion and Mental Health and by "The Journal of Religion and Health."

* Lee, R. B., and De Vore, I., eds., *Man the Hunter,* Chicago, Aldine Publishing Co., 1968.

Restated in biological terms, the legend of the Golden Age probably expresses the fact that, on several occasions during prehistoric life, there existed a high level of fitness between man and his environment. Such fitness was the outcome of Darwinian evolution and was similar to that exhibited by wild animals adapted to the natural conditions under which they have evolved. In man as in animals, biological fitness operates through instincts that operate independently of consciousness and free will. Instincts enable the organism to deal in a decisive and often successful manner with life situations similar to the one experienced by the species during its evolutionary past. But precisely because they are so specialized, instincts are of little if any use for creative change; man can rarely use them to meet imaginatively the unforeseeable and fluid complexities of life. Whereas instincts provide biological security under stable conditions, awareness, free will, and motivation are the attributes that account for man's adventurous liberty and creativity. As man moves his life into new horizons, he depends on thought and freedom to convert adaptive responses into creative processes.

The theory of biological evolution based on natural selection was formulated simultaneously by Charles Darwin and A. R. Wallace. It is now chiefly identified with Darwin, who had the systematic genius and discipline to accumulate and organize the evidence required to demonstrate the biological interrelationships among living things. But Wallace deserves the credit for having recognized that biological evolution—Darwinian evolution—ceased to be an important factor in human life when the human species acquired the brain it now possesses. Ever since the Stone Age, social and cultural adaptive changes have all but eliminated the need for anatomical and physiological evolution. As far as can be judged, this new line of advance set man completely apart from the rest of creation.

It is rather ironical that the most articulate exponent of psychosocial evolution has been Sir Julian Huxley, one of the grandsons of Thomas Huxley, who had been the champion of Darwin's biological evolution a century ago. During the past two decades, Sir Julian has repeatedly discussed the comparative roles of biological and psychological forces in the life of man. In his words, "Man's acquisition of a second mechanism, over and above that of the chromosomes and genes, for securing both evolutionary continuity and evolutionary change, a mechanism based on his capacity for conceptual thought and symbolic language, enabled him to cross the barrier set by biological limitations and enter the virgin fields of psychosocial existence. . . . Evolution in the psychosocial phase is primarily culture; it is predominantly manifested by changes in human cultures, not in human bodies or human gene complexes." In other words, "Evolution in this phase is mainly cultural, not genetic; it is no longer focussed solely on survival, but is increasingly directed towards fulfillment and towards quality of achievement." *

While defending the purely biological doctrine of Darwinian evolution

* Huxley, Julian, *The Humanist Frame,* New York, Harper & Row, 1961.

a century ago, Thomas Huxley also made himself the spokesman of the view that man's future depends on education and therefore on changes that are non-Darwinian because they do not involve the genetic apparatus. With his usually picturesque vigor, he asserted that the newborn infant does not come into the world labeled scavenger or shopkeeper or bishop or duke; he is born as a mass of rather undifferentiated red pulp, and it is only by educating him that we can discover his capabilities. In fact, the concept that early experiences shape the organism applies not only to learning and behavioral characteristics but also to biological attributes. For example, the increase in body size and the acceleration of sexual maturity that have taken place during the past few decades are due to changes in the ways of life during early childhood. The biological and behavioral effects of these changes were observed first in the countries of western civilization, but they are now becoming evident in the Oriental countries that have adopted the Western ways of life, particularly in Japan.

The effects of early environmental factors on the development of individuality are complicated and usually magnified by the fact that man tends to symbolize everything that happens to him and then to react to the symbols themselves as much as to actual stimuli from the external world. All perceptions and apprehensions of the mind can thus generate organic processes of which the environmental cause is often extremely indirect and remote. In most cases, furthermore, the person does not create the symbols to which he responds; he receives them from his group. His views of the physical and social universe are impressed upon him very early in life by ritual and myth, taboos and parental training, traditions and education. These attitudes are not innate, but acquired; they constitute the basic premises according to which the person organizes his inner and outer view of reality; in other words, his conceptual environment.

The fact that the biological and cultural aspects of personality can be shaped according to certain patterns determined by the kind of environment to which the person has to respond is illustrated by the progressive improvement in athletic performances during the past few decades, or by the greater efficiency in reading and other forms of learning ability as a result of practice. Such changes are not genetically determined; they correspond to phenotypic expressions that are the consequences, even though indirect, of conscious human interventions.

During the past century, scientists have emphasized the purely biological aspects of man's interplay with environmental forces and therefore have paid attention only to the deterministic aspects of life. This was justified because the effect of a given situation on a person is always conditioned by his evolutionary and experiential past. But in fact, human beings rarely behave as passive components of adaptive systems. Each person tries to achieve some self-selected end, and this effort conditions his responses to environmental stimuli. While the separate parts of the body machine *react* passively with the environment, the whole man *responds* to the environment in a purposive manner. Response is qualitatively different from reaction in that it implies an active participation of the person usually with a creative outcome.

John Dewey believed that thought is the attribute that enables man to give a creative quality to his adaptive responses. In his own words, "The brain is primarily an organ of a certain kind of behavior, not of knowing the world." * William James also was primarily concerned with the willful, creative aspects of human life, rather than with its determinism. He was interested not in the ultimate nature of things, nor even in their origin, but rather in the consequences of actions. Such an attitude naturally turned his thoughts to the future. According to him, the future was built from the "reserve energies" that he believed to be present in each individual person and that could be brought forth whenever needed for creative adaptation through willful action. It is obviously easier to follow passively one's instincts than to govern one's responses by drawing on one's "reserve energies." But to be human means to be creative. Creation involves choices that often require painful mental effort; hence the worried features in human faces at the time of decisions concerning the future.

Human life is thus determined by three separate classes of determinants: 1] the fundamental characteristics of man's biological nature, which are essentially unchangeable because they emerged during evolutionary development and are inscribed in the genetic code; 2] the environmental forces that each person experiences during his own life and to which he must make adaptive responses; 3] and last but not least man's ability to choose among alternatives and to decide upon particular courses of action.

My reason for emphasizing the conscious, deliberate and creative aspects of adaptation—as against the purely biological ones—is that they account for man's uniqueness, indeed for his humanness.

All men are aware of their kinship to animals. Irrespective of their religion or philosophical allegiance, and whatever the sophistication of their scientific knowledge, they perceive in their minds and feel in their hearts the deep philosophical significance of St. Francis of Assisi's love for his brothers, the beasts, and of Albert Schweitzer's reverence for life. Indeed, most modern men have come to accept, or at least to tolerate, the concept that all living things have evolved one from the other and are therefore biologically related. But human life as we know it today is so far removed from its earthy and animal origins that it poses problems not found in the rest of creation.

There is no evidence that the uniqueness of human life can be explained by anatomical, physiological, or developmental characteristics peculiar to the species *Homo sapiens*. Modern man exhibits specialized expressions or exaggerations of tendencies that exist in one or several other species of primates. As far as can be judged at present, man is characterized not by his biological endowments but rather by what he has created from them; he

* Dewey, John, *Creative Intelligence,* New York, Holt & Co., 1917, p. 36.

differs from the rest of the animal kingdom through his collective achievements over several thousands of generations. In this light, there is much justification for the statement by the Spanish philosopher Ortega y Gasset: "Man has no nature, what he has is . . . history."

Being a reflective and interpretative animal, man uses his intelligence to embody the raw data of experience into his cultures and can thereby transmit acquired knowledge from generation to generation through social processes far more rapid and more efficiently adaptive than genetic mechanisms. He can thus produce new kinds of organizations of experience—scientific concepts, legal systems, moral codes, works of art—that constitute the building stones of psychosocial evolution. The belief that he can plan for the future and should indeed toil for a future transcending his own life span is probably the fundamental basis of his value systems and the ultimate manifestation of his uniqueness. Even if we—that is to say mankind—were to retain perfect biological health, we might soon drift aimlessly toward a state incompatible with the maintenance of the values that make us unique among living forms. We must constantly formulate ethical and esthetic criteria transcending biological necessities and be willing to take a stand at the critical time. In the words of Paul Tillich, "Man becomes truly human only at the time of decision." Freedom to choose among options is the final criterion of humanness.

Man is of course as much influenced by natural forces as are other living things. But he does not willingly submit to nature and constantly tries to escape from his biological bondage. For this reason, the human future is fundamentally different from the ordinary biological future. Unfortunately for the clarity of language, the word "future" is used to denote two very different aspects of things to come. On the one hand, there is a future that inevitably happens because, determined by antecedent forces that operate according to immutable and inexorable natural laws, one might call this the *logical* future that scientists are often able to predict. On the other hand, there is another aspect of the future that is almost unpredictable because it is influenced by individual decisions. History is marked now and then by new departures that correspond to such decisions and that commit individuals and whole societies to new ventures and new attitudes toward life. These departures that generate the *willed* future are the great moments in human history.

Repeatedly in the past, men have used their freedom to create a future of their own choice that could not have been predicted from extrapolations of contemporary trends. For example, the sophisticated administrative structure of the Roman Empire was upset by the meek Christians and then by the Barbarians; the towers and ogives of Gothic cathedrals were rejected by the Renaissance architects; the academic art and bourgeois conventions of the nineteenth century were destroyed by a small band of Bohemians in Paris. Time and again, the logic of historical and technological trends has had to yield to the choices and decisions of individual men. Similarly, one can anticipate that changes in life styles and the influence of a few strong personalities—let alone collective acts of sabotage—will direct our civilization into channels incompatible with the predictions of technocratic futurists. Furthermore, it is almost certain that the kinds of scientific and technological knowledge we are now developing will have much less influence on the future course of civilization than will the new kinds of knowledge and ways of life we shall have to develop if we elect to deal constructively—as we must—with the ecological and social dangers now threatening mankind.

As mentioned at the beginning of this essay, the legend of the Golden Age is extremely ancient and continues to inspire men to turn their gaze backward and to entertain the illusion that they can return to Arcadia and enjoy the Orphic way of life. But even stronger than this purely biological urge, inherited from the distant past, is the belief peculiar to man that he can transform the world and make it a better and happier place. This belief, too, is extremely ancient. Prometheus symbolized man's struggle with the environment, a struggle that eventually led to the technologic and scientific way of life. Increasingly, however, man is becoming not only Promethean but also Faustian, displaying cosmic arrogance and a tendency to believe that his powers are limitless. Technological utopians that we are, we regard ourselves not as tenants or lodgers on the Earth, but as its landlords. We identify progress with increasing mastery of the external world and we search for a better life not by looking backward to Arcadia but by looking forward to a man-made world.

Man's escape from the limitations of biological life is even more strikingly evidenced by what I shall call the Olympian urge. In all parts of the world and long before historical times, countless would-be Olympians have aspired to a godlike quality and have tried to achieve virtue and understanding through spiritual insight and prophetic visions. The power of this Olympian attitude is illustrated not only by the sacrifices of religious martyrs and prophets but also by the prodigious labors of scholars and scientists who have often worked without any hope of worldly rewards for their efforts. Man gives expression to a very ancient heritage when he directs his gaze upward and inward. The parabiological expressions of human life give a real scientific meaning to Paul of Tarsus' statement:

> It is sown a natural body; it is raised a spiritual body. . . . The first man is of the earth, earthy: the second man is the Lord from heaven.
> [I Corinthians 15:44, 47]

Daumier's masterpiece, "The Uprising," symbolizes two of the most appealing characteristics of man: his ability to conceptualize life and his willingness to struggle consciously for an uncertain future. This painting, in the Phillips Gallery in Washington, shows a vigorous and handsome young man on a barricade with outstretched arms and clenched fists. His visionary gaze is lost in the distance toward a future that he will never know, because he will not live long enough; bullets will probably soon strike him down. Certainly it is a vague future that the revolutionary on the barricades sees in his imagination; at most it means Liberty, perhaps Equality and Fraternity. But Daumier's hero is the symbol of Man, the animal with an open future that he creates through faith in the human condition. He is the eternal nomad of the questioning spirit, haunted by the future and blind to danger, the eternal standard-bearer of a worthwhile cause.

Like the classical Greeks, like the cathedral builders, like the rationalists, and like Daumier's revolutionary on the barricade, modern man also makes judgments of values. He knows that it is important to accept sacrifices for the defense of one's homeland and for worthwhile ideals; to help one's fellow-man in need; to work toward improving one's community; to advance knowledge even without hope of financial rewards; to enlarge and enrich the intellectual and emotional perception of the cosmos through science, literature, and the arts. He realizes more and more the truth preached by philosophers for several millennia, that the selfish pursuit of happiness always ends in disappointment.

The awareness that individual human lives acquire value and meaning only when they transcend themselves has taken many different forms. It can be a disenchanted challenge to fate, as when Thomas Wolfe wrote in *You Can't Go Home Again,* "Man was born to live, to suffer and to die, and what befalls him is a tragic lot. There is no denying this in the final end. But we must deny it all along the way." [New York, Harper & Bros., 1940, p. 737] It can be Sören Kierkegaard's call to action, when he wrote, "To venture causes anxiety. But not to venture is to lose oneself." Or it can be the belief expressed by Albert Camus, that while he who trusts in the human fate may be a fool, he who despairs of events is a coward. Whichever way it is expressed, the view that man can transcend his selfish interests, even for forlorn causes, is the mark of a profound and creative faith in the human condition.

The fundamental human value is the freedom to choose, and, if need be, to elect painful effort, dangerous risks, and responsibilities for the sake of some transcendental value. It is this way of life that differentiates man from the rest of creation. It corresponds to a faith more entrancing and more comprehensive than the view of the good life by the Greek philosophers, than the vision of heaven by the medievalists, than the mathematical world conceived by the rational scientists, than the utopian societies imagined by political reformers. It is the largest possible faith, simply because it is open on an endless future with unlimited possibilities.

Man is not only free to act or not to act; he is also usually conscious of the reasons that make him select the cause to which he dedicates his actions. Free will thus implies a motivated choice, which in turn is a matter of faith requiring some vision of the future. It is the possibility to choose that gives its grandeur to the human condition and also constitutes its greatest burden. In every person now and then, and in most persons frequently, there arises the desire to escape from the responsibility of having to make decisions that engage the self and the future of one's fellow-men. But in general, sensible men only daydream of Arcadia; in their waking life they elect to search for adventure or to work for a cause, even if it means struggle and suffering. In a complex but real way, the quality of the adventure or of the cause conditions the quality of the person and of his life. The very last entry of George Orwell's notebook reads "By the age 50, every man has the face he deserves." And in his last novel, *The Fall,* Albert Camus wrote, "Beyond a certain age, everyone is responsible for his visage." These arresting statements express man's responsibility for his own life and his own self.

AUTHORS INDEX

INDEX